Memory in the Cerebral Cortex

Memory in the Cerebral Cortex

An Empirical Approach to Neural Networks in the Human and Nonhuman Primate

Joaquín M. Fuster

A Bradford Book
The MIT Press
Cambridge, Massachusetts
London, England

This book was set in Palatino by DEKR Corporation and was printed and bound in the United States of America.

Library of Congress Cataloging-in-Publication Data

Fuster, Joaquín M.
  Memory in the cerebral cortex : an empirical approach to neural networks in the human and nonhuman primate / by Joaquín M. Fuster.
  p.   cm.
  "A Bradford book."
  Includes bibliographical references and index.
  ISBN 0-262-06171-6
  1. Memory. 2. Cerebral cortex. 3. Neural networks (Neurobiology)
I. Title.
QP406.F87   1994
612.8'2—dc20   94-8307
                                                                CIP

To my convivial and hard-thinking friends of the Helmholtz Club

Contents

Preface

To write another book on memory, one must have truly compelling and persuasive reasons because much—too much—has already been written on the subject. Just recently, several treatises have appeared on the neural representation of memory. Who needs yet another? Indeed, without proper justification, this book can be easily dismissed as another gratuitous demand on the valuable reading time of anyone who wants to keep up with the fast pace of neuroscience.

From my perspective, at least one more compendium is justified because, for all the attention it has received, neural memory remains largely a mystery, though with each passing day the challenge of unraveling it seems more pressing and success closer at hand. Two powerful motives have guided and encouraged me to write this book. One is the need to fill, as well as I can, what I perceive to be a looming interdisciplinary vacuum. The other is the need to organize a private collection of loose insights into the nature of memory from having researched for more than three decades the behavioral neurophysiology of the monkey. Now, almost suddenly, these insights seem to acquire singular relevance in the context of current memory theory and a large body of recent empirical evidence from the human as well as the non-human primate.

Neural memory is an exceedingly broad subject, which can be studied and described at many analytical levels. In fact, memory can be legitimately construed as a property or state of any of the components of the central nervous system; in the hierarchy of the nerve axis, that means any and all of its levels. Yet, given the present state of our knowledge, an all-encompassing view of neural memory would be not only pretentious but surely wrong. Thus, the scope of this book is broad but limited almost entirely to the neocortex, for the "new cortex" is the seat of human experience and the focus of my research experience.

The purpose of this monograph is to present a synthesis of empirical knowledge of the role of primate neocortex in memory. Although much will be said here about the monkey, there should be no doubt in anybody's mind that the book's principal agenda is to understand how the human primate stores and remembers the past and the knowledge that goes with it. We very much need an interdisciplinary review of cortical memory in both human and monkey. Prior works on the same topic have been, for the most part, theoretical or else have relied almost exclusively on neuropsychology—that is, on the study of the effects of brain lesions on memory. Memory theories require empirical testing and, for that, neuropsychology has clear limitations. How serious these limitations are is exemplified by Karl Lashley's epic "search of the engram" (1950). After long and exacting ablation studies, that great psychologist admitted his failure to establish the location of memory in the cortex, although unwittingly he came close to establishing its now undeniable distributed character. It turns out that cortical memory is both localized and distributed, but neither is demonstrable by ablations alone.

It is now possible to overcome some of the problems of ablation by experimental use of reversible lesions. Moreover, the functional organization of the primate cortex has lately become much better known, thanks in large part to single-unit recording in behaving monkeys. New data on neuroanatomy and neurotransmission have also been helpful. Brain-imaging methods in the human are beginning to contribute to our understanding of cortical metabolic changes in psychological processes that are closely related to memory or an integral part of it, such as attention, perception, discrimination, and recall. These developments make the subject of memory approachable in exciting new ways. We can now begin to test the principles and computational aspects of several theoretical models of cortical memory.

The central proposition of the present work is that individual memory is deposited and represented in the neocortex. This does not imply that memory function is restricted to this part of the brain—far from it. We now know that the deposition of memories essentially requires the intervention of certain limbic and subcortical structures. Furthermore, normal behavior is probably determined to a large extent by neural changes that have occurred in noncortical structures as a result of individual experience. However, what we commonly understand as memory—that is, the aggregate of personal experiences of events, objects, names, actions, and knowledge of all sorts, whether or not accessible to consciousness—is represented in the neocortex, particularly within what we commonly call the *cortex of association*. Although presented here in a somewhat novel manner and perhaps with more empirical backing than elsewhere, the concept is not new. Many writers have more or less explicitly proposed it. In fact, as will become apparent, the formulations of some of them have served me well in developing my own concepts. High on the list of my sources of inspiration is the late Friedrich von Hayek (1899–1992), in my opinion the first and unrecognized pioneer of cortical network theory.

The theoretical framework of this book consists of a few basic notions, supported by recent evidence, that not only are useful for sharpening and qualifying the general concept of cortical memory but also suggest further research to substantiate it. Although the supporting evidence is based on the efforts of many investigators, I rely heavily for my argument on results of my own research. It is hoped that this reliance on my own data will not be found excessive or uncritical.

My research has been supported by grants from the National Institute of Mental Health, the National Science Foundation, and the Office of Naval Research. Without their support, this book would not have been possible. I also wish to acknowledge the invaluable help of the many students and collaborators who have shared with me the joys and disappointments of laboratory work. I owe special thanks to my colleagues John Eccles, Howard Eichenbaum, Patricia Goldman-Rakic, Fernando Reinoso-Suárez, Gordon Shaw, Larry Squire, Richard Thompson, and Endel Tulving for their helpful comments and suggestions on the manuscript. I am also grateful to Mary Mettler for helping me assemble a sizable bibliography and to Lynda Newton for a truly splendid job in editing and preparing the manuscript for publication. Last but not least, I thank Elisabeth, my patient wife, for all the vacation time she lovingly allowed me to sequester to bring this work to completion.

Memory in the Cerebral Cortex

1   Introduction

This book is about the *memory of systems, not* about systems of memory. The distinction is crucial, for it clearly detaches the approach of this author from that of others who have explored the subject of neural memory in recent and not so recent times. If there were only one idea that I intend to defend here, it would be the following: Memory is a functional property, among others, of each and all of the areas of the cerebral cortex, and thus of all cortical systems. This cardinal cognitive function is inherent in the fabric of the entire cortex and cannot be ascribed exclusively to any of its parts. Furthermore, as the cortex engages in representing and acting on the world, memory in one form or another is an integral part of all its operations. In this respect, what distinguishes one cortical area from another is its *kind* (i.e., the content and history), of memory; in the temporal domain, it is the *state* of that memory, active or inactive or somewhere between.

Thus, as one of the cognitive functions of the cerebral cortex, memory is global and nonlocalizable. Its most concrete contents, however, those that are inextricable from specific sensory or motor functions (see *phyletic memory,* below), are well-localized. More or less widely distributed over the cortical surface, "mappable" by certain methods, is the rich panoply of individual memories. It is made of myriad idiosyncratic associations between that common fund of specific sensory and motor memory, which already lies in primary areas at birth, and the experience that has accrued thereafter in areas of so-called cortex of association, which means practically anywhere else in the neocortex.

The methodology of cortical memory must be essentially interdisciplinary. Without linkage of disciplines, none of our three major problems—how memory is formed, where it is stored, and how it is retrieved—can be solved. Memory concepts and hypotheses engendered by use of one method must be validated by use of another. Fortunately, this fruitful and necessary interplay of disciplines at various levels of analysis can be expected only to increase in the future. Thus far, it has provided us with virtually all we know about cortical memory, which derives from the efforts of neuropsychologists, electrophysiologists, behavioral scientists, anatomists, neurochemists, and theoreticians of the brain. This book attempts to synthesize the results of those efforts. What follows is a brief outline of the conceptual structure of cortical memory, without the supporting evidence.

A *memory* is basically a network of neocortical neurons and the connections that link them. That network is formed by experience as a result of the concurrent activation of neuronal ensembles that represent diverse aspects of the internal and external environment and of motor action. By this process of coactivation, those ensembles become the network's constituents, the nodes of the network. Networks may vary widely, both in size and constituent ensembles, and are modifiable by further experience—that is, they are open-ended and, throughout life, subject to growth. Because of the multiplicity of actual and potential connections in the cortex, each neuronal ensemble may be part of multiple networks and, thus, part of multiple representations. What most critically defines a network (i.e., a memory representation) is the ensemble of connections that has formed it. Relationship is of the essence and, in this sense, *all memory is associative.* Here, of course, is another departure from conventional thinking. Associative memory, according to a commonly held view, is a special form or system of memory, usually constituted by associations between stimuli and reinforcement and separate from recognition memory, episodic memory, and the like. My view is radically different and at the same time parsimonious: Association is an attribute of all memories, at the root of their genesis as well as their evocation.

The cortical substrate of memory, with its many (potentially infinite) representational networks, is very nearly identical to the connective cortical substrate for information processing, in perception as well as in action. A part of that substrate is made of primary sensory and motor areas and is, to some extent, modifiable after birth. That part of the neural processing substrate is viewed here as the seat of *phyletic memory,* or the memory of the species. It may have been formed in the course of evolution by essentially the same process of coactivation and connective growth that characterizes the development of individual memory in other areas of the cortex. Of course, vastly different time scales and rates of repeated exposure would apply to each.

Perceptual memory is another concept the reader will encounter here, perhaps for the first time. The term is meant to encompass much of the memory acquired and evoked through the senses, from the most concrete to the most abstract. It includes the memory for distinct events, for objects, places, persons, and animals, as well as the factual and conceptual knowledge of the world. It subsumes all that has been characterized by others as declarative, episodic, and semantic memory.

Perceptual memory is mainly represented in posterior cortex—that is, in cortical areas that lie behind the rolandic or central fissure. In the human, that comprises approximately two-thirds of the neocortex.

Another distinctive concept in this book is that of *motor memory,* which consists of representations of motor action in all its forms, from skeletal movement to the spoken language. It too is acquired and evoked through the senses but, once acquired, it is largely represented in the neocortex of the frontal lobe, which comprises roughly one-third of the human neocortex. The most automatic and firmly established aspects of motor memory are represented outside the neocortex, notably in the basal ganglia and the cerebellum. As we shall see, the cerebellum seems to harbor one elementary form of motor memory: classical conditioning.

The cortical networks for representation and processing of action are intertwined with, and somewhat overlap, those devoted to representation and processing of perception. The same principles that apply to the making of perceptual memory apply to motor memory. The single fundamental difference between perceptual networks and motor networks is that the latter, in addition to being representational, are operational: They can and do lead to motor action. However, perception and motor action are functionally interrelated, and both are part of many representational networks. The functional relationships between perceptual and motor memory, and the interplay of their networks, constitute the basis of the *perception-action cycle.* This is the circular course of information processing, serial and parallel, through posterior cortex, through anterior cortex, and through the environment, that shapes and characterizes any sequential structure of novel behavior.

Indeed, this book offers *a new taxonomy of memory.* Just a glance at the table of contents reveals that this taxonomy constitutes the conceptual backbone of the book and determines the manner in which its material is organized. Now, without adequate explanation, the mere idea of a new memory taxonomy is likely to arouse at least the suspicion of cavalier disregard for prior knowledge. However, my taxonomy is not intended to replace or invalidate any other. Though the concept of *phyletic memory* is somewhat nonconventional, it has heuristic value. By extending the structure and functions of memory to primary cortical areas, and by allowing us to treat the entire neocortex as a mnemonic unit, the concept of phyletic memory helps us understand better the interplay between genetic structure and personal experience.

The *perceptual-motor dichotomy* reflects, and to some extent coincides with, a widely accepted dichotomy in neuropsychology—namely, that of declarative versus procedural memory. The latter has proved eminently useful, at the very least for understanding the memory deficits caused by certain brain lesions in the human. This is not the place to discuss the conceptual overlap and differences between declarative and perceptual memory, or between procedural and motor memory. It is appropriate here to point out that my perceptual-motor dichotomy of cortical memory is not based on neuropsychology but on elementary facts and concepts of neural anatomy, development, and physiology. Happily, cortical neuropsychology in the human and the monkey supports this dichotomy.

The emphasis on dichotomies of memory that prevails in our field— and, for heuristic reasons, in this book—is somewhat unpalatable and defies rationality. There is, in nature, no a priori reason for classes or stores of memory to come only in pairs. I believe, however, that my perception-action dichotomy rests on solid ground. It reflects the distinction between the two most basic moieties of structure and function in the nerve axis, one for sensing and interpreting the world and the other for acting in it. This is a deeply rooted dichotomy in the biology of organisms. In this light, that each moiety should have its memory and that in the primate cortex the two should be separated by a deep furrow seem almost trivial facts, yet both, as we shall see, are essential to our discussion.

The classic distinction between short-term and long-term memory is operationally valid but, from the point of view of cortical topography, questionable. These two forms of memory share much of the same cortical substrate and simply reflect different states of that substrate. This, in turn, reflects the psychological reality. There is no such thing as an entirely new experience or memory. All that is apparently new to us happens in the context of old and well-established memory. We interpret the new always in the light of (i.e., in association with) the old. This means that the storage of short-term memories is inextricable from the reactivation of the long-term memories that, by context or similarity, any new experience evokes. Thus, a store for the new that is entirely separate from the store for the old is inconceivable in associative terms which, in my view, are the terms of cortical physiology. It is inconceivable even at the earliest neural stages of new memory formation. So it is that the physiologist of the hippocampus is now discovering, or rediscovering, the importance of context.

The dynamic, nontopographic distinction between short-term and long-term memory serves our methodology well. As we shall see, the selective short-term activation of long-term memory by behavioral means is extremely helpful in estimating its cortical organization, with the help of reversible-lesion, microelectrode, and imaging methods. The same research strategy, of course, is useful to investigate the dynamics of memory.

At any given time in the awake organism, a widely distributed and changing representational network is active in the neocortex. That is *active memory.* Its extent and topography are determined by multiple factors, including the present or recent sensory inputs, the neuronal ensembles that, by association (as a result of prior experience), are activated by those inputs, and the drive or motivation prevalent at the time. The network is largely activated in parallel—that is, through parallel processing pathways—and most of its contituents remain unconscious. A limited portion of the network, which in this book is called the *focus of representation,* is activated mainly by serial processing and is subject to change depending on attention and the nature of what is consciously kept in short-term memory or, to use William James's concept, in primary memory. Presumably, only that portion of the network is conscious.

Working memory, which has aso been called *operant memory,* is an operant concept of active memory, but the two are not identical. Active memory, as defined previously, includes and transcends working memory, for it does not presuppose any mental or cognitive operation. Thus, active memory, which I view as a state rather than a system of memory, subsumes not only working memory but the phenomenal experience of conscious remembering (i.e., primary memory).

This simplified description of the main subjects of this book may prompt the reader to ask a few predictable questions: Is this much conceptual parsimony justified? Can the same principles of organization apply to phyletic as to individual memory and to motor memory as to perceptual memory? How can such uniformity of principles apply to such immensely diverse, idiosyncratic, and complex memories as those of which we are capable? If short-term and long-term memory share the same cortical networks, why is it that in some cases of brain injury, one is lost and the other is not?

Only the reader can judge how persuasive is the argument of this book for my vision of cortical memory and how persuasive are my answers to those questions. Certainly, as I emphasize in the text, many empirical facts are resistant to the generalizations introduced thus far. At this point, however, the reader is asked to consider just one reason why, a priori, a parsimonious explanation of cortical memory is not implausible: that is, the uniformity, indeed parsimony, of the neocortical architecture, which so many writers have found paradoxical for a neural structure of such complex and specific functions. To be sure, there are considerable cytoarchitectonic differences between cortical areas, but these differences are overshadowed by the most distinctive and uniform feature of the primate's neocortex, the stratified and columnar geometry of its elements.

That relative cytoarchitectonic homogeneity, however, is accompanied by *enormous heterogeneity of intrinsic and extrinsic connections.* Almost every day, new intracortical and corticocortical connections are discovered and described in the literature. That connectivity is far from immutable, for the synaptic apparatus of the cortex, especially in associative areas, apparently undergoes considerable changes throughout life. It is undoubtedly the variety and plasticity of cortical connections, especially at the synaptic level, coupled with the idiosyncracy of personal experience that imparts to memories and their networks their immense diversity.

In other words, the structural characteristics of the neocortex are consistent with the notion of a representational system that is relatively simple, redundant and economical in some respects, and highly intricate and diverse in others. On the one hand, the pervasive geometry and cellular composition of the cortex would satisfy the basic requirements for representation of simple sensory and motor features in local networks. On the other hand, the elaborate neocortical connectivity would subserve the representation of individual memories in complex networks that would extend deeply and widely into areas of association.

This is essentially my viewpoint and the substance of this text. Now, having briefly introduced this book for what it is, it seems advisable to point out what it is not. Most definitely, it is not another theoretical essay on the neural substrate of cognition, to join the several now en vogue. Whatever their power of explanation, most of the tenets of those essays are not yet testable. As in some of those writings, however, a hebbian or quasi-hebbian concept of neural memory is adopted here. Such a concept is not only plausible but now has been empirically demonstrated at least in the hippocampus, a piece of ancient cortex very much involved in the formation and retrieval of memory. Also adopted here is a probabilistic, not deterministic, view of the function of cortical neurons in memory acquisition, storage, and retrieval. That, too, is a sensible posture in light of the innumerable facts concerning neural plasticity, redundancy, and recovery from injury. However, few of the concepts of cortical representation advanced in this book can be easily and plausibly treated mathematically. The reason is simple: too many unknown and imponderable variables. Thus, the reader will not find here the microarchitecture of memory and its functional algorithms, other than in cursory hypothetical fashion. What the book offers, instead, is a set of qualitative concepts, based on quantitative empirical evidence, that lead immediately to further memory research and to testable computational models of cortical memory.

Chapter 2 deals with the basic concepts and forms of memory. In chapter 3, there is a discussion of current knowledge concerning the mechanisms of memory acquisition, which is followed, in chapter 4, by a description of the essentials of the cortical substrate of memory, mainly in terms of connective anatomy. The concept of network memory is discussed at some length in chapter 5, with particular emphasis on its developmental and methodological aspects. The cortical organization of perceptual memory is the subject of chapter 6 and that of motor memory the subject of chapter 7. Chapters 8 and 9 deal with dynamic aspects of memory, the first with memory retrieval and attention, the second with active memory. Finally, chapter 10 is devoted to certain relationships between consciousness and memory. In almost every chapter, questions concerning the pathology and abnormalities of memory are discussed.

2 Basic Concepts and Taxonomy of Memory

Broadly defined, *memory* is the capacity of an organism to retain information about itself and the environment in which it lives. In these broad terms, memory need not involve the nervous system at all. An antigen, or even a scar, is memory of sorts. Neural memory is special in several ways; among them is its capacity not only to retain information but also to utilize it for adaptive purposes. In this sense, neural memory is analogous to immunological memory. In this sense also, neural memory becomes connatural with learning, from which it is operationally difficult to distinguish it, although the term *learning* usually refers only to the process of acquiring memory.

A further qualification of neural memory is its potential to be recalled and used in circumstances different from those in which it was acquired; how different the circumstances depends on the organism and the nature of the information. In the human, memory becomes synonymous with past personal experience, and its recall may be conscious—that is, part of phenomenal (i.e., subjective) experience and communicable by language.

INDIVIDUAL VERSUS PHYLETIC MEMORY

The central nervous system contains and retains not only information experienced by the individual organism but also information accumulated by its ancestry in the course of evolution. Essentially, this information consists of the basic architecture and connections of the brain at birth. This fund of structural memory, which includes the primary sensory and motor neocortical systems with their genetically determined layout, can be properly characterized as *phyletic memory,* or memory of the species. It is an inherited endowment of memory that the organism brings with it to the world and which is, of course, eminently adaptive. It contains all the adaptive power that natural selection has gathered in prior evolution.

An unprovable but seemingly reasonable tenet in this monograph is that the phyletic memory of sensory and motor systems—that is, their connective structure and architecture, as well as their representational properties—have developed in evolution by essentially the same mechanisms of association by co-occurrence and contiguity that contribute to the formation of individual memory in higher cortical systems, although the time scale of the two developments would be immensely different. Whereas individual memory develops through a life span, phyletic memory would have developed through millions of years and innumerable generations. Another difference would be exposure. Whereas individual memory can result from a single exposure, phyletic memory may be the result of countless repetitions of the same experiences by countless individuals of the same species. Clearly, we are not dealing with inheritance of changes acquired during a lifetime; Lamarckism is out of the question.

Also different, in this conceptual scheme, are the anatomical substrates and the contents of the two forms of memory. In the structure of primary systems, phyletic memory contains the innate capacity to respond to and to reenact (to recall) the elementary features of sensation and movement that are common to the repertoires of all members of the species. (Note that the concept of *feature* is applied here to movement as well as sensation.) Individual memory is contained in higher cortex, mostly (but not exclusively) in so-called cortex of association. This, of course, does not negate the genetic structural foundation of this cortex, which is as firm and elaborate as that of primary cortex, probably all the way down to the synaptic level, where structurally subtle but functionally critical differences may exist between the two. At any rate, the transition between the two types of memory—phyletic and individual—is probably much smoother, both structurally and functionally, than we have been led to believe. Indeed, one probably blends into the other. Developmentally, it is appropriate to view individual memory as an expansion of phyletic memory. As a result of experience, phyletic memory would become individualized epigenetically by expanding, through synaptic changes, into the connective substrate of higher cortex. In the awake organism, there is a constant dynamic interaction between phyletic and individual memory.

Sherry and Schacter (1987) offer different concepts of the role of evolution in memory and of the relationship between what we call phyletic and individual memory. Those authors depart from the notion of multiple and specialized memory systems to handle the various forms of human memory, some of which are described in later sections of this chapter. Based on distinctions between habit and explicit memory, for example, they postulate that there are certain functional incompatibilities between those systems, each incapable of performing the functions of others. These authors envision that *incompatibility* as the theoretical reason for the evolutionary differentiation of memory systems.

Instead of incompatibility, this book emphasizes *complementarity*. Focusing on the distinctions between perceptual and motor memories, an argument can be made for the gradual and parallel evolution of two mutually complementary systems, one for memory of sensory experience and the other for memory of action. The argument becomes especially compelling in light of the relative segregation, yet also the functional interaction, of neural structures—cortical areas in particular—devoted to sensory processing and to motility.

Another proposition in this book is that all memory is essentially *associative*. Individual memories are formed by the facilitation, or perhaps creation, of synaptic connections between neurons that represent different sensory or motor features if and when such features co-occur in the internal or external environment. The temporal coincidence or continuity of attributes, which determines synaptic association, may be accompanied by spatial contiguity. It is important to emphasize that, in this view, the association may be between sensory features, between motor features, or between sensory and motor features. This view is meant to apply to classical and instrumental conditioning as well as to the higher forms of individual memory.

Furthermore, it is maintained in subsequent chapters that the neurons and connective links that constitute individual memories make up cortical networks of widely differing distribution and proportions. They may cover large expanses of associative neocortex and also cortical areas of functional transition between primary cortex and cortex of association. The informational content of memory networks resides essentially in the links themselves, in the associative relationships among their neuronal elements. It is not so much that a memory trace is contained in a network; rather, the memory trace *is* the network. It is one of innumerable networks, separate from others or interconnected with them and, like them, subject to activation and change, growth and attrition.

The generalities presented thus far, ahead of the evidence, have undoubtedly suggested to the reader a reductionist approach that openly conflicts with the evidence that memory is not simply a unitary or dual phenomenon but that there are many different kinds and systems of it (Broadbent, 1983; Tulving, 1987). Thus, before proceeding further, let us briefly review some conventional or current classifications of individual memory and some of the rationale that supports them.

Every definition and classification of memory described in the literature tends to reflect the methodology of the writer. Consequently, definitions and classes of memory in human psychology tend to differ from those in animal psychology and neurobiology. The reported differences in memory types are largely attributable to differences in the criteria used for definition, which receive varying emphasis depending on the methodology employed. (For a historical review of the issue, see Squire,

1987). *Memory systems* have been distinguished according to several attributes or criteria, the principal of which are the following: (1) the content or kind of information those systems mediate and store; (2) their principles of operation—that is, of storage and retrieval, of acquisition and utilization of relevant information; (3) their storage capacity; (4) the duration or persistence of their information storage; and (5) the putative neural structures and mechanisms involved in their operations.

In addition to emphasizing two basic forms of information content (perceptual and motor memory) and the role of the cerebral cortex in storing memories of both, this book considers critical one aspect of memory that has generally been neglected, the *state of memory*—in other words, whether a memory trace (a network) is active or inactive; whether, at a given time, it is open to new acquisition and recall; whether it controls behavior and is possibly conscious. Neglect of such distinctions of state may lead to spurious distinctions of memory types or systems. As we shall see, some of the differences between so-called memory stages, most of which are based on the assumption that memory moves from one brain store to another, are reducible to differences in the state of one and the same memory store.

SHORT-TERM VERSUS LONG-TERM MEMORY

Traditionally, a widely accepted dichotomy in the human has been that of short-term and long-term memory (James, 1890; Broadbent, 1958; Norman, 1968; Baddeley, 1988). An essential criterion of distinction between the two is their temporal persistence—in other words, the length of time during which a memory is retained and retrievable. That length of time may be seconds to minutes in short-term memory and up to years in long-term memory. Information capacity is another distinction between the two: The capacity of short-term memory is limited, whereas that of long-term memory supposedly is not. Another difference, it has been claimed, is that the retrieval of long-term memory is facilitated by specific cues, whereas that of short-term memory is not.

Considerable support for the differentiation of these two types of memory has come from the study of amnesic patients with various forms of brain lesions. Whereas patients with Korsakoff's disease, for example, suffer from severe impairments of long-term memory, they show unimpaired capacity to retain information for the short term. Patients with lesions of medial temporal lobe structures including the hippocampus, such as the celebrated case of H.M., are impaired in the acquisition of new information while their capacity to recall long-term memories remains unimpaired (Scoville and Milner, 1957; Corkin, 1984; Squire, 1987). Also unimpaired is their capacity to retain information in immediate or recent memory.

Such findings have reinforced the notion of two interactive memory systems, one for short-term and the other for long-term memory. The first, relatively fragile (with low resistance to such factors as distraction), would have storage of limited capacity and short duration. The second, sturdier, would have unlimited capacity and long persistence. New information would stay in the first before being transferred to the second. This constitutes a dual-system memory model. More elaborate views of sequential-processing memory systems have been proposed by Murdock (1982) and by Atkinson and Shiffrin (1968) with their modal models. Essentially in all these models, sensory information, after the initial encoding in some kind of sensory memory, would be transferred to a limited-capacity short-term memory store and from there to their ultimate long-term store.

The dual-system and multistage models of memory processing have been challenged by Craik (1983) on the basis of evidence that long-term memory is highly dependent on the solidity of initial encoding and rehearsal. Craik argues that memory is largely a function of the depth and elaboration of that initial encoding. The efficacy of retrieval would depend on how well the information had originally been acquired and not on the operation of hypothetical intermediate stages. Consequently, the idea of memory transfer from temporary (i.e., short-term) to permanent storage would be unnecessary. This kind of argumentation, like the argumentation for multiple memory stores, is inconclusive because it is based mostly on constructs of cognitive information processing and only superficially on the underlying neural structures and mechanisms. The fact remains, however, that damage to different noncortical structures seems to affect short-term and long-term memory differently.

Several kinds of short-term memory have been described, again mainly on the basis of storage-time distinctions and phenomenal or neuropsychological data. The shortest of short-term memories would be *iconic memory* (Coltheart, 1983), which is the capacity to retain a sensory image for up to 1 second after presentation. It can be blocked or erased by backward masking—that is, by interposing within that period a strong and competing stimulus (Sperling, 1960). According to Neisser (1967), iconic memory matches closely the sensory image that has elicited it. *Immediate memory* would last a few seconds longer. It coincides with what is commonly understood as short-term memory; the distinction between the two is unclear because it is based largely on a temporal criterion that depends strictly on the particular operations for testing one and the other.

Then there is an interesting notion of short-term memory, known as *primary memory*, that derives exclusively from phenomenal experience. The concept was introduced by William James long ago (1890) but unquestionably has current validity. James defined primary memory as the memory of the immediate past still in consciousness and the object of selective attention. Its duration would be under the subject's control and modifiable by such operations as thinking and rehearsal. Like consciousness and attention, it has, at any given time, limits of content and capacity. The concept of primary memory is useful to understand the selectivity of the short-term activation of perceptual and motor memory networks for the control of behavior. In any event, the distinction between a phenomenologically defined primary memory and any operationally defined short-term memory is difficult because of differences in the defining criteria.

There is, however, an operational definition of short-term memory that transcends the temporal criterion and that is directly relevant to many of the issues discussed later in this book: *working memory*, a concept of short-term memory that derives from cognitive psychology (Baddeley, 1983). It is essentially a temporary storage used in performance of cognitive behavioral tasks, such as reading, problem solving, and delay tasks (e.g., delayed response and delayed matching to sample), all of which require the integration of temporally separate items of information (cross-temporal integration). This form of short-term memory has also been called *operant* or *provisional* memory and is, as we shall discuss later, one of the important functions that the prefrontal cortex performs (Fuster, 1989) in cooperation with other cortical, and possibly subcortical, structures.

In the absence of a better understanding of neural mechanisms, the various concepts of short-term memory just described will remain useful, at least for generating hypotheses by which to explore those mechanisms. Nonetheless, the distinctions between them are tenuous. It is possible, indeed probable, that all classes of short-term memory thus far identified are based on the sustained temporary activation (that is, increased firing) of the neural elements—most probably pyramidal cells—of any given cortical network. Which network, or part thereof, is activated at a given time, and to what degree would depend on the nature of the information coming through the senses, on the behavior in progress, and on the sector of long-term memory associated with, and evoked by, either of them. Depending on such factors as repetition, novelty, and motivation, new information that has temporarily activated the network may be incorporated into it, thus expanding long-term memory with new associations.

Be that as it may, it seems important here to delve further into the distinction between two common usages of the expression *short-term memory* which, because of differences in methodology, may be assumed to refer to separate neural substrates though, in reality, they may not. In one view, short-term memory is the gateway to long-term memory, in other words, a storage stage or site and its content before that content becomes consolidated. In the other view, short-term memory is the temporary retention of an item of information, new or old, for behavior in the near term. This behavior may be part of ordinary life, whether in the form of motor action or logical reasoning, or it may be simply, for example, the answering of queries from a psychologist testing mnemonic function. Its ad hoc property in the context of current behavior is what characterizes this second kind of short-term memory, which is essentially what we have called working memory.

The confusion between those two concepts of short-term memory and the functions they imply stems from the fact that they cannot be easily separated by experiment from each other and from long-term memory, either at the psychological or at the neural plane. A new item of working memory may become consolidated into long-term memory depending on such factors as its saliency, relevance, and rehearsal. Thus, it may behave as short-term memory in the conventional (gateway) sense. At the same time, all kinds of short-term memory traces have inherent associative connections with long-term memory. This is most evident when the material in short-term memory is verbal. It is obvious to anyone that the acquisition and recall of verbal material is determined and facilitated by that material's associations with items in long-term memory. The role of those associations is most obvious in the retrieval of that material (Buschke, 1975). A person must be familiar with a word, or at least the symbols used for the word, to be able to retrieve it easily from short-term memory. Long-term memory also plays a critical role in the acquisition and recall of nonverbal memory. It is practically impossible to dissociate an item from the context in which it is acquired or recalled, and that context itself usually carries associations with long-term memory.

At the neural plane, the distinction between consolidating and working short-term memory is also difficult and confusing. Consolidating short-term memory probably always involves extracortical structures, most likely limbic, to effect consolidation in the cortical network (see chapter 3). That network naturally also contains representations of the context into which the new engram is formed. The second kind of short-term memory may or may not involve limbic structures. What serves as working short-term memory may have already previously been formed and consolidated in the network. It is a part of that network which is activated ad hoc, for the occasion, as behavior dictates. In either case, the cortical substrate for both forms of short-term memory may be the same, although the physiological relationship between the process of cortical memory consolidation and that of temporary activation of a working memory remains unclear. Without evidence to the contrary, both kinds of short-term memory can be assumed to involve the activation of a cortical network with a solid component of long-term memory and a more or less prominent component of new or transiently relevant memory. For this reason in this book, with its focus on the neocortex, I make no major effort to distinguish between these two kinds of short-term memory, in terms of either their cortical base or their dynamics.

It is a reasonable presumption that all types of short-term memory mentioned earlier, including immediate and primary, as well as long-term memory essentially share the same cortical substrate. The basic differences between them would lie in the degree and distribution of neuronal activity within that substrate. Other than iconic memory, which may involve only the brief activation of a sensory or parasensory cortical area (a piece of phyletic memory?), short-term memory probably, and essentially, involves the sustained activation of a vast cortical network. That activation of a vast network is the physiological basis of what we understand to be *active memory.*

It follows from previous discussion that the activated network may represent not only features of new information but also features or events of the organism's past history with which that information is associated. This old, associated part of the activated network may comprise a substantial sector of long-term memory which is otherwise in a latent condition—that is, relatively inactive until the new information is met. Such notions will be critically discussed in the context of network memory theory (chapter 5) and the behavioral neurophysiology of cortical networks (chapters 6 through 9). It is appropriate to note here that, from a purely functionalist point of view, the notion of short-term memory simply as an activated sector of long-term memory has received considerable support from cognitive scientists (Norman, 1968; Wickelgren, 1975). It has been most effectively defended by Cowan (1988) after extensive review of psychological data.

The physiologically more concrete idea that short-term memory involves the temporary electrical activity of an interconnected neuron assembly (net, cage-work, or lattice) was first proposed by Hebb (1949), who specified that the activity within one such assembly is maintained by reverberating circuits. The existence of such circuits had been previously surmised from anatomy by Lorente de Nó (1938) and, for a time, gained considerable popularity. Hebb (1949) further postulated that the reverberating activity leads to structural changes within the assembly that, by themselves, constitute long-term memory. These basic concepts remain valid but need modification and further research. On the basis of recent evidence (to be discussed later), it is necessary to expand greatly the assembly of Hebb to the dimensions of a cortical network that transcends any given cytoarchitectonically identified area. The concept of reverberation remains unproved but plausible.

DECLARATIVE VERSUS NONDECLARATIVE MEMORY

In recent years, cognitive scientists and neuropsychologists have recognized important distinctions between different types of long-term memory. From detailed observations of what certain amnesic patients can or cannot do or remember, new categories of memory have emerged depending on the kinds of information (knowledge) that memory contains and the behavioral operations it controls. The terminology used by different authors varies, but there seems to be considerable agreement on the main concepts behind another major dichotomy of memory. One entity of that dichotomy is what has been called *declarative memory*, and the other is *procedural memory* (Cohen and Squire, 1980; Cohen, 1984; Squire, 1986; Cohen and Eichenbaum, 1993). The two concepts have evolved to include or exclude various kinds of memory contents. Zola-Morgan and Squire (1993), two of the pioneering and most articulate proponents of the dichotomy, have expanded and modified the concept of procedural memory, which they now characterize as *nondeclarative* (or *implicit*) memory.

Declarative (or *explicit*) memory is the memory of events and facts; it is what is commonly understood as personal memory. One part of it contains the temporally and spatially encoded events of the subject's life, for which reason it has alternately been called *episodic memory* (Tulving, 1983, 1987). Another part contains the knowledge of facts that are no longer ascribable to any particular occasion in life; they are facts that, through single or repeated encounters, the subject has come to categorize as concepts, abstractions, and evidence of reality, without necessarily remembering when or where he or she acquired it. This is what Tulving (1987) has called *semantic memory*. The distinction between these two forms of declarative memory, episodic and semantic, is appealing and suggestive of two separate memory systems, but the empirical evidence for corresponding neural systems is weak. This may be because these two implied memory systems are neurally inseparable, reflecting what is phenomenally obvious—namely, that the two kinds of declarative memory derive from, and blend into, each other without sharp transition. The presence or absence of temporal and spatial tags, and the categorization of evidence in the form of events or facts, do not clearly separate episodic from semantic memory. Even if they can be separated as distinct entities, they unquestionably maintain a dynamic interaction through life. Both can be conceived as different levels of categorization of information in one and the same memory store (see chapter 5). In neural terms, the two may be based on the same cortical network, although perhaps different parts of it, different levels of the representational hierarchy for explicit information. Nonetheless, it seems unwarranted to claim a separate cortical system or process for each.

Nondeclarative (*implicit*) memory, the counterpart of declarative memory, is a somewhat difficult concept to grasp. It encompasses a wide variety of skills and mental operations that, in addition to short-term memory, some amnesic patients have *not* lost, though they have lost the capacity to form new permanent declarative memory (Squire, 1987; Zola-Morgan and Squire, 1993). The deficit of these patients is epitomized by the thoroughly investigated case of H.M., a patient who, for the treatment of severe epilepsy, underwent a large bilateral excision of medial structures of the temporal lobe, including a large part of the hippocampus, the parahippocampal gyrus, and the amygdala (Scoville and Milner, 1957; Corkin, 1984). After surgery, the patient lost his ability to remember practically anything that happened to him since the operation, yet he remained able to retain new information for a short time and to learn new motor tasks, although he forgot the events and circumstances surrounding his performance of them. It was this remarkable ability to learn and perform sensorimotor tasks—including mirror reading—in the face of severe memory difficulties, which H.M. shared with other amnesics (Cermak et al., 1973; Brooks and Baddeley, 1976), that led Cohen and Squire (1980) to postulate a different form of memory, which they called *procedural*. Eventually, as noted earlier, it was renamed *nondeclarative* (Zola-Morgan and Squire, 1993), a concept meant to include that of procedural memory without being restricted to it. It seemed to have its substrate in other than medial temporal lobe structures.

The scope of procedural or nondeclarative memory was increased early on by the finding of a peculiar mnemonic ability, known as *priming*, that is preserved also in amnesic patients (Tulving et al., 1982; Squire, 1987; Tulving and Schacter, 1990). Priming is the facilitation of the recognition of a stimulus (usually a word) by prior exposure to another stimulus (the so-called priming stimulus) with which the recognized stimulus has a relationship of associated meaning or similarity. The facilitation takes place despite the subject's inability to recognize that association or to remember the priming stimulus. Because priming improves a perceptual skill, it was included in procedural memory (Squire, 1987). However, it is useful to consider that unconscious or nonexplicit elements of perception—of the priming stimulus and of the retrieved material—may have access to a common and preexisting declarative base of knowledge. Thus, priming can be understood as a phenomenon of perceptual processing outside of what I later call the *focus of representation* (and thus probably unconscious), yet part of the operations of perceptual (declarative) memory activation. On other grounds, Tulving and colleagues (1982) excluded priming from the sphere of procedural memory and placed it in a different perceptual memory system, separate from semantic as well as declarative memory. For these and other reasons, Squire and Zola-Morgan (1988) also removed priming from procedural memory but still left it as part of nondeclarative or implicit memory.

If the distinction between declarative and nondeclarative memory is somewhat difficult in the human, it is even more so in the animal.

Attempts have been made, by lesion studies, to trace in the monkey the parallel of the human memory dichotomy and to better establish the neuroanatomical base for the two types or systems of memory. These attempts have been only partly successful. Monkeys with hippocampal and amygdalar lesions were found impaired in the performance of tasks that have been inferred to test declarative memory, such as delayed nonmatching to sample (DNMS) with trial-unique stimuli (Mishkin, 1978; Zola-Morgan and Squire, 1985). The same lesions did not appear to impair motor skills (Zola-Morgan and Squire, 1984). Later, lesions of several other brain structures, but not the amygdala, were found to produce deficits in DNMS performance. As a result of these experiments, an array of structures—including the hippocampus, the parahippocampal gyrus, the perirhinal and entorhinal cortices, and certain nuclei of the diencephalon—has been thought to constitute a system for the formation of declarative memory (for review and rationale, see Zola-Morgan and Squire, 1993). Whereas this conclusion harmonizes with some of the pathological and psychological findings in human amnesics, it remains tentative, primarily for methodological reasons. Among them is the still uncertain value of DNMS as an animal model of declarative memory in the making. At any rate, many researchers, including Squire and his colleagues, are increasingly espousing the notion that, regardless of what parts of the brain contribute to its consolidation, declarative memory is established and maintained in the neocortex (see chapter 3). Otherwise, the search for brain lesions that would affect the postulated forms of nondeclarative memory has been so far inconclusive.

A double dissociation of structures for declarative and nondeclarative memory has yet to be found. As an example of the problems to be resolved, *habit*, one of the many definitions of procedural memory (Mishkin and Petri, 1984) and thus part of nondeclarative memory according to some, is also part of all the tests of declarative memory adopted for animals, including DNMS. Almost the same comment can be made about *reference memory* (Olton et al., 1979; Kesner et al., 1987), another term that has been used to designate the memory of "how" (vs. "what")—in other words, the procedural memory of the formalities of a behavioral task. In summary, only with great difficulties can the two memories, declarative and nondeclarative, be tested apart from each other in the animal, either in behavioral or neural terms.

Despite those methodological difficulties, concepts such as declarative, episodic, semantic, and procedural memory remain valid and useful to anyone attempting to clarify the cortical substrate of memory. Here I will summarize my ideas concerning the relevance of these concepts to a discussion of cortical memory, as well as the relationships between the taxonomies of memory from which they derive and my own.

In my view, declarative memory (the knowledge of "what") includes almost all that is here construed as perceptual memory and is thus distributed largely in posterior (i.e., postrolandic or postcentral) cortex. However, declarative memory, as it is commonly understood, does not include those aspects of perceptual memory that we call *phyletic*; in other words, it does not include the cortical components of the sensory apparatus. Conversely, perceptual memory, as formulated in this book, includes both kinds of declarative memory, episodic and semantic, but without a line of demarcation between the two, either structurally or physiologically (see chapters 5 and 6).

Clearly, procedural memory (the knowledge of "how") represents the highest, most abstract aspects of motor memory and, at the same time, some of the most automated, however complex and concrete. Again, it does not include phyletic memory, whereas motor memory does. Most, if not all, procedural and motor memories, as proposed in this book, have a base in frontal cortex when they are being formed. After extensive motor learning, the most automated and concrete aspects of motor memory are relegated to noncortical components of the motor system. However, the most abstract aspects of motor memory, including some procedural memory, retain their cortical base.

PERCEPTUAL VERSUS MOTOR MEMORY

In this text, I adopt the distinction between perceptual and motor memory as the basis for organization and discussion of the book's content. I do so for the following reasons:

1. The proposed dichotomy is of fundamental biological significance and makes allowance for phyletic memory at its root.

2. In the cerebral cortex of the primate, the territories for perceptual and motor memory are anatomically well demarcated, the first in posterior and the second in frontal cortex.

3. In both these cortical territories, the development of perceptual or motor memory follows neuroontogenetic gradients, from primary cortex (phyletic memory) to cortex of association.

4. In both posterior and frontal cortex, the representation of, respectively, perceptual and motor memory is hierarchically organized.

Thus, the proposed division of memory not only makes profound biological sense but is based on a conceptually attractive symmetry of anatomical, developmental, processing, and representational orders in the two sectors of the cerebral mantle that serve the two most basic domains of neural function: *sensing* and *acting*.

Neither the concepts nor the terms of perceptual and motor memory are new. Because of their intuitive appeal, both have been used in a number of contexts and, for this reason, it is difficult to trace their historical origin. As far as I know, however, they have never been described together, as two generic and complementary classes of memory, each grouping a large variety of mnemonic functions and stores with deep evolutionary and developmental roots. Nor have these two kinds of memory been viewed as two vast and mutually interactive sectors of neural memory that are eminently suited to fulfill together the adaptive needs of the organism. This view has been neglected because of the prevailing tendency to treat memory functions and systems separate from perceptual and motor functions and systems. This tendency ignores the reality that both perceptual and motor processes are firmly anchored in memory and intimately dependent on it. In fact, it is practically impossible to dissociate memory from either perception or movement. In many respects, perception and action are phenomena of memory and, conversely, memory is an intimate part of perceptual and motor processing.

Perceptual memory is the knowledge of the world and of the self acquired through the senses. It includes the primary sensory qualities themselves, objects, events, facts, and concepts. Like declarative memory, it may be defined by temporal and spatial attributes (episodic memory), or it may not (semantic memory): It may be the memory of classes of percepts and thus devoid of space and time tags. My preference for the adjective *perceptual* to describe this kind of memory stems from its essentially sensory origin in terms of both function and neural processing substrate. The latter, as noted previously, includes primary sensory cortex, the seat of phyletic perceptual memory. In functionalist terms, the substrate for perceptual memory is almost identical to what Tulving and Schacter (1990) have called a *perceptual representational system* (PRS).

Motor memory (MacKay's [1954] *kinemnesis*) is not identical to procedural memory but subserves several forms of knowledge formerly attributed to it. It includes motor learning, motor skills, and classical conditioning. These do not carry time or place tags. The higher and more developed forms of motor memory represent classes of movement with a substantial *temporal dimension*. Another feature of highly developed motor memories is their *schematic character*. As we shall see, the prefrontal cortex is critical for the storage and behavioral utilization of those highly developed motor memories.

Both perceptual and motor memories may be in either *active* short-term condition or *inactive* long-term condition. As already mentioned, and as far as the neocortex is concerned, the distinction between short and long term probably is one of functional state rather than of content or store. This is consistent with a substantial body of neural data (to be discussed in subsequent chapters) and seems true for perceptual as well as motor memory.

There is, as we shall see, a well established *cortical substrate* for perceptual memory and another, not so well-established but increasingly recognized, for motor memory. In the primate, the first lies in the neocortex behind the central (rolandic) sulcus, the second in the neocortex in front of that sulcus. Because of the presence of sensory and parasensory association areas in occipital, parietal, and temporal regions, the argument for localization of perceptual memory in posterior neocortex is relatively easy and not too controversial. There is a wealth of evidence for it, ranging from data on human agnosias to microelectrode studies in monkeys performing sensory memory or discrimination tasks. When it comes to the cortical localization of motor memory, however, the argument is more difficult and often meets with skepticism. A couple of obvious reasons come to mind. First, the phenomenal experiences of motor memory are commonly anchored in sensation, kinesthesia at the very least. We remember actions by the sensations they produced or by which they were accompanied. Motor memories are practically inseparable from sensory memories (in chapters 4, 7, and 9, we'll see why). Only in the very abstract do motor memories detach themselves from sensation, as do some perceptual (e.g., semantic) memories. Second, the methodology for studying the cortical correlates of movement, let alone the motor engram, is more complicated and messier than that for studying the cortical correlates of sensation and its cognitive aspects. It is much easier to time-lock brain activity to a discrete stimulus than to a usually not so discrete motor action, which may be only loosely contingent on a stimulus. The difficulties increase considerably when we deal with the cognitive aspects of movement.

One of the most significant developments of modern neurobiology is the reemergence of the frontal lobe cortex as the part of the cerebral mantle essentially devoted to the organization of motor action and all its related cognitive functions, including memory. The entire dorsolateral frontal cortex, from the central sulcus (rolandic fissure) to the pole of the frontal lobe, can be considered *motor cortex* in the broadest sense of the term—neocortex, that is, devoted to action in the most ample terms, including skeletal movement, ocular movement, spoken language, and even perhaps certain kinds of internal action such as logical thinking. The motor attributes of the frontal lobe were first proposed by Betz (1874), the Russian neuroanatomist who extrapolated to the telencephalon the posterior-anterior sensorimotor dichotomy that prevails along the nerve axis, from the spinal cord on up. However, the concept has rarely been considered much more than a meaningless overgeneralization. One of my objectives in subsequent chapters is to revive that principle and to substantiate the idea that the frontal lobe cortex is the seat of motor memory and, in large part because of this, is the supreme organizer of action.

3 Principles of Neural Memory Formation

Ramón y Cajal (1923) was probably the first to propose formally the connective foundation of neural memory. He did it in his initial theoretical paper, presented in 1894 at an international medical congress in Rome. There, as he recounts in his autobiography, he offered an

explanation of the adaptation and professional skill, that is, of the functional proficiency due to exercise (physical education, operations of speech, writing, piano playing, mastery of fencing, etc.) . . . by the creation of new cellular appendices . . . capable of improving the adjustment and the extension of contacts, and even of organizing completely new relations between previously independent neurons (Ramón y Cajal, 1923, p. 288).

The concept was not entirely new, however, for a similar concept—as Ramón y Cajal acknowledges—had been advanced by Tanzi (1893) independently 1 year before.

Many years later, Hebb (1949) formulated his famous principles of memory formation by facilitation of contacts between neurons. It is interesting to note that whereas Ramón y Cajal, in his 1894 report, had obviously referred to the importance of such contacts for motor skills, Hebb made his proposals in the context of perception, attempting to explain perceptual integration and the transition from perception to memory. One concerned himself primarily with motor memory, the other with perceptual memory. Both pointed to the synapse as the locus of plastic change in the formation of memory (figure 3.1).

HEBB'S POSTULATE

Hebb stated his best-known neurophysiological principle as follows:

When an axon of cell A is near enough to excite a cell B and repeatedly or persistently takes part in firing it, some growth process or metabolic change takes place in one or both cells such that A's efficiency, as one of the cells firing B, is increased (Hebb, 1949, p. 62).

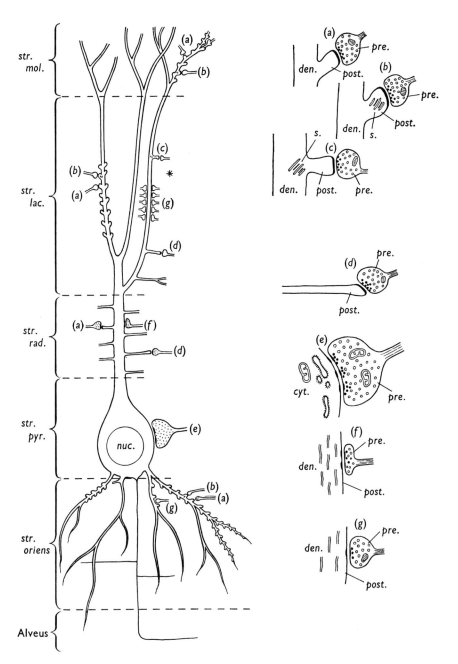

Figure 3.1 Schematic diagram of a pyramidal cell and different types of synapses on it, as observed by electron microscopy in the hippocampus. Note the variety of synaptic terminals and points of contact (*a* through *g*). (From Hamlyn, 1962, with permission.)

This elementary principle has now received considerable empirical support, at least insofar as many cellular and electrophysiological phenomena have been observed that are compatible with it, in invertebrate as well as vertebrate animals. Changes in the strength of preexisting synapses were shown first and most clearly to occur during learning in mollusks (Kandel, 1976) and crayfish (Krasne, 1978), which have relatively simple and well-identified neuronal circuits. For example, in two forms of nonassociative conditioning of the gill-withdrawal reaction of the *Aplysia* mollusk—namely, sensitization and habituation—changes in ion conductance lead to the increase and decrease, respectively, of neurotransmitter release from presynaptic neurons, which in turn result in more or less synaptic transmission. In both *Aplysia* (Hawkins et al., 1983) and *Hermissenda* (Alkon, 1984), ion conductance changes have also been noted to take place and to produce persistent synaptic alterations during classical conditioning. Conductance changes similarly appear to play a role in the increased excitability of motor cortical cells of the cat in eyelid conditioning (Woody, 1982; Aou et al., 1992).

Long-term potentiation (LTP) in the mammalian brain is the outstanding electrophysiological phenomenon of persistent change in synaptic strength as a result of impulse transmission across synapses. Viewed by many as the biophysical basis of Hebb's postulate, that phenomenon has been extensively investigated in the hippocampus, an ancient cortical structure with simple and well-understood connectivity (figure 3.2). The phenomenon was first described in the hippocampus of the rabbit by Bliss and Lømo (1973). In essence, what they observed is that the brief tetanic stimulation of the perforant path induces a potentiation of synaptic excitability of granule cells in the dentate gyrus that can last for several hours (figure 3.3). LTP has now been observed in other species and brain structures, and its duration has been found to extend, in some instances, to days and even weeks (Swanson et al., 1982; Teyler et al., 1989).

Nevertheless, the cellular mechanisms by which, according to Hebb, the repeated impulse conduction from cell A to cell B may lead to permanent change are not yet known precisely. The intracellular reactions underlying ion conductance and neurotransmission changes described in invertebrate learning and in LTP are not fully understood. Several plausible hypotheses have been advanced to substantiate Hebb's idea and to explain LTP (Huttunen, 1973; Stent, 1973; Lynch and Baudry, 1984; Brown et al., 1990), but none has been conclusively proved. In essence, however, what matters in terms of memory theory is that changes do occur in synapses as a result of use (i.e., as a result of repeated transmission of excitation across them). Figure 3.4 illustrates different varieties of use-dependent synaptic changes based on experimental evidence of LTP generation, some of which are discussed in the next section.

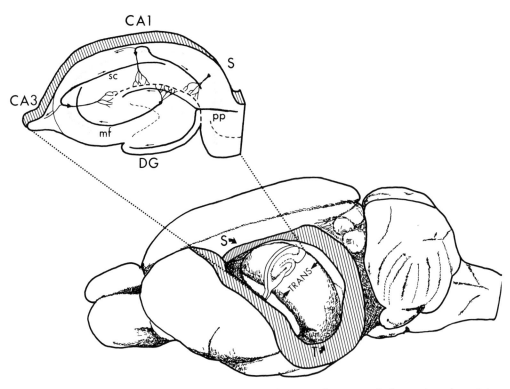

Figure 3.2 View of the hippocampus of the rat after removal of a portion of overlying neocortex. The hippocampus, or Ammon's horn, is a C-shaped part of phylogenetically ancient cortex extending from the septal region (S with arrow) to the temporal region (T). (*Top left*) Section of the hippocampal formation along its transverse axis. CA1, CA3, pyramidal fields; DG, dentate gyrus; mf, mossy fibers; pp, perforant path; S, subiculum; sc, Schaffer collaterals. (From Amaral and Witter, 1989, with permission.)

SYNCHRONOUS CONVERGENCE

Even if Hebb's postulate is proved correct, it alone is not sufficient to completely explain the essence of associative learning and memory, which is the facilitation produced by *simultaneity of inputs* impinging on a cell or group of cells. The optimal associative effect of simultaneity of inputs on a given neuron should be that the neuron, after exposure to two or more concomitant stimuli, would fire in response to any one of those stimuli, even though originally that stimulus was not sufficient to make it fire (see figure 3.4A).

Hebb was aware of the need for additional explanation and attempted to provide it by qualifying his basic assumption. Aware of the evidence that different axons terminate on a cell's surface in close proximity of one another (Lorente de Nó, 1938), Hebb explained the effect of input synchrony by summation of excitation of the same synaptic "knobs." If that summation were sufficient to fire the cell, then, after repeated

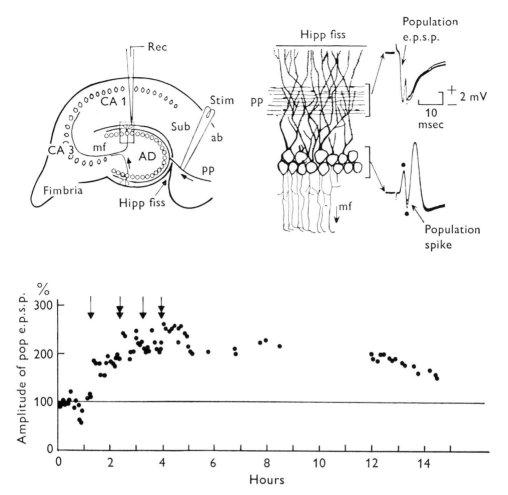

Figure 3.3 (*Top left*) Section of hippocampus showing the placement of stimulating electrode (Stim) and recording microelectrode (Rec). (*Top right*) Enlargement of recording location, the apical dendritic field of the dentate granular cells; (*far right*) population response potentials recorded from the synaptic layer (*above*) and from the cell body layer (*below*). The graph in the lower part of the figure shows the potentiation of the population response (e.p.s.p., excitatory postsynaptic potentials) by stimulation trains at 15/sec for 15 seconds (*single-headed arrows*) and 100/sec for 3 seconds (*double-headed arrows*). ab, angular bundle; AD, dentate; CA1, CA3, pyramidal fields; Hip fiss, hippocampus fissure; mf, mossy fibers; pp, perforant path; Sub, subiculum. (From Bliss and Lømo, 1973, with permission.)

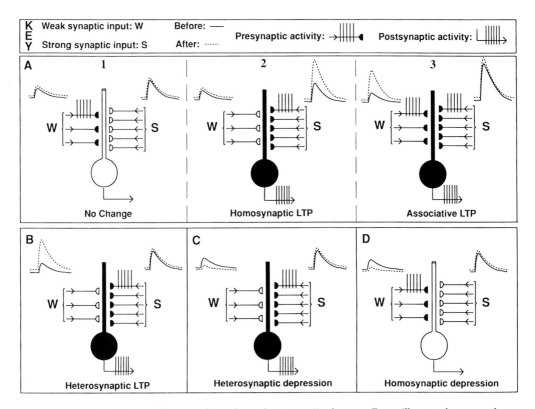

Figure 3.4 Diagram of use-dependent synaptic changes. Every illustrated neuron, from A to D, receives a weak synaptic input (W) and a strong one (S), strength defined by number of afferent fibers. The schematic potential traces above each input reflect the amplitude of the excitatory postsynaptic potential produced by a single stimulus of that input before (solid curve) and after (broken curve) tetanic high-frequency stimulation of one or both inputs. Filled (black) elements indicate excitation during tetanic stimulation. (*A*) Associative LTP: Whereas tetanic stimulation of W alone does not induce LTP (A1), that of S may induce homosynaptic LTP (A2); concurrent stimulation of W and S (A3) causes associative LTP (enhancement in W). (*B*) Heterosynaptic LTP (tetanic stimulation of S alone causes LTP in W). (*C*) Heterosynaptic depression. (*D*) Homosynaptic depression. (From Brown et al., 1990, with permission.)

summations, the basic rule should hold for any isolated input. Following this line of reasoning, Hebb also repostulated what he called an "old idea," which he found necessary to explain perceptual integration by convergence of inputs:

[A]ny two cells or systems of cells that are repeatedly active at the same time will tend to become "associated," so that activity in one facilitates activity in the other . . . [W]hat I am proposing is a possible basis of association of two afferent fibers of the same order—in principle, a sensori-sensory association (Hebb, 1949, p. 70).

It was up to Marr (1969) and Stent (1973) to develop this idea further and to provide concrete backing, at least theoretically. I mention here what should be recognized as *Hebb's second rule* to emphasize the critical importance of the synchronous association of those "fibers of the same order" for understanding the formation of phyletic as well as individual memory. Groups of synaptic terminals of the same order converging on a neuron and excited together would become strengthened as a group. Hebb's second rule would thus coincide with what later was called the *principle of cooperativity* (Miller, 1991).

To better appreciate it in contrast to lack of synchronicity, let us briefly follow Stent's (1993) argument in its essentials. His reasoning begins with the observation by Wiesel and Hubel (1965) that cross-eyed kittens, whose striate cells do not receive synchronous inputs from corresponding points of the two retinas, fail to develop normal responses. Stent argues that the lack of synchronicity leads to a situation in which one input (from one eye) will find the cell in striate cortex unprepared to fire because of the postsynaptic voltage and neurotransmitter changes just induced in it by the other input. This will lead to the failure of either input to create the necessary metabolic changes in the cell that will induce synaptic efficiency. In fact, synaptic efficiency will be reduced by asynchrony. Conversely, synchrony of inputs creates synaptic efficiency.

The concept having to do with sensorisensory association, which is essentially Hebb's second rule, has received support from experiments of invertebrate physiology. Carew et al. (1984) directly tested in *Aplysia* the first rule—that is, the postulate that for associative changes to occur, use of a synapse must contribute to spike generation in the postsynaptic neuron (cell A acting on cell B). These investigators found that the generation of action potentials is neither sufficient nor necessary for the postsynaptic effect and the behavioral conditioning that result from association of two stimuli (conditioned [CS] and unconditioned [US]). In fact, learning occurs even if the motor neuron is prevented from firing by a hyperpolarizing current. The critical factor that *does* lead to strengthening of the connection between sensory and motor cell is the coactivity of two sensory cells impinging on the latter (figure 3.5). Thus, the postsynaptic change and facilitation depend on presynaptic co-occurrence of excitatory sensory inputs. The importance of synchronous convergence of inputs for synaptic strengthening has been further substantiated by recent experiments (Buonomano and Byrne, 1990). Synchronous convergence explains several previous observations in *Aplysia* (Hawkins et al., 1983; Walters and Byrne, 1983) and is fully in accord with Stent's (1973) reasoning.

Further evidence of the role of synchronous convergence has been obtained in LTP studies. In some, LTP has been shown to have associative properties apparently based on that kind of convergence. For example, by repeated simultaneous stimulation of two hippocampal inputs, it has been possible to "condition" LTP—in other words, to

HEBB'S RULE

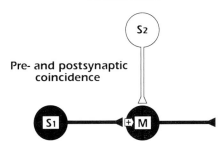

Pre- and postsynaptic coincidence

HEBB'S "SECOND RULE"

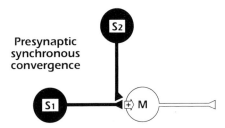

Presynaptic synchronous convergence

Figure 3.5 *(Top)* Scheme of Hebb's postulate indicating in black the two cellular elements (S_1 and M, for his cell A and cell B) that need be concurrently excited for synaptic facilitation to occur. *(Bottom)* Scheme of what is here called Hebb's *second rule* (two presynaptic elements, S_1 and S_2, concurrently excited), as epitomized by the LTP scheme A3 in figure 3.4 and endorsed by data from *Aplysia* (see text).

induce it by stimulating only one of those inputs, which formerly was incapable of inducing it by itself (McNaughton et al., 1978; Levy and Steward, 1979; Barrionuevo and Brown, 1983; Larson et al., 1986; White et al., 1990) (see figure 3.4A). A striking example of associative LTP has also been observed in the cortex of the cat by Iriki and coworkers (1989). Tetanic stimulation of sensory cortex was shown to induce LTP in motor cortical cells, presumably via corticocortical connections, whereas that of the ventrolateral nucleus (VL) of the thalamus did not. Pairing the two stimulations (sensory cortex and VL) induced motor cortical LTP demonstrable by potentiation of response to single stimuli applied to either sensory cortex or thalamus (figure 3.6). Associative LTP was found only in superficial cortical layers. Baranyi and colleagues (1991), by intracellular recording and microinjection, have subsequently clarified some of the membrane conductance changes associated with motorcortical LTP.

There is no empirical evidence that two inputs must coincide precisely in time to produce effective association. Because the electrochemical changes induced by one input on the postsynaptic membrane have a certain duration, the other input need not arrive in perfect synchrony

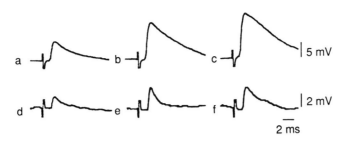

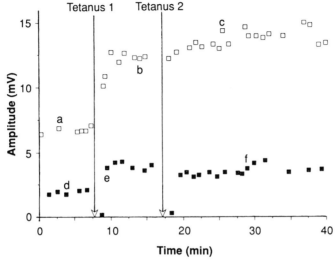

Figure 3.6 Excitatory postsynaptic potentials (EPSPs, top) and time course of associative LTP (bottom) in a motor cortical neuron: a,b, and c show EPSPs by thalamic stimulation before and after combined tetanization of the ventrolateral nucleus and the somatosensory cortex; d,e, and f show EPSPs from somatosensory cortical stimuli under the same conditions. (From Iriki et al., 1989, with permission.)

to induce interactive effects (such as temporal summation) and thus to lead to associative changes. In certain parts of the mammalian cortex—though not in striate cortex, if Stent is correct—the inputs may conceivably be separated by up to hundreds of milliseconds and still interact to that effect. Furthermore, there is evidence that the *temporal order* of stimuli—nonsynchronous by definition—is critical for some kinds of associative learning. The principle of synchrony, however, may not be violated in these cases, for a given temporal order of stimuli can act as *one* stimulus and become associated with another. For the moment, it seems appropriate to assume some unspecified latitude to the postulated synchrony and accept that in some systems, including neocortex, the simultaneity of inputs may be imperfect yet effective. In other words, *near-synchrony* within a certain range of time may be sufficient for learned association; neither the perfect coincidence in time of arrival nor the temporal overlap of the inputs may be an absolute requirement.

Now let us resume briefly the argument for phyletic memory, attempting to extend back into phylogeny the principle of synchronous convergence. It is useful to reason from ontogeny into phylogeny and vice versa. If, as we shall discuss further in the next chapter, synchrony or near-synchrony of inputs is important for the normal functional development of the connective cortical apparatus of the visual system, it is reasonable to suppose that such synchrony was also important for the phylogenetic development of that apparatus and of other sensory systems as well. Some general considerations concerning the structure of the physical world and its impact on sensory systems in evolution are relevant here to support this argument.

Within discrete parts of the environment surrounding an organism, equal physical properties are more likely to occur simultaneously or almost simultaneously than are unequal ones, basically because of the spatial and temporal extensiveness of any given feature (e.g., a color, a tone, a straight edge). Note the observation made long ago by the philosopher James Mill (1829, p. 79) that "resemblance" can be reduced to a special case of co-occurrence, a special case of what he called synchronous order. It also is appropriate to invoke David Hume's dictum that causality is nothing but constant coincidence. Stryker (1991) has this dictum in mind when he argues for the neural basis of the perceptual constancy of slightly differing views of the same object taken in succession. In any event, it can be assumed that equal and spatially or temporally contiguous qualities will more likely and more often impinge simultaneously or nearly simultaneously on discrete sectors of the senses than will unequal and discontiguous ones. Thus, in the course of evolution, where probability assumes a determining role, the synchronies inherent in the physical world may have contributed to the convergence of similar and simultaneous inputs on sensory cells. By synchronous association, a basic connective structure could have been created such that those cells were made representative of those inputs and responsive to them. At the same time, it is apparent that those cells, interconnected and clustered in groups to represent certain prevalent features, became organized into an internal order topologically representing the environment or the body surface, especially in sectors of sensorium that are representable in spatial coordinates (i.e., retinotopically or somatotopically). The relevant point here is that synchronous convergence may indeed have been the principal driving force in organizing the connectivity of the primary sensory systems with which the organism is born.

That primary and innate organization, which we can consider the product of "neural Darwinism," would be the base upon which the rest of the processing and representational organization is built postnatally.

Whether or not the principles of its phylogenetic formation agree precisely with those that Edelman (1987) proposes for the formation of neural networks (see chapter 5), it seems plausible that the same principles contribute to the development, in postnatal life, of the synaptic structure of higher stages of the sensory processing and representational hierarchies. Beyond the formation of cell groups for representation of simple features, synchronous convergence presumably contributes to the formation of groups of cells for complex features, which are composites of associated simple features (e.g., complex cells), and then composites of composites (e.g., hypercomplex cells). Thus, basically the same principle of association by synchrony that in phylogeny possibly served to fashion the structure of sensory systems may serve the organism after birth, by selective enhancement of synaptic contacts, in the making of ever higher and more individualized layers of a sensory hierarchy. It is not unreasonable to imagine, on the motor side, a mirror image of comparable processes and a comparable hierarchy, a motor hierarchy also generated in phylogeny by synchronous convergence and growing in the same manner through ontogeny and through the rest of a life span.

SYNCHRONOUS DIVERGENCE

As we have noted, in the scheme of Hebb (1949) and in those of other theorizers, convergence leads to the formation of cell groups, or assemblies, that represent composites of common features from different parts of the sensory field. (Hebb used cortical visual areas 17, 18, 19, and 20 as the ground for his speculation.) It is a process of synthesis that, theoretically, continues up the hierarchy and forms ever more synthetic groups to represent classes of information and classes of classes and so on. There is abundant convergence of cortical pathways to support this process. However, this process alone would lead to something akin to the proverbial grandmother cell and to an infinite regress. Both outcomes are absurd and, of course, incompatible with experimental evidence.

Simply on those grounds, it would seem that the process of synthesis by synchronous convergence should be accompanied by a converse process, one of analysis by *divergence*. Evidence of this can be found in the patterns of connection of cortical sensory pathways, epitomized by the visual system (Van Essen, 1985). As we proceed up the visual hierarchy, we find divergent as well as convergent paths. Figure 3.7 emphasizes the divergence of interareal connections in cortical stages of the system's hierarchy. Divergent connections presumably assist feature analysis, for these connections lead from striate cortex (V1) to areas specializing in the analysis of different features (e.g., color, movement).

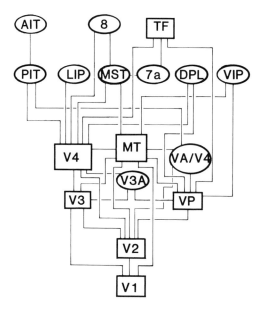

Figure 3.7 Connectivity between cortical areas of the visual system. (From Van Essen, 1985, with permission.)

Thus, sensory information, as it proceeds through the cortex, is probably not only synthesized but dispersed for further analysis, and then the outcomes of analysis are synthesized again, and so on.

Synthesis and analysis can accordingly be traced *pari passu* at all stages up a hierarchy. The first process would combine attributes into syntheses of attributes represented by cell groups that receive the converging inputs of the component features. The second would analyze the features of compound stimuli and distribute the outputs to higher-level cell groups that would, in turn, form new syntheses with those outputs, and so on. At no point would there be a need for an all-encompassing synthetic representation ("grandmother cell"), because most or all of the component features of that ultimate theoretical synthesis would be distributed among many other syntheses at the same or different levels of the hierarchy, each synthesis made of inputs from different analyzers.

Both convergence and divergence of connections are cardinal features of a number of computational models of learning that have been developed on hebbian principles and incorporate temporal synchronicity in the makeup of neural networks. For in-depth review of such models, the reader is referred to specialized compendia, such as that by Levine (1991) or Churchland and Sejnowski (1992). The functional architecture of some models will be discussed in chapters 5, 6, and 9, as it pertains to my theoretical approach or to our data.

NEW MEMORY ON OLD MEMORY

If our basic assumptions of memory formation are correct, processing and representation are practically inseparable at all levels, from the lowest to the highest. The cortical cell groups and networks that represent previously stored information are the same ones that will process and incorporate new information as it comes through the senses. The anatomical substrate created by previous processing will serve to process (i.e., analyze and synthesize) the new information. New associations will be formed with the old ones and, as a consequence, the new representations will contain a part of the old. It is a dynamic process of continuous interaction between novel experience and memory stores, in which the new serves to retrieve the old (including phyletic memory) and the old serves to interpret, analyze, and synthesize the new. Not only will a given experience activate the pathways and cell groups formed by the elements that the experience has in common with others from the past, but also it will serve to form connections between features or events that co-occur in the present. In conclusion, sensory processing and memory representation probably share largely the same cortical substrate. Representations are formed by accretion of new experience (i.e., new or newly reinforced synaptic connections) on a preexisting architecture which, in subsequent chapters, is viewed as consisting of widespread cortical networks.

It is important to understand that, in that accretion of new memory on old, the same principles of association by co-occurrence and synchronous convergence may apply as in the association of new external inputs among themselves. Indeed, an activated network of old memory may be construed by itself as a source of internal inputs. Those internal inputs from old memory may impinge on certain cortical ensembles in conjunction with new external inputs. Thus, the new and the old can synchronously converge on those ensembles and, in that way, new associations between the two may be engendered.

The same can be said for inputs from the internal milieu. Such inputs have their source in the visceral and humoral sphere and can reach the cortex through limbic and thalamic stations. They too can co-occur and converge with all sorts of other inputs, internal and external. This may be the basis for the formation of cortical associations between sensory experience and the basic drives of the organism.

In any event, the commonality of the cortical substrates for processing and representation has a respectable empirical base that will be discussed in more detail later. It is mentioned here to draw the attention of the reader to two fundamental points that derive from the breadth and complexity of cortical processing hierarchies. The first is the immense variability of the potential size and distribution of cortical memory traces. The second is the inherently dynamic and changing character of those cortical representations that participate in the processing of any new information the organism encounters, however minute and discrete that new information may be, and however well controlled by the zealous investigator.

LIMBIC SYSTEM AND MEMORY CONSOLIDATION

Now let's consider the manner in which new information, by the processes of synchronous convergence and divergence, can induce permanent synaptic changes in the cortex. As noted previously, the precise biophysical mechanisms underlying those changes at the level of the single cell are not yet understood. Substantial evidence, however, indicates that for these changes to become the permanent base of memory, the electrical activation of cell groups, or the neurochemical processes induced by such activation, must persist for some time. This evidence derives from demonstration of what has been called a *period of consolidation*. Such a period has been inferred from data showing that, for some time after a stimulus, its retention can be blocked by certain interfering measures, such as electroconvulsive shock (Glickman, 1961; McGaugh and Herz, 1972). Conversely, certain chemical substances have been shown to enhance memory retention when administered during a given period after learning (see below, Chemical Enhancement of Memory). The duration of the inferred consolidation, however, appears to vary with the kind of information to be retained, with the form of interference, and with the chemical administered. The time during which information becomes consolidated has been utilized to define operationally short-term memory. Of course, this process of consolidation would be the aspect of short-term memory that, in chapter 2, was referred to as the *gateway to long-term memory*. Like the other aspects or kinds of short-term memory, namely active and working memory, the consolidation of new memory may be based on the temporary activation of a cortical network at some level. In fact, memory consolidation may consist in the formation of a stable network as a result of that activation (see chapter 5).

In any case, some form of dynamic consolidation process—electrical, chemical, or both—appears necessary in cortical neuron populations for memory to endure. The concept of such a process is what led Hebb (1949) to postulate his dual-trace memory mechanism. According to him (he was discussing memory formation at lower levels of the cortical visual hierarchy, i.e., striate and peristriate cortex), activity would persist for a time in the cell group, or assembly, by reverberation within its neuronal circuits; this is what Hebb considered the basis of short-term memory. As a consequence of that activity, metabolic changes would take place that establish the memory trace permanently in the assembly. Whether Hebb's assembly coincides with what physiological studies have identified as a column, a minicolumn, or any other form of module with equipotential elements is debatable. Obviously, at higher levels, the representational ensembles (networks) for complex information are much larger than any of those modules and overstep the limits of any anatomically defined neocortical area. Anyway, the fact that recurrent or reverberating activity through reentrant circuits has not been demonstrated by available means does not exclude it as a possible mechanism of persistent representation at one or another level of a sensory or motor processing hierarchy. In chapter 9, we will consider reentry as an essential feature of an empirically tested computational model of active memory.

At higher levels of sensory and motor hierarchies, where representations are not restricted to small cell groups and are presumably widely distributed in associative networks, the principles of memory formation may be essentially the same as at lower levels, but a new element seems to appear: the role of limbic structures, especially the hippocampus, in memory acquisition and consolidation. At what level of a hierarchy those limbic structures begin to intervene and how they do it is still largely unknown. A plausible assumption is that limbic influences, acting on neurons of nonprimary (associative) neocortex, complement or enhance the basic processes of synchronous convergence and divergence in the formation of new associations, and thus new memory, by the strengthening of synaptic junctions. Fair (1992) proposes that this strengthening of synapses, which according to him probably takes place especially in cortical layers III and V, is achieved by reverberating activity between associative cortex and the hippocampus. The evidence for propositions of this kind has been growing in recent years but remains very sketchy. It consists of anatomical, neuropsychological, and neurochemical data that will be presented in brief next.

Studies of fiber connections in the monkey have provided considerable support for the notion that all corticocortical pathways originating in primary sensory areas send connections to limbic structures at one stage or another of their progression (Van Hoesen, 1982; Amaral, 1987). There seems to be a general flow of neocortical sensory input into the limbic system, especially the hippocampus (see chapter 4). This is clearly evident in the visual (extrastriate) pathway, which has been most thoroughly investigated; areas 19, 20, and 21 (inferotemporal cortex) send projections to limbic structures. It is also true, however, for other associative areas of posterior cortex and for prefrontal association areas 9 and 46, which presumably constitute higher stages of the motor hierarchy or, perhaps more precisely, the cortical region where sensory hierarchies meet the motor hierarchy.

All those cortical pathways into limbic structures appear to be reciprocated by pathways in the opposite direction (Amaral, 1987). The reciprocal connectivity between neocortex and hippocampus may be crucial for memory consolidation, and so it deserves special mention. None of that connectivity is direct. Both the afferent and efferent connections of the hippocampus with neocortex flow in stepwise fashion through the limbic cortex of the inferomedial aspects of the temporal lobe—that is, through perirhinal, parahippocampal, and entorhinal areas (figures 3.8, 3.9). Thus, through that inferomedial temporal cortex, which seems to act as a funnel for connections in both directions, the hippocampus has reciprocal input-output relationships with multiple neocortical areas of association. Just as there is a corticolimbic flow of connections, there is a limbic-cortical counterflow. Given that all connective steps in sensory cortical pathways are reciprocal, it is reasonable to suppose that such a limbic counterflow may influence perceptual functions all the way back to sensory cortex.

Neuropsychological observations indicate that the amygdala and even more so the hippocampus are important for memory formation. As

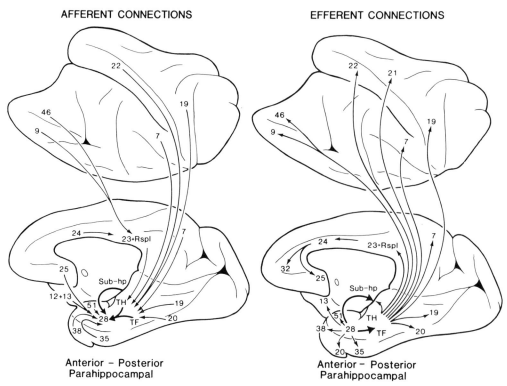

CORTICAL CONNECTIONS OF THE PARAHIPPOCAMPAL GYRUS

Figure 3.8 Afferent and efferent connections of the parahippocampal gyrus, including perirhinal and entorhinal areas, with the neocortex. The entorhinal cortex (area 28) constitutes a major node of bidirectional linkage between neocortical areas of association and the hippocampus. Rspl, retrosplenium; Sub-hp, subicular-hippocampal pathways. (From Van Hoessen, 1982, with permission.)

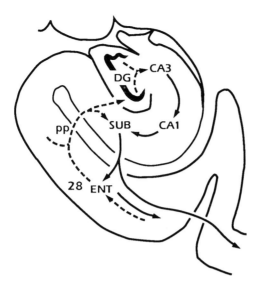

Figure 3.9 Diagram of a cross-section of the hippocampal formation depicting its intrinsic connectivity and pathways of extrinsic connection with the neocortex through the entorhinal area (28). CA1, CA3, pyramidal fields; DG, dentate gyrus; ENT, entorhinal area; pp, perforant path; SUB, subiculum.

previously noted (see chapter 2), midtemporal lesions in the human were shown to induce *anterograde amnesia*—that is, a severe impediment to form new memories (Scoville and Milner, 1957; Squire, 1987). Using behavioral paradigms supposed to test the formation of new declarative visual memory in the monkey (e.g., delayed nonmatching to sample), experimental lesions of amygdala or hippocampus also were shown to induce what appeared to be an anterograde memory deficit (Mishkin, 1978; Zola-Morgan and Squire, 1985). The deficit was cumulative, in that it was maximal after combined amygdalar and hippocampal lesions and of lesser magnitude after lesions of either amygdala or hippocampus. This, paradoxically, suggested an equivalent role in memory formation for two structures that, despite their anatomical contiguity, have different phylogenetic and embryological origins and markedly different architecture. That cumulative deficit raised unsettling questions about the value of the behavioral tasks utilized for testing the formation of declarative memory and the experimental lesions performed to impede it. Those questions have now been partly clarified. Zola-Morgan and colleagues (1989) have shown that the most critical structures injured in those earlier experiments may have been the perirhinal and parahippocampal areas 35 and 36, at the base of the temporal lobe, which provide the intermediate link between entorhinal and inferotemporal cortex. This evidence implicates the hippocampus, rather than the amygdala, in memory formation. In fact, later experiments with selective lesions (Zola-Morgan et al., 1991) do so more directly, while con-

Principles of Neural Memory Formation

firming the traditionally accepted role of the amygdala in emotion and in the evaluation of the motivational significance of external stimuli and events (Gloor, 1960; Fuster and Uyeda, 1971; LeDoux, 1992a,b, 1993).

Precisely because of its emotional role, however, the amygdala cannot be excluded from memory processes. Indeed, the amygdala may contribute to the hippocampus and cortical networks the neural inputs from the affective sphere that human psychology makes us suspect are so important for the formation and solidity of new memory. This role of the amygdala in memory has been substantiated by interactions between this structure and neurotransmitter systems in the learning process (see the next section).

A recent experiment (Zola-Morgan and Squire, 1990) suggests that the role of the hippocampus in memory consolidation is time-limited. Hippocampal lesions interfered with monkeys' ability to perform visual discriminations learned within 4 weeks before surgery, whereas they apparently did not interfere with more remotely acquired discriminations. It is as if, after memory acquisition, the hippocampus exercised its consolidating role mainly within a time window of 4 weeks. As time passes and a given memory is consolidated, probably in neocortex, that role would wane.

It seems reasonable to infer, from animal experiments as from clinical data, that limbic structures play a critical role in the consolidation of memory traces. Mishkin's (1982) conceptualization of the amygdala and the hippocampus as critical components of a memory system remains plausible in very general terms. It is not yet clear, however, despite the electrochemical evidence discussed next, precisely how those structures take part in memory consolidation; nor is their role in memory retrieval clear, though it is a role we presume and that will be discussed in later chapters.

NEUROTRANSMITTERS AND MEMORY CONSOLIDATION

Neurons throughout the cerebral cortex are under the influence of several neurotransmitter systems of subcortical origin that may intervene decisively in the formation of new memory. Clearly, the modulation of cortical neurons by these systems, which regulate the states of sleep, wakefulness, and alertness, can be supposed a priori to influence the synaptic changes that underlie the consolidation of memory. Thus far, however, the available evidence is inconclusive regarding precisely which systems affect that process and how they do it.

By indirect evidence, it appears that the *cholinergic system*, with its source in the nuclear complex of Meynert at the base of the diencephalon, is critically implicated in memory. The evidence derives from neuropathological investigation of patients suffering from Alzheimer's dementia, a disease characterized, from its inception, by disorders of memory. In early stages of the disease, the most common deficit is one of attention and fixation of new memory. Later, long-term memory also is affected. On autopsy of some Alzheimer patients, severe lesions of the cholinergic nuclear aggregates of the basal diencephalon have been reported (Whitehouse et al., 1982). Pathological alterations have also been found in the hippocampus and the entorhinal cortex (Hyman et al., 1984); in light of the issues discussed in the previous section, those pathological alterations have been linked to the troubles these patients have in memory formation. A recent study of functional imaging shows that the hippocampus is one of a few brain structures most consistently hypometabolic in Alzheimer's disease (Perani et al., 1993). The general conclusion may be drawn that the memory disorders of Alzheimer patients are somewhat attributable to the impairment of the cholinergic neurotransmitter system, the hippocampus, and its cortical links to associative cortex.

A substantial body of animal learning literature, reviewed by Decker and McGaugh (1991), indicates that the cholinergic system exerts its role in memory not alone but by interactions with other neurotransmitter systems. Here I will provide only the essence of the evidence they review from the work of many laboratories. Most of the experiments have been performed on rats trained in one or several of the following tasks: active avoidance, inhibitory avoidance, radial arm maze, Morris water maze, match to sample, and nonmatch to sample. By using agonists and antagonists of acetylcholine (ACh), norepinephrine (NE), dopamine (DA), serotonin, γ-aminobutyric acid (GABA), and several opioids, performance has been shown to be improved or impaired, thus indicating a role of the neurotransmitters in question in the acquisition or retention of memory (see the next section for some specific substances). Using the appropriate combinations of chemicals, two neurotransmitter systems can be manipulated concurrently; in this manner, several synergistic or antagonistic effects of neurotransmitter pairs have been observed. Most prominently, interactive effects on memory have been demonstrated between the cholinergic system, on the one hand, and an NE, DA, serotonin, GABAergic, or opiate system on the other. By local chemical injections into the amygdala of trained or learning animals, McGaugh (1992) and his colleagues have obtained evidence of some such interactions within that structure. From their observations, they conclude that cholinergic, noradrenergic, opiate, and GABAergic systems interact within the amygdala, and the end result of these interactions is to regulate the release of NE, thus supporting the role of the amygdala in memory formation.

The amino acid *glutamate* is probably the most pervasive of all intrinsic excitatory transmitters in the central nervous system. It is especially abundant in the hippocampus and the cerebral cortex (Westbrook and Jahr, 1989). Glutaminergic synapses work on two broad categories of receptors: quisquilate or kainate (Q/K) and *N*-methyl-D-aspartate (NMDA). When activated by glutamate, both groups of receptors depolarize the postsynaptic membrane by opening ion channels (see figure 3.10). In recent years, *NMDA receptors* have attracted considerable interest for having peculiar properties that make them highly relevant to neural plasticity and the formation of memory (Dingledine, 1983; Cotman and Iversen, 1987). Those properties can be summarized as follows: (1) NMDA receptors are voltage-dependent—that is, they are activated by glutamate only beyond a certain level of depolarization of the postsynaptic membrane, at which level Mg^{2+} ions are expelled from membrane channels, and Ca^{2+} current, along with Na^+ current, is allowed to flow into the cell. Furthermore, that current increases as a function of the degree of depolarization. (2) The NMDA-induced current and postsynaptic potentials are longer in duration (a few hundreds of milliseconds) than those induced by non-NMDA receptors.

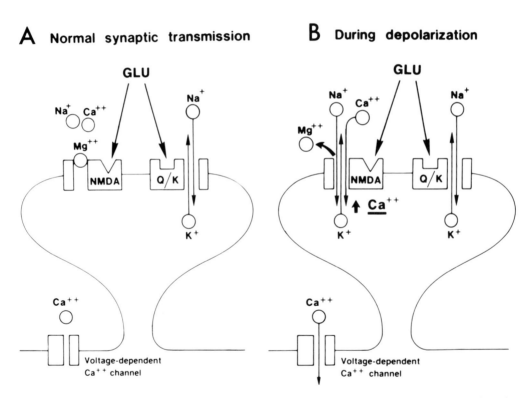

A **Normal synaptic transmission**   **B** **During depolarization**

Figure 3.10 During low-frequency synaptic transmission (A), glutamate (GLU) released from the presynaptic terminal acts on both NMDA and Q/K receptors. Na^+ and K^+ flow through the Q/K receptor channel but not through the NMDA receptor channel because the latter is blocked by Mg^{2+}. (B) During high-frequency depolarization (tetanus), the NMDA channel is unblocked, allowing Ca^{2+} to flow through it. These phenomena would be the basis of LTP. (From Nicoll et al., 1988, with permission.)

Because of the long course of the currents they generate, NMDA receptors are well suited for temporal integration and thus, possibly, for mediating synaptic changes as a result of synchronous or near-synchronous convergence of inputs. By activating NMDA receptors, the strong stimulation of one pathway can depolarize the membrane enough, and for a long enough period, to potentiate the response of the cell to weaker stimuli arriving through other pathways during that time. This seems to be the case in LTP.

There now is considerable evidence that the activation of NMDA receptors is responsible for the induction of LTP in the hippocampus (see Nicoll et al., 1988, for review). The first such evidence was the observation that an NMDA antagonist blocks the development of LTP in the CA1 region of the hippocampus during high-frequency tetanic stimulation of the Schaffer commissural pathway (Collingridge et al., 1983). This has also been seen to occur in the dentate gyrus, on stimulation of the perforant path (Errington et al., 1987). The role of NMDA receptors in LTP appears, to some extent, to be regulated by GABAergic inhibition, inasmuch as the release of postsynaptic cells from inhibition facilitates their LTP (Wigstrom and Gustaffson, 1985).

It is not known how LTP ultimately results in the permanent synaptic changes that presumably lead to enhanced transmittance. It has been postulated that these changes are mediated by protein metabolism (Lynch and Baudry, 1984; Routtenberg, 1985). There is some evidence that glutamate, possibly through NMDA receptors, can activate second messenger systems in the postsynaptic cell, whereby protein changes would be induced for maintenance of LTP and concomitant structural changes of the synaptic apparatus (Collingridge and Bliss, 1987; Westbrook and Jahr, 1989; Schuman and Madison, 1994). Recent evidence implicates nitric oxide (Böhme et al., 1993) and amino-methyl-isoxazoleproprionate (AMPA) glutamate receptors (Maren et al., 1993), in addition to NMDA receptors, as coadjuvant or intermediary agents in the protein metabolic changes underlying hippocampal LTP and its behavioral manifestations.

Experiments with LTP have also suggested an important role of NMDA in the formation of associations by synchronous convergence (see Cotman et al., 1988, for review). As noted earlier, weak inputs to hippocampal cells are potentiated if they arrive while a strong LTP-inducing input is present. At least one NMDA antagonist has been shown to impede the learning of a spatial task if perfused in the hippocampus (Morris et al., 1989). NMDA is also implicated in visual and olfactory plasticity (cf. Cotman et al., 1988), as well as in the formation of motor programs in the spinal cord (Grillner et al., 1987).

In conclusion, NMDA receptors, especially in the hippocampus, appear important for use-dependent synaptic strengthening and, therefore, in learning and memory. The underlying mechanisms, however, remain obscure. Even more uncertain than their role in the hippocampus is the role of NMDA receptors in the cerebral cortex, where they are exceedingly common (Cotman et al., 1987). One apparent clue to their involvement in corticocortical association is the finding that their greatest concentration is in cortical layers II and III, which are the last to myelinate in the course of ontogeny (see chapter 4) and where corticocortical fibers predominantly terminate (Jacobson and Trojanowski, 1977a,b; Jones, 1981; Van Essen and Maunsell, 1983; Schwartz and Goldman-Rakic, 1984; Andersen et al., 1985). This is in accord with electrophysiological findings (Pumain and Heinemann, 1985; Thomson et al., 1985; Cotman et al., 1987). It is entirely possible that, in associative learning and memory, the NMDA receptors of cortical pyramidal cells are activated by confluence of glutaminergic inputs from hippocampus and from concomitantly activated cortical areas. Such activation of cortical NMDA might be the basis for synaptic changes at the root of memory formation.

Whatever the neurochemical mechanisms involved, the fundamental role of the hippocampus in the consolidation of memory is becoming increasingly evident. In their recent book, Cohen and Eichenbaum (1993), based mainly on extensive review of neuropsychological evidence, propose that the critical function of the hippocampus is the processing of relationships between representations. I would again suggest that the hippocampus probably exercises this function by somehow reinforcing the synaptic substrate of temporally coincident representations in the neocortex. Thus, by virtue of this role, the hippocampus would be the solidifier of the self-organizing neuronal network that, in chapter 5, is envisioned as the seat of the engram.

CHEMICAL ENHANCEMENT OF MEMORY

Can memory be enhanced by chemical means? There is as yet no simple answer to this question. It seems beyond dispute that, as indicated previously, under certain conditions a number of substances can facilitate some of the neural processes involved in memory formation. The precise pharmacological mechanisms by which they do so are not fully understood, however, and their action is not demonstrably specific only to memory. Most of the chemical agents in question have a variety of neuropharmacological and psychopharmacological effects beyond that of enhancing memory, and some of these effects are known to be detrimental to certain other organismic functions.

General CNS stimulants, or disinhibitors, were the first drugs to qualify as memory enhancers. Lashley, as early as 1917, noted that caffeine and strychnine accelerated the rat's rate of learning. Strychnine and picrotoxin, when administered *after* learning trials, were shown to improve performance of learned tasks (McGaugh and Petrinovich, 1959; Breen and McGaugh, 1961). From these findings, it was inferred that those drugs somehow facilitate the consolidation of memory and, consequently, its retrieval.

There has been a long series of investigations identifying neurotransmitter agonists or antagonists as facilitators of memory. Among the *monoaminergic agonists* so characterized have been the amphetamines and other re-uptake inhibitors of norepinephrine, dopamine, or serotonin (see the review by McGaugh, 1989). These substances have also been noted to facilitate learned animal performance when administered posttrial.

Probably no group of memory enhancers has received as much attention as those that act on cholinergic modulator systems. One of the reasons for this is the previously mentioned evidence that the cholinergic system of basal diencephalic origin (nucleus of Meynert) may be critically impaired in neurodegenerative disorders, such as Alzheimer's disease (Whitehouse et al., 1982; Coyle et al., 1983), that are accompanied by severe amnesia. Another reason is the evidence that certain cholinesterase inhibitors, such as *physostigmine*, have been noted in some instances to alleviate the amnesic troubles of the elderly and the Alzheimer patient (see the review by Bartus, 1990). As Bartus indicates, however, the therapeutic use of these substances is severely limited for the following reasons: (1) extremely short half-life, (2) poor penetration of the blood-brain barrier, (3) high incidence of untoward effects, and (4) narrow therapeutic window. In any event, for reasons outlined earlier, to single out acetylcholine as the neurotransmitter mediator of memory formation seems simplistic.

Finally, a relatively new class of chemical substances, the so-called *nootropics* (aniracetam, piracetam, etc.) warrant mention. These substances were developed specifically to alleviate the cognitive troubles of the aged (for review, see Bartus, 1990). They are unrelated to neurotransmitters and have been reported to facilitate consolidation of memory (especially avoidance conditioning) when administered long after learning trials (Cumin et al., 1982; Mondadori and Petschke, 1987). One of them, CGS5649B (Ciba-Geigy, Ltd.), has been claimed to do so even when given 24 hours after trials (Mondadori et al., 1991). Nefiracetam (DM-9384, Daiichi Pharmaceutical) has been shown to enhance classical eye-blink conditioning in older rabbits (Woodruff-Pak et al., 1993). Significantly, some nootropic agents have been reported to enhance LTP (Staubli et al., 1990). All nootropic agents seem to have in common their dependence on the integrity of steroid metabolism. Adrenalectomy and other forms of interference with that metabolism render them ineffective as memory enhancers. Because steroids act as modulators of gene transcription and synthesis of proteins, it is tempting to speculate that nootropics facilitate the biophysical changes that take place in cortical neurons as a result of the synaptic transactions that underlie the formation of memory. One does well to keep in mind, however, that nootropics have thus far been tested only on a narrow range of animal learning tasks, and no evidence is available yet of their effectiveness in primate, let alone human, memory.

4   Anatomy of Cortical Memory

Cortical memory is not a type or system of memory different from those mentioned in chapter 2. It most likely includes all of them. The term, however, is not meant to exclude noncortical structures from the process, storage, or content of any of those memory types or systems. Rather, it is meant as a generic term for the involvement of the cerebral neocortex in all those kinds of memory, however they are defined and by whatever criterion. What follows is a brief description of the general principles of cortical organization, as it is currently understood and as it bears on the structure of memory networks. The emphasis here is on connectivity and on the constitution of cortical hierarchies for processing and storage of perceptual and motor memory.

BASIC ARCHITECTURE OF THE CORTEX

It has been known for a long time (Ramón y Cajal, 1904) that the basic structure of the neocortex is remarkably similar throughout. All of it is characterized by the striking horizontal and vertical regularities of its cells and fibers (figure 4.1). As noted by numerous observers, the structural uniformity of the neocortex is patently at odds with the highly specialized nature of its functions. This uniformity alone argues loudly for ascribing functional specialization to a less conspicuous attribute of cortical organization: the connectivity of cortical neurons. In fact, the architectonic differences between cortical areas are ontogenetically determined by afferent connections and develop *pari passu* with them. On these grounds, Creutzfeldt (1977) has singled out thalamic afferents as the crucial determining factor of cortical functions. Indeed, functional specificity may not be determined only by thalamocortical afferents but by corticocortical connections as well. Furthermore, the possibility should be considered that some of the connective links between associative cortical areas, which I so much emphasize in this book, are established through the thalamus (Reinoso-Suárez, 1984). With these ideas in mind, it is now appropriate to take a close look at cortical connectivity.

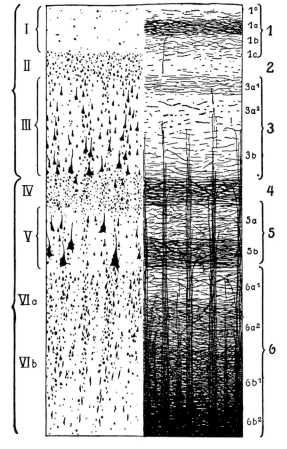

Figure 4.1 Cellular and myelin structure of the cerebral cortex, according to Brodmann and Vogt. (From Economo, 1929, with permission.)

The analysis of the laminar organization of the neocortex, with its characteristic six layers, reveals several strata of horizontally running fibers. Prominent among them are the basal dendrites and the horizontal top-layer ramifications of the apical dendrites of pyramidal cells, all of them offering contacts to incoming axon collaterals and terminals from neighboring or distant cells (figures 4.2, 4.3). The recurrent collaterals from pyramids usually follow a horizontal or oblique course and spread around as much as 2 to 3 mm. Their effect on other local neurons seems to be partly inhibitory, probably through interneurons (Renaud and Kelly, 1974; Hess et al., 1975).

Then there are the arrays of fibers that run vertically, perpendicular to the cortical surface. Prominent among them are the apical dendrites of pyramidal cells which group themselves in bundles approximately 100 μm thick (Fleischauer, 1978; Szentágothai, 1978a,b; Roney et al., 1979) (see figure 4.3). Corticocortical afferents from afar commonly terminate on those apical dendrites in layers I to III. In addition, there are

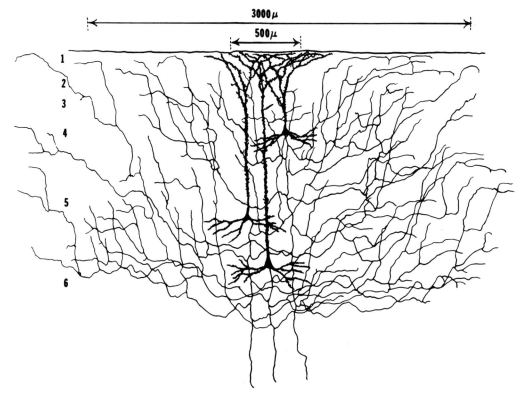

Figure 4.2 Cortical pyramidal cells surrounded by recurrent collaterals. Dendritic spines appear as rugosities on the surface of apical dendrites. (From Scheibel and Scheibel, 1970, with permission.)

the vertical plexuses of thalamic afferents ascending to layer IV (to contact stellate cells), as well as the axons from pyramidal cells, in layers III, V, and VI, descending to the white matter with subcortical or cortical destination (Lorente de Nó, 1938; Scheibel and Scheibel, 1970). In sum, the geometry of cortical connectivity contains, implicitly, the potential for extensive parallel processing along vertical arrays of neural elements as well as for corticocortical association. Both will be needed to support the role of cortical networks in perception, movement, and memory.

One of the most significant characteristics of the functional neuro-anatomy of sensory cortical areas is their *modular organization.* In these areas, neurons that specialize in detecting a given sensory feature, such as visual orientation, are arranged in columns (50 to 80 μm wide, depending on the area or feature) that traverse the cortex orthogonally to its surface (Mountcastle, 1957; Hubel and Wiesel, 1968; Asanuma, 1975). Thus, the column, or minicolumn, could be conceptualized as the ubiquitous and irreducible functional unit of cortex (Mountcastle, 1978). Outside of primary sensory areas, however, the modular organization is less clear. Also less clear is the intrinsic connectivity of a

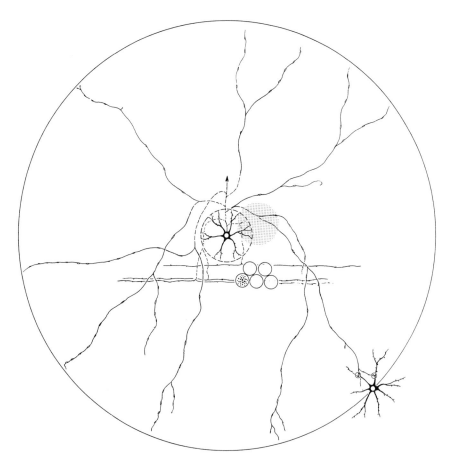

Figure 4.3 Diagram of two pyramidal cells viewed from the surface. The large circle, with a diameter of approximately 3 mm, indicates the zone within reach of the collaterals of the cell in the center. The small circles (approximately 100 μm in diameter) correspond to dendritic bundles. (From Szentágothai, 1978b, with permission.)

column, even within primary sensory areas. Nonetheless, as a general rule, most of the thalamic and some of the cortical afferents to a column terminate on the neurons of its layer IV, whereas most corticocortical fibers originate and terminate in cells of supragranular layer III (some terminate in layers V–VI) (figure 4.4). Important outputs to cortical or subcortical locations emerge from layers III, V, and VI.

The point that bears emphasize here is that, whether we consider the single pyramidal cell or the columnar module as the functional cortical unit, corticocortical inputs and outputs are pervasive in the neocortex. It is reasonable to suppose that therein, in addition to thalamic input, lies the heterogeneity of connectivity that defines cortical function and the content of memory. Later we shall consider the details of that connectivity when we discuss cortical hierarchies. Before that, let us

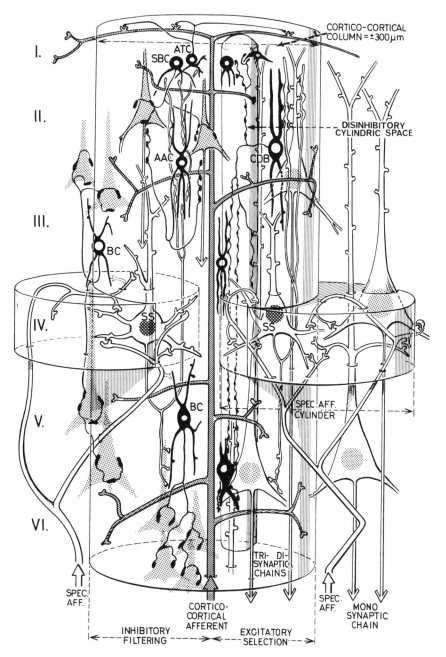

Figure 4.4 An idealized column of cortex comprising and defined by the terminal branches of a corticocortical afferent axon (three functional assumptions are noted in the diagram). The column is flanked by sections of two specific (thalamic) afferent cylinders. AAC, axoaxonic cell; ATC, axonal tuft cell; BC, basket cell; CDB, cell *à double bouquet*; SBC, small basket cell; SS, spiny stellate cell. (From Szentágothai, 1983, with permission.)

consider the cortical substrate of phyletic memory and its margin of plasticity.

PHYLETIC CORTICAL MEMORY

As in most matters regarding evolution, the reasoning behind the concepts of phyletic memory and of its expansion into individual memory are somewhat teleological and only sparsely supported by empirical knowledge. There are, however, two lines of experimental evidence that support those concepts, albeit indirectly and with the help of retrospective reasoning from ontogeny into phylogeny. The first is the evidence that, in certain periods of the life of the organism, even its inherited substrate for primary sensory and motor processing exhibits plasticity and depends on experience for the development of its structure and functions. Second is the anatomical and physiological evidence of at least some cortical information processing along ontogenetic gradients, from early-maturing sensory areas to late-maturing areas of association. The first line of evidence will be briefly discussed in this section and the next, the second in later sections.

Sensory Phyletic Memory

At birth, the primary sensory systems of the mammalian brain are almost entirely developed anatomically (Lund and Bunt, 1976; Wise and Jones, 1976; Rakic, 1977). The basic architecture of the adult sensory cortex has been attained, its neural elements are in place, and its connectivity is virtually complete. However, several important structural changes are yet to occur. After an overproduction of cortical cells and synapses, both will decrease in numbers postnatally and eventually will stabilize at adult levels (Rakic et al., 1986), in a process similar to the one observed in neuromuscular junctions (Changeux and Danchin, 1976). The same is true, throughout the cortex, for neurotransmitter receptors (Lidow et al., 1991). Axonal and dendritic arborization will also undergo some postnatal growth. In any case, whereas the sensory cortex of the neonate would appear, on cytoarchitectonic grounds, to be ready for normal function, experimental data show that it is far from ready, at least with regard to vision.

To achieve its full functional development, the visual cortex needs visual experience during a critical period of early life. In the absence of that critical experience, that cortex will remain functionally defective and normal vision will not be attained or, if it is, it will be only after considerable training. Some analogous and indirect evidence of this, beyond the perinatal period, derives from the study of vision in the congenitally blind human who has undergone correction of congenital cataracts (Senden, 1960). More direct evidence derives from studies of the behavioral and electrophysiological effects of early visual deprivation in cats and monkeys (Wiesel and Hubel, 1965; Hubel and Wiesel, 1970; Blakemore and Van Sluyters, 1974; Blakemore et al., 1978). The functional underdevelopment resulting from sensory deprivation is accompanied by faulty development of fine structure, especially as it pertains to the arborization of thalamic (lateral geniculate) axons that reach cortical layer IV (Wiesel, 1982). In the visually deprived adult, thalamic terminals fail to show the normal patterns of segregation by ocular dominance columns. (figure 4.5, right).

Many questions remain unresolved concerning the ontogeny of structure and function of primary sensory cortex. One such question is the role of competition of inputs in the development of synaptic terminals and contacts. This question has been raised by several findings, among them the abnormalities and asymmetries of axonal terminations and of neuronal responsiveness in the visual cortex of monocularly deprived animals (LeVay and Stryker, 1979; Wiesel, 1982). Inputs obviously compete in early ontogeny for the development of synapses. The sparing of synapses from the normal perinatal attrition—after overproduction—

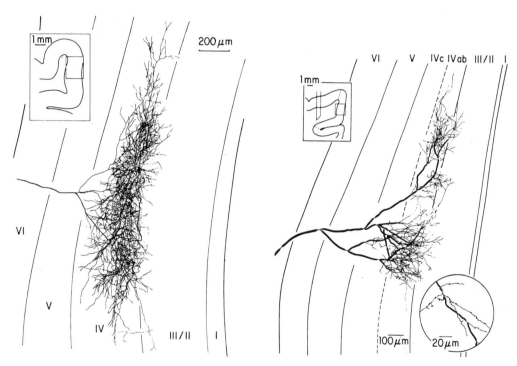

Figure 4.5 Arborization of a geniculocortical axon in the visual cortex of a 17-day-old kitten (*left*) and an adult cat (*right*). In the mature animal, the arbor is subdivided into clumps, corresponding to ocular dominance columns, separated by gaps filled by afferent terminals from the other eye (here unstained). With posnatal monocular deprivation, the gaps are filled by expansion of afferents from the nondeprived eye. (From LeVay and Stryker, 1979, with permission.)

depends on the availability of input. Moreover, in the partial absence of normal inputs, the growth of axons and synaptic terminals takes place apparently at the expense of those that have not been "protected" by input (Wiesel, 1982). Correlated neural activity from both eyes seems important for the normal development of axon collaterals between ocular dominance columns in striate cortex (Löwel and Singer, 1992).

In conclusion, visual experience during a critical postnatal period is essential for the development of a normal visual cortex and, consequently, for normal adult vision. Postnatal plasticity and the role of sensory input for morphological and functional development have also been shown in somatosensory cortex (Van der Loos and Woolsey, 1973; Kalaska and Pomeranz, 1979) and olfactory cortex (Wilson et al., 1987) but, in these cortices, critical periods have not been demonstrated as clearly as in visual cortex. Nevertheless, these findings are in agreement with the general principle that, for the final maturation of a sensory cortical substrate that is phylogenetically predetermined and almost invariant in structure and function from one individual to another, the organism needs exposure to sensory input. It is reasonable to infer that during a certain critical period after birth, the organism does with the environment what phylogeny has previously done through millions of years: acquires the capacity, which here we call *phyletic memory*, to distinguish and recognize the elementary sensory features of the world that it will later combine in connective cortical networks for construction of individual memory. *That critical period of new experience at the beginning of life might be like a necessary rehearsal of phyletic memory before individual memory can be formed.*

Motor Phyletic Memory

All this would apply to sensory phyletic memory, especially of the visual modality, for which there is the most empirical evidence. The question now is, do similar principles apply to motor phyletic memory? Is there a critical period of motor experience necessary for the structural and functional maturation of primary motor cortex? Despite serious methodological difficulties in approaching these questions, there is enough evidence to suggest that they can be affirmatively answered. Let us summarize some of it.

The ethological literature (Tinbergen, 1951; Lorenz, 1970) contains ample evidence that animal organisms are born with the ability to perform a variety of patterns of motor behavior, some of them fairly complex although stereotypical. These patterns can be conceptualized as innate *templates of movement*, driven by instinct and ready to be expressed in appropriate conditions of the internal and external milieu. For their normal development, some of them require the presence of these conditions within a certain period of time after birth; thus, they are subject to a critical period. One notable example, which here deserves a small digression, is the song of birds, a species-specific behavior with a reasonably well-known neural substrate (Konishi, 1985). To develop their song, birds have to hear the song of conspecific birds within a critical postnatal period (Marler, 1981; Konishi, 1985). They also need to hear their own song; in other words, they need auditory feedback. Even deaf birds, however, can develop rudimentary song patterns. The available evidence on these issues (Nottebohm, 1991) points to the presence, at birth, of innate patterns of song production that become perfected with imitation and auditory feedback. In the normal bird, the size of the song-controlling motor nuclei correlates with the richness of the song and is subject to seasonal fluctuations in accord with hormonal factors that influence its expression. Plasticity in avian song systems, however, is not limited to neonatal life but has been shown to extend into adulthood, with evidence of continuing neuronal replacement within those systems (Alvarez-Buylla et al., 1990).

Mammals also display innate behaviors that seem minimally dependent on sensory input. Human infants display a variety of movements, some reflex and others instinct-driven, that eventually become the components of complex sequences (Piaget, 1952; Bruner, 1973). For good reasons, which need not be discussed here, it has been postulated that all complex skills develop on a matrix of unlearned movement (Adams, 1984), much as perception develops on a matrix of elementary sensations.

It is not clear to what extent that primitive motility, the postulated basis of phyletic motor memory, is supported by the motor cortex in the mammalian brain, nor is it clear whether the development of that cortex undergoes a critical period. There is, however, evidence of early plasticity in both cerebellar cortex and primary motor cortex (reflecting, to some degree, subcortical plasticity). Mice that, during a postnatal period, perform a great deal of motor activity develop much more dendritic arborization of Purkinje cells than do mice deprived of the opportunity to perform it (Pysh and Weiss, 1979). In adult life, structures of the cerebellum, including the cerebellar cortex, have been implicated in certain aspects of motor memory (Thompson, 1986). Adult rats that have undergone unilateral ablation of motor cortex as neonates show low-threshold ipsilateral movements by microstimulation of the motor cortex of the intact hemisphere (Kartje-Tillotson et al., 1985); this is not the case in normal adults. These observations suggest that, after the neonatal ablation, the plasticity of the intact motor cortex enables it to compensate for the loss of the contralateral cortex, which is normally in charge of those movements. Peripheral manipulations of the motor system of the rat in early development have been shown to result in reorganization of motor cortex (Donoghue and Sanes, 1987, 1988). In the monkey, Lawrence and Hopkins (1976) showed that the development of fine finger motility correlates with the development, at an early age (within the first 4 weeks), of corticospinal fibers from primary motor cortex. They also demonstrated, by bilateral removal of somatosensory areas, that the development of finger motility does not depend on sensory input.

These findings, as a whole, speak for the presence of considerable early plasticity in motor systems, including motor cortex, with suggestions of postnatal critical periods. They are fully consistent with the notion of the parallel development of phyletic motor memory and phyletic sensory memory.

LATE PLASTICITY OF PRIMARY AREAS

After critical ontogenetic periods, cortical cells, axons, and dendrites have largely finished their growth and natural recession and they do not conspicuously manifest further morphological plasticity. It is for this reason that some theorists, such as Edelman (1987), speak of a first and fixed repertoire of cell groups and connections (see chapter 5). Further changes, according to him, would occur by stimulus selection of preexisting and preconnected cell groups of that first repertoire and by strengthening of their synaptic contacts. Thus, a secondary repertoire would emerge as the substrate for perception and memory.

In any case, some degree of plasticity of cortical neurons can be demonstrated experimentally not only in early ontogeny but beyond, whether due to growth of new connections or facilitation of old ones. In addition to the plastic phenomena already mentioned in the early development of striate cortex, having to do with the critical period for vision, it has been observed that cortical neurons in animals raised in an enriched (i.e., sensorially stimulating) environment show more dendritic branching and spines than in animals raised in an impoverished (i.e., sensorially poor) environment (Diamond et al., 1966; Floeter and Greenough, 1979; Withers and Greenough, 1989). Those animals are behaviorally superior in performing a number of tasks (Rosenzweig, 1984). Conversely, visual deprivation in early life leads to degeneration of dendritic processes in visual cortex (Cragg, 1967; Globus and Scheibel, 1967; Valverde, 1971).

Also in early development, by selective experimental sections and lesions, it is possible to reroute sensory pathways in such a manner that the afferents of one modality are forced to innervate the primary cortex of another (Roe et al., 1990; Sur et al., 1990). This causes the cortical neurons of one modality to respond to events of another (*cross-modal plasticity*). However, the structural and functional outcome of these manipulations is closely dependent on the developmental stage at which they are conducted. The later that is, the less effective are these manipulations in changing the connective organization of sensory systems. In sensory cortex, even by early manipulations, only the microcircuitry may be affected but not the laminar organization or the efferent and callosal connections. This is another indication that, not long after birth, the sensory derivative of the original cortical matrix, or *protocortex* (O'Leary, 1989), has been largely, though not completely, committed in both structure and function.

Be that as it may, the plasticity of somatosensory cortex has been well documented in young as well as adult animals (Van der Loos and Woolsey, 1973; Kalaska and Pomeranz, 1979; Merzenich and Kaas, 1982; Wall, 1988). In owl monkeys, the cutting of afferent innervation from a part of the hand leads to a remarkable rearrangement of the receptive fields of nerve cells in areas 3 and 1, where hands and fingers are represented (Merzenich and Kaas, 1982; Kaas et al., 1983). That rearrangement includes the expansion of fields of representation for areas of the skin with preserved innervation, at the expense of those for deafferented areas (figure 4.6). In the rhesus monkey, 12 years after extensive deafferentation of the upper extremity, massive rearrangements have been observed in cortical somatosensory maps, such as an expansion of the face map by 10 mm or more (Pons et al., 1991). Behavioral tactile stimulation has been seen to produce a converse effect: expansion of the cortical fields representing the stimulated skin areas (Jenkins et al., 1990). The remapping of somatosensory cortex by lesion or stimulation provides evidence of competitive forces that are latent under normal conditions of physiological equilibrium between areas but become manifest when that equilibrium is altered. Further evidence of somatosensory cortical plasticity in the adult animal has been obtained in owl monkeys trained to perform tactile frequency discriminations (Recanzone et al., 1992a,b). As the monkey learns to perform such discriminations, an expansion of hand representation areas has been observed in primary somatosensory cortex. In the human adult, Mogilner and colleagues (1993) have observed somatosensory plasticity by means of magnetoencephalography. Two subjects submitted to an operation for webbed fingers (syndactyly) showed, within weeks after surgery, evidence of cortical reorganization correlating with the function of their newly separated fingers.

Recanzone and associates (1993), by microelectrode recording, have begun to substantiate the plasticity of the primary auditory cortex of the owl monkey. Their study shows that animals trained to perform fine auditory discriminations undergo a tonotopic reorganization of that cortex. The cortical representation area, as well as the sharpness of tuning and the magnitude of cell responses, are greater for behaviorally relevant acoustic frequencies in trained monkeys than in control monkeys.

Adult plasticity has also been shown in the motor system, including motor cortex. In the cat, Keller and coworkers (1990) note that the

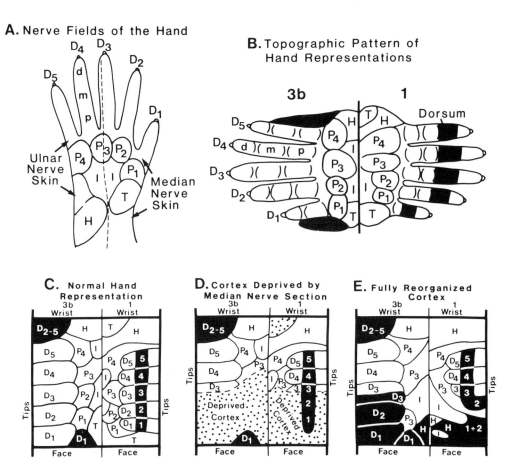

Figure 4.6 Reorganization of the receptive fields of neurons in somatosensory cortex of the owl monkey after section of the median nerve. (*A*) Nerve fields of the owl monkey's hand. (*B* and *C*) Schematic pattern of normal hand representation in cortical areas 3b and 1. Deafferented portions of those two areas (*D*) are filled, several months after deafferentation, by expanded representation of skin surfaces innervated by the ulnar nerve (*E*). (From Merzenich and Kaas, 1982, with permission.)

unilateral lesion of deep cerebellar nuclei induced a deficit in motor performance that was followed by recovery after some 40 days; histological examination after recovery revealed the sprouting of terminal corticocortical connections from somatosensory to motor cortex (especially in layers II to V). Evidently, the axon terminals had developed new synapses to motor neurons, presumably in order to establish surrogate function.

In experiments highly reminiscent of those that Merzenich and his colleagues conducted on the somatosensory cortex of the monkey (figure 4.6), Sanes and coworkers (1990) have demonstrated the reorganization of the motor cortex of the adult rat after motor nerve lesions.

Again, the central representation of peripheral sectors increases to fill the vacuum left by denervation; remarkably soon after denervation, the thresholds for eliciting movement by electrical stimulation of motor cortex decrease around the areas representing the denervated sectors (Donoghue et al., 1990). It has been demonstrated that intracortical microstimulation in the adult rat results in remapping of motor cortex, albeit transiently (Nudo et al., 1990). Microstimulation of the cat's somatosensory cortex has been shown to induce long-term potentiation (LTP)—as manifested by increased-amplitude excitatory postsynaptic potentials (EPSPs)—in neurons of area 4 (Sakamoto et al., 1987). Also in the cat, it will be recalled (see chapter 3), motor cortical LTP is conditionable by association of somatic cortical input with thalamic (ventrolateral nucleus) stimulation (Iriki et al., 1989).

In the monkey, neurons of motor cortex can also be conditioned, in that they show increases of firing frequency in response to the conditioned stimulus in an instrumental conditioning situation (Fetz and Baker, 1973; Schmidt et al., 1978). This does not necessarily mean, however, that the plastic changes of conditioning have occurred in those very cells; such changes may have occurred in neurons that precede them in the motor or sensory circuitry. Whether or not these changes occur in motor cortex, it is important to note that they probably require intact inputs to that cortex from sensory cortex. An experiment by Pavlides and colleagues (1993) strongly suggests the need for those inputs. These investigators tested monkeys for their ability to learn new skills with one of their hands after ablation of the hand area in contralateral somatosensory cortex. The animals had severe difficulties acquiring the skills, whereas they had no difficulty doing so with the hand contralateral to the intact hemisphere. Significantly, after they had learned the skills with this hand, the lesion of the monkeys' contralateral cortex did not induce any deficit on the established performance. Pavlides and his colleagues conclude that the corticocortical projection from somatic to motor cortex is critical for learning new skills but not for the performance of existing ones.

In conclusion, despite the evidence of early stabilization of cortical connectivity, some plasticity persists in adult life, even in primary cortical areas. After critical ontogenetic periods, changes of connectivity from learning and experience may consist mostly of changes in synaptic strength, but the possibility remains that some of these connective changes are due to axonal or dendritic growth. At any rate, the transitions between developmental stages are not sharp, and the development of the cortical processing apparatus, even in the adult, may reflect basically a continuation of changes of connectivity as a result of interaction with the environment.

SENSORY CORTICAL HIERARCHIES

The evidence for cortical processing and representational hierarchies is well documented in primates, and most of the following discussion is based on data from the macaque monkey. For this reason, it is appropriate to begin this discussion by depicting the two most commonly utilized cytoarchitectonic maps of the lateral cortex of the monkey's brain, the maps by Brodmann (1909) and by Bonin and Bailey (1947) (figure 4.7). Both areal nomenclatures will be used, to some extent interchangeably, in the ensuing text. Figure 4.8 shows the approximate location of sensory and motor areas according to physiological criteria. Figure 4.9 does the same for primary areas on a cytoarchitectonic map of the human cortex.

Sight, Sound, and Touch

Studies of cytoarchitecture and connectivity demonstrate the existence of major neocortical pathways for the three sensory modalities of vision, somesthesia, and audition. (Taste and olfaction have receiving areas in

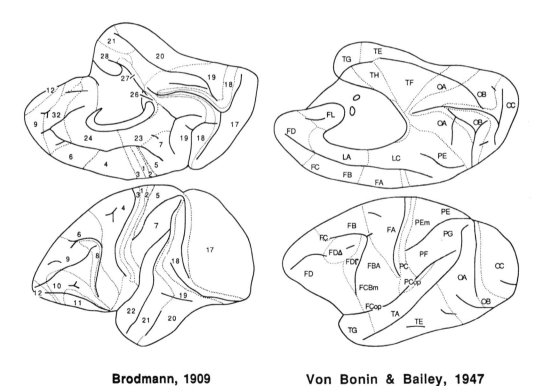

Brodmann, 1909   **Von Bonin & Bailey, 1947**

Figure 4.7 Cytoarchitectonic cortical maps of the macaque monkey: the map of *Cercopithecus* by Brodmann and of *Macaca mulatta* by Bonin and Bailey. (Slightly modified, from Cavada and Goldman-Rakic, 1989a, with permission.)

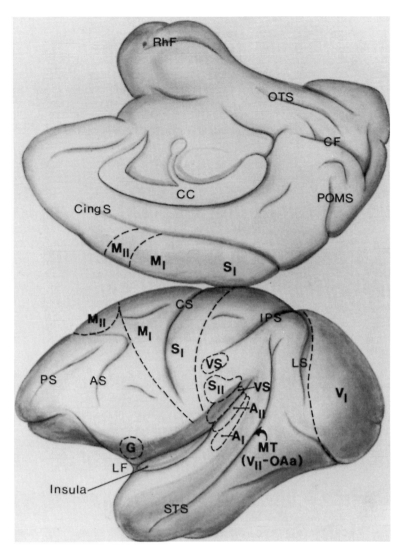

Figure 4.8 Functional map of primary and secondary sensory and motor areas in the macaque. A$_I$, primary auditory area; A$_{II}$, secondary auditory area; AS, arcuate sulcus; CC, corpus callosum; CF, calcarine fissure; Cing S, cingulate sulcus; CS, central sulcus; G, gustatory area; IPS, intraparietal sulcus; LF, lateral fissure; LS, lunate sulcus; M$_I$, primary motor area; M$_{II}$, supplementary motor area; OTS, occipitotemporal sulcus; POMS, medial parieto-occipital sulcus; PS, principal sulcus; RhF, rhinal fissure; S$_I$, primary somatosensory area; S$_{II}$, secondary somatosensory area; STS, superior temporal sulcus; V$_I$, primary visual area; V$_{II}$-OAa, secondary visual area. (From Pandya and Yeterian, 1985, with permission.)

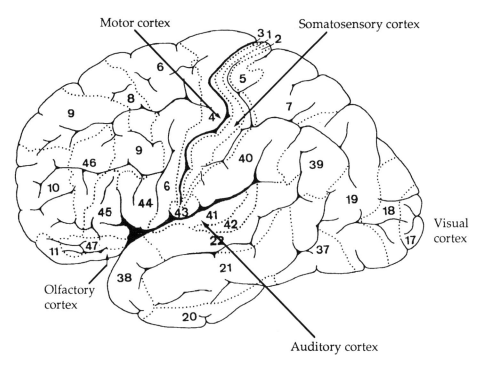

Motor cortex

Somatosensory cortex

Visual
cortex

Olfactory
cortex

Auditory cortex

Figure 4.9 Brodmann's map of the lateral aspect of the human cortex, with primary sensory and motor areas indicated.

limbic or paralimbic cortex.) Those pathways, made of interconnected areas and the fibers that link them, originate in primary sensory cortex and course by interlocking steps into the association cortex of the parietotemporal and prefrontal regions (Jones and Powell, 1970; Van Essen and Maunsell, 1983; Pandya and Yeterian, 1985) (figure 4.10). The number and functions of the areas in each pathway are far from clear, but a few general points seem evident. One is that the connective links between areas are, in practically all instances, reciprocal; this means that a given area not only projects forward to the next but receives projecting fibers from it. In general, fibers feeding forward originate in supragranular layers, especially III, and terminate in layers III and IV of the subsequent area (layer IV also receives thalamic input). Conversely, backward (reciprocal) fibers originate in infragranular layers (V–VI) and terminate in both supragranular and infragranular layers of the precursory area (Jones et al., 1978; Rockland and Pandya, 1979; Pandya and Seltzer, 1982; Galaburda and Pandya, 1983; Seltzer and Pandya, 1984). Interestingly, backprojections from prefrontal onto posterior (parietal) cortex are reported to originate mainly in layer III (Schwartz and Goldman-Rakic, 1984), similar to forward projections that originate in areas behind the central sulcus.

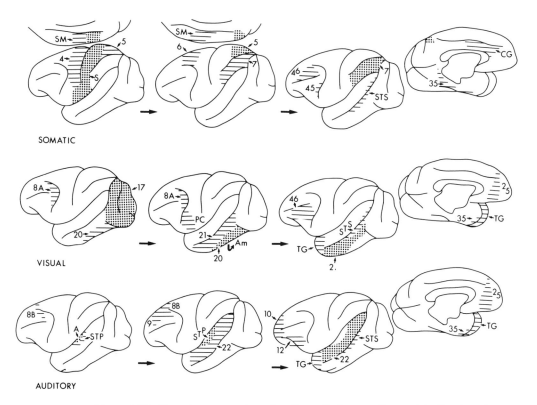

Figure 4.10 Stepwise progression of corticocortical connections originating in primary somatic, visual, and auditory areas, as determined by silver staining after ablation. Each ablated area is shown by dotted shading and its area of projection by horizontal stripes. (From Jones and Powell, 1970; slightly modified by Amaral, 1987, with permission.)

The areas that constitute the pathway for a given modality are not necessarily linked in linear fashion, one after the other; complex patterns of converging and diverging fibers can be traced between areas at various stages of the pathway. An area may receive projections from several areas and project to several others. Most importantly, the connectivity is not as orderly and stereotypical as some have mistakenly claimed; connections may skip one or more stages of any given pathway in both directions. These patterns of connectivity indicate that the potential exists in the anatomy of the cortex not only for serial but also for extensive parallel processing of sensory information (Goldman-Rakic, 1988). To reiterate what was noted in the previous chapter, these intricate patterns of connectivity—some converging and some diverging—also indicate the potential for both sensory synthesis and sensory analysis. Because of the interconnections between nonsuccessive steps, the synthesis and the analysis may take place simultaneously at different levels and distant regions.

By considering the generally forward flow of the cortical pathways originating in primary sensory areas and the cytoarchitecture of the areas that constitute those pathways, it is possible, despite the noted complexities, to make a schematic map of successively linked association areas, such as that by Pandya and Yeterian (1985) (figure 4.11). In it, three successive association areas are delineated for each of three sensory modalities. Thus, according to the scheme, there would be a first-order, second-order, and third-order unimodal association area for vision, audition, and somesthesia. This scheme has heuristic value and accommodates certain psychological and physiological data, which will be discussed in chapter 6, but undoubtedly oversimplifies a very complex arrangement of anatomical and functional areas and connections. However, no more detail is needed at this time.

Another general point is that the connective progression from primary sensory cortex to association cortex seems to take place from early-maturing areas to late-maturing ones, at least to judge by order of myelination, which is one of the indices of maturation. The fact that cortical areas mature at different rates has been known since the early 1900s (Flechsig, 1901, 1920; Campbell, 1905) (figure 4.12). In the human, the intrinsic and extrinsic axons of primary sensory areas as well as motor areas of the cerebral cortex are among the first to myelinate; those of functionally transitional areas—of unimodal association—do so next; and those of associative polymodal areas of the parietotemporal and prefrontal regions myelinate last. Some of these areas (e.g., prefrontal) do not become fully myelinated until puberty (Kaes, 1907; Yakevlev and LeCours, 1967). This seems to be the order of cortical myelination also in the rhesus monkey (Gibson, 1991). Furthermore, in both the human (Conel, 1939; Brody et al., 1987) and the monkey (Gibson, 1991), myelin has been noted to develop last in cortical layers II and III. Because these supragranular layers, as mentioned earlier, are the source and termination of profuse corticocortical connections, it is reasonable to infer that these connections are late in becoming fully functional. To the extent that cognitive development depends on such connections, their late myelination would seem to support the development of higher cognitive functions, including memory. Supporting this conjecture is the recent observation, by Lamantia and Rakic (1990), that the sectors of corpus callosum connecting primary sensory cortices are rich in large myelinated axons, whereas those that connect association cortices contain mainly thin unmyelinated ones, presumably late in becoming functional. However, it should be emphasized that nowhere in the nervous system is myelination a precondition for axonal involvement at some level of function.

Also by other criteria, such as cell and dendritic size, axonal arborization, and synaptic contacts, primary areas have been noted to mature

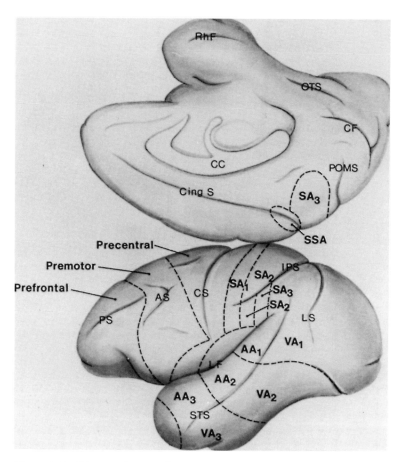

Figure 4.11 Diagram showing the approximate location of parasensory association areas. Visual (VA), auditory (AA), and somatic (SA) areas of association are marked by subscript 1, 2, or 3 to designate, respectively, first, second, or third order. AS, arcuate sulcus; CC, corpus callosum; CF, calcarine fissure; Cing S, cingulate sulcus; CS, central sulcus; IPS, intraparietal sulcus; LS, lunate sulcus; OTS, occipitotemporal sulcus; POMS, parieto-occipitomedial sulcus; PS, principal sulcus; RhF, rhinal fissure; SSA, supplementary somatic area; STS, superior temporal sulcus. (From Pandya and Yeterian, 1985, with permission.)

Anatomy of Cortical Memory

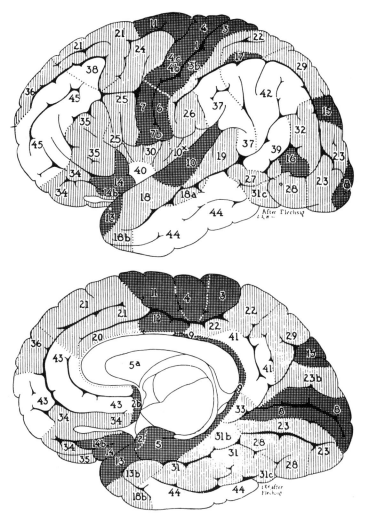

Figure 4.12 Ontogenetic map of the human cortex. The numbers refer to order of myelination. (From Flechsig, modified by Bonin, 1950, with permission.)

before association areas. One good example of late maturation, as defined by those criteria, is the dorsolateral prefrontal cortex (Huttenlocher, 1979). It is not clear, however, by any criterion, that ontogenetic maturation follows precisely the order of corticocortical connectivity that we encounter in the monkey. In fact, this has been disputed on the basis of fine cytoarchitectonic study (Pandya and Yeterian, 1990). Furthermore, the studies of synaptogenesis in the monkey indicate that synapses are formed nearly in synchrony throughout the cortex (Rakic et al., 1986; Bourgeois et al., in press), as are the receptors for various neurotransmitters (Lidow et al., 1991). Their numbers show an overproduction in all areas between the ages of 2 and 4 months and then a gradual and also nearly synchronous attrition to adult levels. Clearly, these data challenge the view of regional differences of maturation rates suggested by myelination data. However, the two sets of findings can be reconciled; they are certainly not incompatible. Synapses may be in place at the same time everywhere in the cortex, but their functional efficiency may not develop at the same rate in all areas. That efficiency may depend on myelination of presynaptic fibers, which may take place at different rates in different areas. In any event, the correlation between maturational and processing gradients remains, in the primate, a plausible inference of general validity, though questionable and still far from established fact.

Is ontogeny, here too, reflecting phylogeny in some way? With respect to cortical connectivity, the principle may be upheld but, again, only on very broad grounds. Evolutionary studies support the notion that association cortex undergoes relatively greater phylogenetic development than primary cortex. As far as the development of anthropoid apes and hominids is concerned, endocranial casts provide evidence of a large and disproportionate growth of the parts of the cerebral mantle that contain areas of association, especially those with polymodal convergence (Eccles, 1989). Particularly striking is the development of the frontal lobe, the bulk of which accommodates the prefrontal cortex. This general evidence is certainly in agreement with some of the data thus far available on the ontogenetic development of cortical areas.

From the physiological perspective, it is obvious that the constituent areas of sensory cortical pathways are not merely relay stations but stages for specialized representation and analysis of sensory information. A brief discussion of functional anatomy is appropriate here, especially with regard to vision and somesthesia, the sensory modalities with cortical systems that are most extensively investigated.

The notion of hierarchical processing of visual information along the primary visual pathway, within what could be ascribed to phyletic memory, was a direct inference from the studies of Hubel and Wiesel (1962, 1968) on the properties of single units in the structures of the visual pathway of the cat and the monkey. From the retina, through the lateral geniculate body, to the striate cortex (V1), successive populations of neurons, topologically organized with respect to the visual field, engage in the analysis and synthesis of the various features of visual objects (form, color, orientation, etc.). At certain stages in the pathway, simple features are analyzed and encoded within the confines of retinotopically arranged groupings of cells; at higher stages, more complex features are analyzed and encoded, presumably by synthesis of inputs from preceding stages, and so on up the processing hierarchy.

Those processes continue beyond striate cortex in areas of the circumstriate belt and the temporal cortex—that is, in the areas that constitute the so-called extrastriate cortical pathway for vision: V2, V3, V4, and inferotemporal cortex or area TE (Van Essen and Maunsell, 1983; Van

Essen, 1985) (see figures 3.7, 4.13). A separate pathway proceeds into posterior parietal cortex, presumably for the processing of motion and visuospatial information (Ungerleider, 1985). In extrastriate cortex, important changes occur. The processing does not necessarily continue seriatim through successive areas. Instead, it splits into several channels that progress through different areas or subareas, each specializing in the analysis of one or more visual features and, at some points, it merges again into areas beyond. The ensemble forms a general pattern of successive converging and diverging channels that suggests a trend of serial and parallel processing (see chapter 3), as well as synthesis and analysis, toward ever higher stages of the hierarchy. A most important point needs to be reemphasized: All connective steps are reciprocal, therefore allowing for reentry and for "top-down" influences at every stage.

Another fundamental change supervening in extrastriate cortex is the breakdown of retinotopy. Features are no longer analyzed, as in V1, in an organization of cell modules that topologically reflects the retina and, therefore, the visual scene. Instead, ever more special and complex features seem to take precedence over visual location. As the trend reaches the inferotemporal cortex (Gross, 1973), retinotopy practically disappears. In this cortex, the cells have very large receptive fields and, for them, it matters little in what part of the visual field the feature or combination of features falls that is going to activate them selectively (Desimone and Gross, 1979; Desimone et al., 1984). Furthermore, some of the cells become susceptible to the behavioral relevance of stimulus features (Fuster, 1990) and apparently become capable of retaining them in short-term memory (Fuster and Jervey, 1982; Miyashita and Chang, 1988; Fuster, 1990). It seems reasonable to suppose that it is in extrastriate cortex, possibly inferotemporal cortex, that visual phyletic mem-

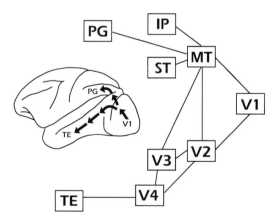

Figure 4.13 Scheme of the two postulated cortical visual pathways. (From Ungerleider, 1985, with permission.)

ory meets individual memory or, more precisely perhaps, where the former becomes individualized. I will discuss these matters further in chapter 6.

The functional evidence of processing hierarchies for other sense modalities is less substantial. In the monkey's parietal cortex, indications of such a hierarchy for somesthesia have been found in the responses of single units to somatic stimulation (Duffy and Burchfiel, 1971; Iwamura et al., 1985, 1993; Pons et al., 1985). In primary somatic cortex (SI), which comprises Brodmann's areas 3a, 3b, 1, and 2, and progressing into areas 5 and 7 of posterior parietal cortex, some general trends of neuronal responsiveness have been discovered that conform to a somatic processing hierarchy, as suggested by the flow of cortico-cortical connections (Pandya and Yeterian, 1985). Those trends of parietal neuron response along connective gradients are characterized by increasingly larger receptive fields, reactivity to simultaneous stimulation of multiple areas of the body surface, and reactivity to simultaneous stimulation of skin and deep-tissue receptors. The analogies with the visual system are remarkable. The posterior parietal cortex, especially area 5, would be the functional analog of the inferotemporal cortex and perhaps provide the transition from somatic phyletic memory to somatic individual memory (see chapter 6). Accordingly, units in area 5 seem to exhibit short-term memory properties for tactile stimuli similar to those that inferotemporal units exhibit for visual stimuli (Koch and Fuster, 1989).

In recent years, anatomical, physiological, and neuropsychological studies have emphasized the importance of another connective pathway: from SI into SII, the latter in the parainsular cortex of the lateral fissure (figure 4.14). The functions of SII cortex are not well understood but are believed important for somesthetic integration (Pons et al., 1987). By selective ablations of SI and microelectrode recording in SII, Pons and colleagues (1992) investigated the contributions of subareas of SI (3a, 3b, 1, and 2) to the responsiveness of SII neurons to tactile features. They concluded that in the monkey, and presumably all primates, most tactile information is processed in series, though along parallel modality-specific channels (cutaneous, "deep" sense, etc.), from SI to SII. This deviates from the general mammalian plan, according to which all tactile information is processed in parallel, concomitantly through SI and SII. The primate, therefore, seems to reflect an evolutionary shift from parallel to serial processing within the cortical substrate for tactile analysis. It remains to be seen whether, in light of prior discussion in this chapter, the same shift also takes place in ontogenetic development. In later chapters, we shall consider the advantages of serial processing for haptic perception and selective attention.

Recently, Schneider and coworkers (1993) obtained evidence of another tactile area, the granular insular (Ig) area, which seems to consti-

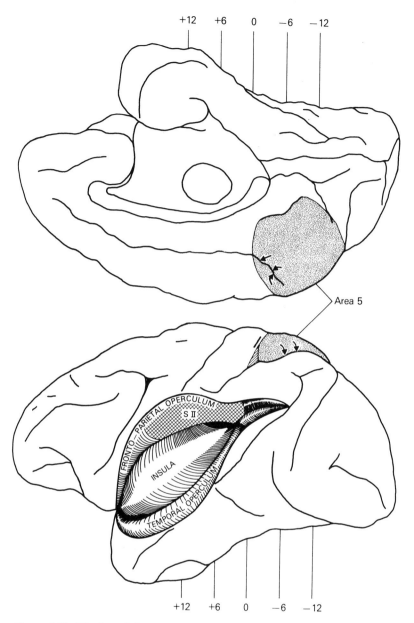

+12 +6 0 −6 −12

Area 5

FRONTO-PARIETAL OPERCULUM
S II
INSULA
TEMPORAL OPERCULUM

+12 +6 0 −6 −12

Figure 4.14 The lateral fissure opened for exposure of the cortex of area SII and the insula. (From Murray and Mishkin, 1984, with permission.)

tute an intermediate step in the pathway from SII to the limbic system. Cells in Ig respond to stimuli of several sensory modalities. However, the large majority of them respond exclusively to tactile or deep-tissue somatosensory stimuli. They have large receptive fields suggestive of high-level integration.

Now let us return to the more general aspects of cortical connectivity. Between unimodal association areas, especially in and around the superior temporal and intraparietal sulci, intermediate areas can be found that receive connections from adjacent areas and, therefore, convergent inputs from more than one modality (figure 4.15). By this definition, these intermediate areas may be called *polymodal*. In addition, the three association pathways of visual, somatic, and auditory origin *converge on paralimbic cortical areas* at the base of the temporal lobe. All three send fibers to entorhinal and parahippocampal cortex (see figures 3.8, 4.16) and, through it, as discussed in the preceding chapter, have access to the amygdala and the hippocampus. Again, these connections are reciprocal. Some higher-order modality-specific areas of associative cortex project directly to the amygdala (Turner et al., 1980).

In addition to maintaining reciprocal connectivity with limbic structures, sensory association areas send long fibers to the cortex of the frontal lobe, especially prefrontal areas, through the subjacent white matter. Several unimodal and polymodal postcentral areas project to frontal cortex and receive reciprocal projections from it (Jones and Powell, 1970; Jacobson and Trojanowski, 1977a; Schwartz and Goldman-Rakic, 1984; Andersen et al., 1985; Pandya and Yeterian, 1985; Cavada and Goldman-Rakic, 1989b; Barbas, 1992) (figure 4.17). There is topological order (i.e., segregation) in these connections with regard to both origin and termination.

Topology between areas is maintained at a much greater and more detailed level than that suggested by the sketches of connectivity in figures 4.16 and 4.17. Here it seems necessary again to correct the misleading impression of prevalent serial processing that, for all their heuristic value, these figures may convey. Indeed, topological order can be found even in the connectivity between discrete and distant cortical areas, indicating the importance of parallel processing in and between such areas. A good example is the connectivity between posterior parietal (area 7) and prefrontal areas (figure 4.18). A double anterograde tracing study by Selemon and Goldman-Rakic (1988) has shown a remarkable degree of correspondence between these areas. There is now substantial evidence indicating that those areas and the connections that link them play fundamental roles in oculomotor attention and memory (Mesulam, 1981; Goldman-Rakic, 1987; Andersen et al., 1990). These functions are almost inconceivable without both serial and parallel processing: hence the significance of topological order in connections between hierarchical stages and, as in this case, between the

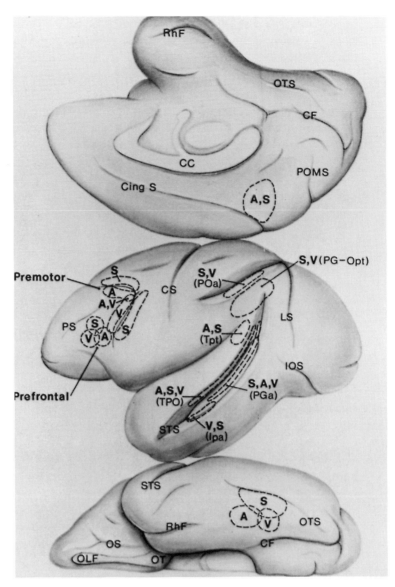

Figure 4.15 Diagram showing sensory convergence areas. A, auditory; S, somatic; V, visual. IOS, infero-occipital sulcus; O, olfactory tubercle; OLF, olfactory bulb; OS, orbital sulcus. Other abbreviations as in figure 4.11. (From Pandya and Yeterian, 1985, with permission.)

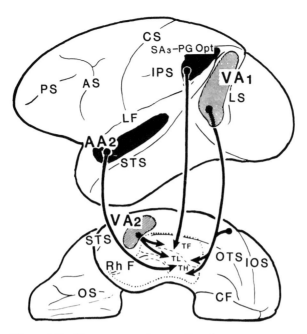

Figure 4.16 Convergence of connections from sensory association areas on the parahippocampal gyrus. Abbreviations as in figures 4.11, 4.15. (From Pandya and Yeterian, 1985, with permission.)

perceptual hierarchy of posterior cortex and the motor hierarchy of anterior cortex.

The connections from distant areas to the prefrontal cortex illustrate also the principle of convergence that is important for integration and synthesis. In the prefrontal cortex of the monkey, notably the area of the sulcus principalis, axon terminals from contralateral prefrontal and ipsilateral parietal cortex have been found to innervate alternating bands of cortex in a pattern of columnar interdigitation (Goldman-Rakic and Schwartz, 1982) (figure 4.19).

Obviously, the aggregate of long corticocortical connections from postcentral cortex arriving in separate or adjacent fields of frontal cortex constitutes the principal access of sensory processing hierarchies to the motor processing hierarchy. The access of those connections to frontal fields indicates the availability of diverse sensory inputs to the cortex of the frontal lobe for the integration and control of behavioral action.

To complete this section we must refer, albeit briefly, to the pathways and areas of representation for the two sensory modalities that have not been discussed thus far: taste and olfaction. Interestingly, their pathways reach both limbic system and frontal lobe more directly than the pathways for the other sensory modalities.

Anatomy of Cortical Memory

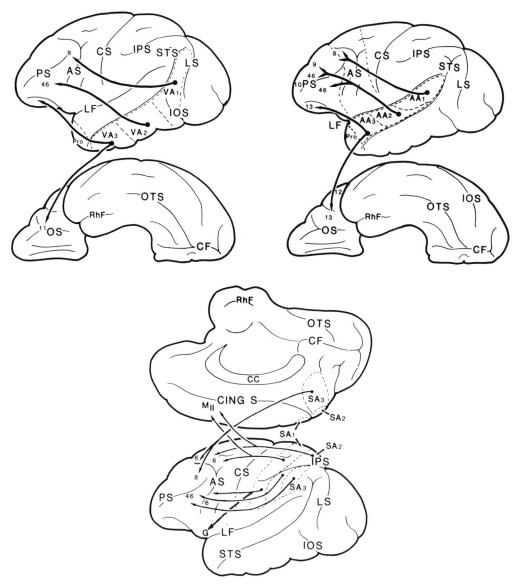

Figure 4.17 Projections from posterior sensory association areas to frontal cortex. Abbreviations as in figures 4.8, 4.11, 4.15. (From Pandya and Yeterian, 1985, with permission.)

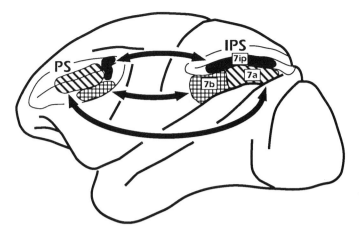

Figure 4.18 Reciprocal connectivity between parietal area 7 and dorsolateral prefrontal cortex. IPS, intraparietal sulcus (opened); PS, principal sulcus (opened). (Slightly modified from Cavada and Goldman-Rakic, 1989a, with permission.)

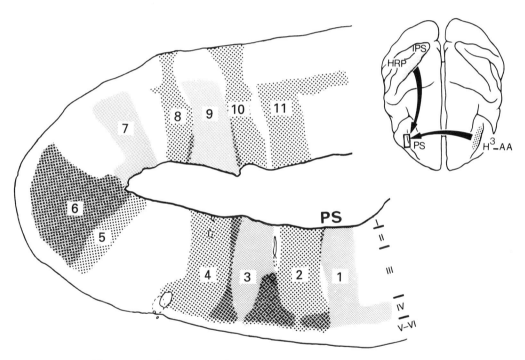

Figure 4.19 Convergence of projections from parietal and contralateral prefrontal cortices on the cortex of the sulcus principalis (PS), traced by double-label (HRP and H^3-AA) axon-transport method. IPS, intraparietal sulcus. Parietal terminal zones (1, 3, 6, 7, and 9) are marked by fine shading, callosal (contralateral) terminal zones (2, 4, 5, 8, 10, and 11) by coarse shading. (From Goldman-Rakic and Schwartz, 1982, with permission.)

Taste and Smell

The senses of taste and smell are supposed to be phylogenetically older than the others and, perhaps because of their ancient origin, have their cortical representation in phylogenetically older, paralimbic cortex. In primates, gustatory input is collected by the nucleus of the solitary tract in the brain stem and, through the ventromedialis posterior (VMP) nucleus of the thalamus, is conveyed to the primary sensory cortex for taste, which lies in the frontal insula and operculum, in the depth of the sylvian fissures (see figures 4.14, 4.20). Input from the olfactory bulb goes directly to the primary olfactory cortex (olfactory tubercle and prepiriform cortex).

The gustatory cortex of the insula and operculum has been found to project to a caudolateral area of orbitofrontal cortex, at the base of the frontal lobe (Rolls et al., 1989b) (see figure 4.20). Beyond that cortex, taste pathways are uncertain, but taste units have been recorded in hypothalamus (Burton et al., 1976), medial orbitofrontal cortex (Thorpe

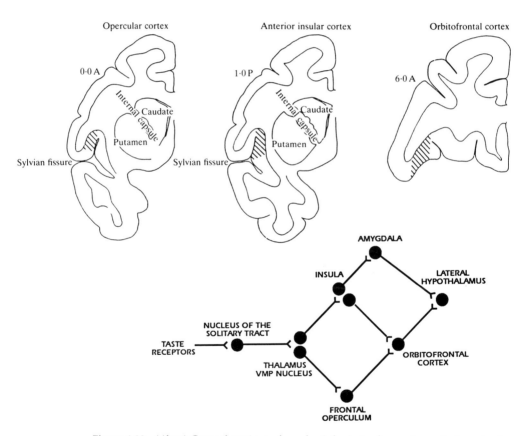

Figure 4.20 (*Above*) Coronal sections of monkey's brain to show primary taste cortex in the frontal operculum and insula. (*Below*) Schematic diagram of taste pathways. (Slightly modified from Rolls, 1989, with permission.)

et al., 1983) and the amygdala (Sanghera et al., 1979). Thus, assuming that the caudolateral orbitofrontal cortex is essentially cortex of association, the processing of taste information follows the same general pattern of neural progression as that of the three modalities discussed thus far, only perhaps with fewer cortical stages. Here again we have primary sensory processing, secondary or associative processing, and output to limbic structures, which reciprocate with backprojection.

In the olfactory system, things are somewhat different. Olfactory information is transmitted directly from olfactory bulb to prepiriform cortex. The output from this cortex then is processed through thalamus (nucleus mediodorsalis) and, from there, is projected to a medial orbitofrontal area. Thus, the main difference between the gustatory and olfactory systems seems to be that, in the latter, a thalamic stage succeeds, rather than precedes, primary sensory cortex; in olfaction, therefore, a thalamic nucleus is interposed between sensory cortex and the association cortex of the orbitofrontal region.

MOTOR CORTICAL HIERARCHY

The motor counterpart of the sensory hierarchies of posterior cortex just outlined is a hierarchy of areas for motor processing that also can be readily recognized in the cortex of the frontal lobe of the monkey. Here the processing goes in the opposite direction—that is, from association cortex (prefrontal cortex) to primary cortex (MI). Direct connections have been described from prefrontal areas to premotor areas (Künzle, 1978; Arikuni et al., 1986; Goldman-Rakic, 1987; Bates and Goldman-Rakic, 1993) and from premotor areas to MI (Pandya and Vignolo, 1971; Muakkasa and Strick, 1979). Again, the connectivity between the areas concerned is reciprocal, but another apparent difference from sensory hierarchies should be noted. All three major steps (prefrontal, premotor, and motor) of the frontal motor hierarchy project to subcortical structures and receive reentrant connections from them. Long reentrant connective loops have been identified that originate in frontal areas, course through the basal ganglia and the lateral thalamus, and return to frontal areas (DeLong and Georgopoulos, 1981; Alexander and Crutcher, 1990c) (figure 4.21). In accord with the general rule of corticocortical reciprocity, frontal areas send projections to all the areas of postcentral cortex from which they receive them (Pandya et al., 1971; Mesulam et al., 1977; Pandya and Yeterian, 1985; Cavada and Goldman-Rakic, 1989a, b; Barbas, 1992) (figure 4.22) and, again, that connectivity appears to be topologically orderly (see figure 4.18).

Unlike the sensory processing in postcentral cortex, it should be noted that frontal motor processing appears to go against ontogenetic and phylogenetic trends. Indeed, prefrontal and premotor cortices appear to develop after primary motor cortex, at least according to the myelo-

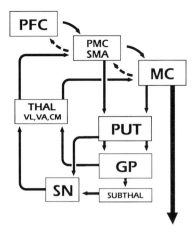

Figure 4.21 Reentrant connective loops between cortical and subcortical structures involved in motor control. CM, center median nucleus; GP, globus pallidus; MC, motor cortex; PFC, prefrontal cortex; PMC, premotor cortex; PUT, putamen; SMA, supplementary motor area; SN, substantia nigra; SUBTHAL, subthalamic nucleus; THAL, thalamus; VA, anteroventral nucleus; VL, ventrolateral nucleus.

genetic criterion. Furthermore, fine cytoarchitectonic analysis reveals the progressive development of cortical architecture from areas 4 to 6 and 6 to 9 (Vogt and Vogt, 1919; Sanides, 1964)—thus from motor to premotor and from there to prefrontal cortex.

From the functional point of view, another distinction should be noted between cortical motor processing and sensory processing. Whereas the latter goes primarily from the particulars of sensory analysis to the synthetic generalities of perception (Merzenich and Kaas, 1980), motor processing seems to do the reverse—that is, to progress from the generalities of the temporal structure of behavior presumably represented in prefrontal cortex (Fuster, 1989) to the particulars of movement, to the microgenesis of the action (Brown, 1987). This progression of processing from the general to the particular, down the frontal motor hierarchy, is reflected in the patterns of frontal cell discharge in anticipation of motor acts that are contingent on prior events and are preceded by a substantial period of preparation (see chapters 7 and 9). Prefrontal cells fire with the longest lead time before movement. They are succeeded by premotor cells and these, in turn, by cells in MI. It is as if an excitatory volley successively recruited in cascading fashion the three stages of the descending motor hierarchy before the movement was to take place. Implicit in this seriatim recruitment, as I argue in chapters 7 and 9, is the order by which motor representations in those three cortical stages come to control the motor act.

At the top of the motor hierarchy, the prefrontal cortex represents the most global and temporally extended aspects of the behavioral structure, the schema of which that motor act may be only one com-

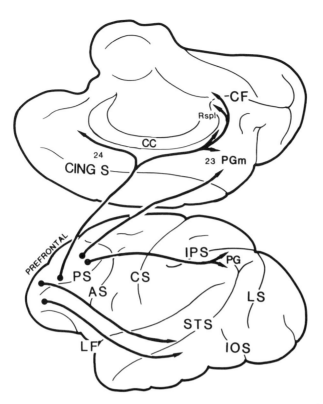

Figure 4.22 Schematic diagram of some of the projections from prefrontal cortex to medial and postcentral cortex. Abbreviations as in figures 4.8, 4.11. (From Pandya and Yeterian, 1985, with permission.)

ponent. Furthermore, because that motor act may be contingent on prior events (i.e., stimuli) that are part of the same behavioral structure, the prefrontal cortex may have to maintain those events in short-term memory. For that, prefrontal neurons make use of their long connections with posterior (sensory) cortex. It is presumably to mediate cross-temporal contingencies with short-term active memory (see chapter 9) that the prefrontal cortex is reciprocally connected with practically every region of the posterior neocortex, perhaps with the exception only of primary visual and auditory cortices (Pandya and Yeterian, 1985; Barbas, 1992). To sum up, as a consequence of their role in short-term (working) memory for the act, as well as the motor preparation for it, prefrontal cells are the first to be activated and are activated for a longer time before that act.

Premotor cells come next, for they are involved in more specific and concrete aspects of movement. They represent global schemes of action defined by trajectory and goal, irrespective of the particular sector of musculature to achieve them. As they are recruited for organization of the act, their activity increases, with a lead time that is intermediate between those of prefrontal and motor cortex cells.

Finally, the cells in motor cortex (MI) come in. They represent the most specific and concrete aspects of the act by spatial and temporal definition. They perform their task by a population code closely determined by the trajectory of the act and the muscular sector of the motor apparatus to be mobilized. They have, as we shall see, a brief prospective memory for the act, which they precede with their activation by a mere fraction of a second.

INTERHEMISPHERIC CONNECTIVITY

In both posterior and anterior neocortex of the primate, callosal connections can be traced from practically any given area to the homologous contralateral area or other areas of the other hemisphere (Pandya et al., 1969; Pandya and Vignolo, 1971; Goldman and Nauta, 1977; Jacobson and Trojanowski, 1977b; Cavada and Goldman-Rakic, 1989a, b; McGuire et al., 1991). The role of these commissural connections is not clear, but the data from split-brain and stimulation experiments suggest that they are used for the transfer or expansion of memory from one hemisphere into the other (Doty, 1965; Sperry et al., 1969; Sperry, 1974, 1982). In primates, especially the human, where considerable hemispheric specialization of function has been demonstrated (Rubens, 1977), those connections certainly provide the memory substrate with associative possibilities beyond those present within one hemisphere. Let us briefly review the facts as they relate to cortical memory.

Of course, the most relevant anatomical fact is that the neocortices of the two hemispheres are linked by the massive array of commissural fibers, myelinated and unmyelinated, that constitute the corpus callosum. By and large, those fiber connections run in both directions and link homotopical locations of the two hemispheres, though some connections are heterotopical. That mutual connective correspondence, well established in the monkey, applies to all areas: primary and associative, sensory and motor, from the occipital to the frontal pole. In principle, homotopical areas of the two hemispheres can be supposed to cooperate in basically the same functions. This cooperativeness, however, has some notable exceptions.

Because of the decussation (crossover) of fibers in peripheral stages of the visual, auditory, and somatic pathways (not olfactory), it turns out that sensory inputs from each visual half-field, ear, and hand are led more or less exclusively to contralateral cortex. This has remarkable implications for sensory processing and representation. For one thing, it implies that sensory functions for each side of the environment are lateralized, to some extent, in the contralateral cortex. This fact led Sperry to his pioneering work on hemispheric specialization (for reviews, see Sperry et al., 1969; Sperry, 1974, 1982). The essence of his methodology—which, in humans has been medically justified—is to sever cerebral commissures, including the corpus callosum, and to present information only in one hemisector of sensorium, thus obliging the subject to use the cortex contralateral to the input side for a variety of cognitive tests. In this way, that hemicortex can be "made aware of information unbeknownst to the other," and the cognitive functions of the two hemicortices can be challenged independently of each other. In this manner, Sperry's group determined that a memory can be lateralized—that is, circumscribed to one hemisphere.

By the same methodology, and by neuropsychological study of the effects of unilateral cortical lesions, evidence has been obtained that there is a degree of hemispheric specialization of higher cortical functions, including those that involve the storage and utilization of knowledge (for reviews, see Harnad et al., 1977; Eccles, 1989). Of course, the best-established forms of specialization are those related to language, which are mostly the purview of the left (dominant) cortex, but others, such as calculation and nonverbal ideation, have also been noted to be localized, to some degree, in one hemisphere (Sperry, 1974).

To summarize, the important points here, in terms of memory function, are the following: (1) The two hemispheres can store different memory contents; (2) cortical memory networks, by way of collosal fibers, can span both hemispheres; and (3) the activation of memory networks in retrieval, attention and active memory can traverse the corpus collosum, and may be maintained by reentrant transcallosal circuits.

INDIVIDUALIZED ANATOMY OF CORTICAL MEMORY

The scheme of corticocortical connections outlined previously for the monkey's brain is certainly incomplete. More detail will be provided as needed in subsequent chapters. Surely, however, many more corticocortical connections are yet to be discovered than are described in this book. As more and more of them are described, it is difficult to avoid the unsettling impression that a wiring diagram of such complexity as that of the primate cortex will never be known entirely.

The problem of defining cortical connectivity is aggravated by the suspicion, confirmed by experienced anatomists, that there is considerable variability among animal subjects of the same species and that the quantification of connections by any of the available analytical methods (axon transport, immunology, etc.) is, to some extent, dependent on subjective judgment. Thus, innumerable inconspicuous connections may be dismissed in one's analysis as atypical or artifactual. Yet those inconstant and tenuous connections may be a very important part of our story, which has not received enough attention; both the variability and the subtlety of those connections may be enormously significant as far as memory is concerned. Both may be structural manifestations of possibly much more postnatal plasticity than is generally recognized and of the essentially dynamic nature of the cortical networks that represent individual memory. This may be so even as we ignore another probably critical part of the story that remains unrecognized in most neuroanatomical studies—namely the microscopical counts of synapses and of possible nonsynaptic contacts (Bach-y-Rita, 1993) that web the cortical networks together.

In this book, I adopt the position, at least in principle, that those cortical networks, with all their individual variance and peculiarities, have their substrate in the sensory and motor processing hierarchies of the cerebral cortex that I have outlined. Memories, I maintain, are not only the result of information processing in those cortical hierarchies but also the guide under which that processing takes place. That is presumably why representation and processing are difficult to separate methodologically. The anatomy of memory is largely the anatomy of perception and movement. At the lower levels of the jacksonian organization of memory that I propose, sensory and motor systems would contribute phyletic memory—that is, the immediate recognition of sensory features and the concrete means to interact motorically with the world, as the species has learned to do. At higher levels, beyond primary areas, the cortex of association would contribute individual memory, the aggregate of stored experience that the organism has accumulated about its particular world, as well as the ways it has learned to deal with it. In subsequent chapters, the theoretical and empirical basis for these contentions is discussed.

What I have presented in this chapter is only the crudest of schemes, a structural framework that may accommodate memory no better than a road map accommodates the life and history of a nation. For now, it may suffice to guide our research and to help us establish some general principles of memory function. We are still very far, however, from being able to understand and describe the fine, unique, customized anatomy of our individual memories.

5   Memory Networks

In the previous two chapters, I have presented an overview of the basic mechanisms of memory formation as we currently understand them and the framework of cortical connectivity on which memory grows and finds support. That connectivity offers the potential basis for the operation of two fundamental principles of processing and representation: *convergence* for synthesis and *divergence* for analysis. The first would serve the more general aspects of memory formation and storage (perceptual binding, categorization, abstract concepts, semantic memory, etc.), the second its most concrete aspects (segregation, discrimination, episodic memory, etc.). I have discussed the place of limbic structures, especially the hippocampus, in the consolidation of cortical memory and some of the possible neurochemical processes involved in it. I have also discussed the cortical contribution to phyletic memory and the plasticity of its connective endowment. Finally, I have outlined in the primate cortex the connective substrate of sensory and motor hierarchies for processing and representation of perceptual and motor information. In this chapter, I discuss, in general terms, how those connective hierarchies are filled with content, how cortical memory is formed, and how it is recalled (i.e., activated). Above all, the essence of this chapter is theory and methodology. My first priority here is to set a level of discourse for cortical memory that leads to useful ideas and neurally testable hypotheses.

A LEVEL OF DISCOURSE FOR CORTICAL MEMORY

Possibly by now the reader has already concluded that my approach to memory is thoroughly *associationist*, to use an old term, or *connectionist*, to use a new one. Perhaps the reader has also concluded that I have chosen this approach without due regard for flourishing contemporary currents in molecular biology, cognitive science, and information-processing theory. These conclusions are not entirely correct. Certainly, I place in the neural connection the emphasis I believe it deserves, for association is apparently at the basis of all memory, and our recognition of the crucial role of the synapse in learning and memory is growing rapidly. However, I am fully aware of the relevance of other methodologies or schools of thought (schools flourish when empirical progress stagnates, as Hopfield has aptly remarked). Memory is clearly an interdisciplinary subject. Thus, my position on neural memory is eclectic but carries what I consider to be a useful bias. Before defining that bias any further, it seems appropriate to justify the eclecticism by pointing out the merits and limitations of some of those other methodologies. This should help define the level of the present discourse.

Theoretically, neural memory is reducible to molecules. Leaving aside the tempting but preposterous analogy of memory and the genetic code and the no less preposterous—and disproved—notion that memory is encoded *in* proteins, there is no denying that the synaptic changes that determine and support memory ultimately are reducible to molecular changes in the nerve cell. There is, however, no imaginable and practical method of defining a memory by chemical means, whereas we are beginning to be able to do so by electrical means. Even if it were feasible, the molecular analysis of a memory would not be any more useful for understanding its content and operations than is chemical analysis of the ink for understanding the written message. That level of analysis would simply be too low for the purpose.

Yet continued advancement in *molecular neurobiology* certainly will provide definitive knowledge about the genetics and ontogeny of the cerebral foundation of memory, including the cortex and the hippocampus. It will provide much-needed information on the vicissitudes of chemical substances, such as the neurotransmitters, which assist in the formation of memory networks. Molecular neurobiology may not help us understand the structure of memory, but undoubtedly it will help us understand its infrastructure. It may also help us grasp the chemical alterations of that infrastructure that either hamper or facilitate memory processes in general.

Cognitive science—literally "the science of knowledge"—is an important methodology for the study of memory, especially human memory. Analysis of the mental operations of higher cognitive functions is relevant and useful because memory is one such function that serves all others, including, of course, perception and language. Language is an aid to *psychophysics*, a branch of psychology that explores the laws of perception. Insofar as perception is intimately related to and influenced by memory, psychophysics can be useful to the study of cortical memory.

Cognitive science and psychophysics in and of themselves, however, do not contribute to our understanding of neural memory. They are, at best, helpful for building a self-contained body of lawful relationships, a "functionalist" view (Churchland, 1986) of memory that may relate only indirectly to the way the brain stores and retrieves information.

There is, however, a field of cognitive science and psychophysics, best characterized as *cognitive neuroscience,* that contributes much to the analysis of neural memory. It includes the study of memory in the development of the nervous system and of its alterations as a result of brain lesions. These studies are the basis of the neuropsychology of memory and of much of our discussion in chapter 2.

In the past half century, with the advent of the digital computer, there has been a remarkable proliferation of information-processing models of memory with varying degrees of neural plausibility. For a brief and clear historical review, the reader is referred to Anderson and Hinton (1981). For more extensive and detailed reviews, the reader is referred to Anderson and Rosenfeld (1988), Shaw and Palm (1988), and Levine (1991). The most successful models, those that best approximate human memory in their operations, are the models of distributed and self-organized associative memory. The term *associative memory* is used here generically to include two accepted meanings of the word *associative:* (1) to define a learning process, much as we have discussed in chapter 3, and (2) to define a recognition process, by which a memory is recalled on the basis of a fraction of it—in other words, from a stimulus or from another representation that is somehow associated with it (Kohonen, 1977, 1984).

Among the associative models of memory, those that best approximate the operations of the brain are based on the assumption of modifiable connections between representational elements that may be construed as neurons or groups of neurons. Their common organizational architecture is a matrix or network of connections between representational elements that constitute its "nodes." The principle of simultaneous convergence in network formation is the foundation of most models of cortical associative memory (cf. Palm, 1982; Levine, 1991). Another important principle shared by most of those models is that of parallel access to the network: hence the concept of the associative memory network with parallel access and processing (Hinton and Anderson, 1981). Prominent among the network memory models are the self-organizing models of Kohonen (1977, 1984) and Edelman (1987), the word-recognition and categorization models of Anderson (1977) and of McClelland and Rumelhart (1985), and the connectionist models of Feldman (1981) and Ballard (1986). In addition there are the correlational or holographic models (Gabor, 1968; Pribram, 1969; Willshaw, 1981) which are not, strictly speaking, network models but are models of distributed associative memory with reduplication of information in multiple locations.

Although they differ in their architecture and computational aspects, all the models mentioned thus far do considerable justice to neuroscientific knowledge. They conform to most of the constraints and requirements imposed by neural structure and function, at least as presently known. Although their development is largely attributable to and supported by computer science and artificial intelligence, none assumes that the brain works like a digital computer (though earlier models did; see, for example, Pitts and McCulloch, 1947) or that neural memory is anything comparable to computer memory. They all respect—in fact, assume—the enormous capacity of the brain for parallel processing, unlike conventional computers. They all acknowledge, implicitly or explicitly, an important distinction between computer memory and neural memory: The latter, unlike the first, is primarily content-addressable—that is, accessible by exposure to its content. Finally, almost all of them base their postulated memory networks in the cerebral cortex.

So, which is the best model of cortical memory? The question must remain open until we know more about how the brain works. One serious problem with most models is the difficulty they pose to most anyone attempting to evaluate the soundness of their computational algorithms. Aside from the complexity of some of those algorithms, it is not yet possible to verify the validity of some of their basic assumptions, although some of their predictions are physiologically testable. Nonetheless, that a given model can reach, through a set of formulas, the same solution as does the brain in, say, the recognition of a word does not mean that the brain arrives at that solution in the same way. Besides, most models have difficulty accommodating two fundamental features of cortical processing and memory—namely, the probabilistic nature of the first and the robustness of the second. Anyone who has dealt with the facts of cortical neurophysiology knows that variance is the rule; no certain output comes from any input, as the information theorist would like or expect. That is why the structural rigidity of those models and their deterministic algorithms appear so artificial and difficult to reconcile with the redundancies, the dynamics, and the plasticity of the brain.

The robustness of memory is demonstrated by its resistance to brain injury; certain cortical injuries may not affect memory at all or, if they do, they affect it only temporarily. With the possible exception of holographic models, all models have difficulty with this fact. Nevertheless, we cannot reject any of them outright on these or any other grounds. We should expect, however, that they will become structurally less rigid and less algorithmic, more probabilistic, and more dynamic in order to accommodate fully the properties of real cortical networks in memory. In any event, all the models mentioned are, to a large degree, compatible with one another and with empirical evidence. All have desirable and mutually complementary features. The model of self-organized associative cortical memory by Kohonen (1977, 1984), with its laminar network organization, is particularly attractive. The dynamic memory system proposed in this book is in some ways similar to it.

None of the models mentioned thus far takes into proper consideration all three critical issues of neurobiological memory: (1) the anatomical connectivity of the mammalian neocortex beyond primary areas (in other words, the real neural architecture of individual memory networks); (2) how a cortical memory network develops from its genetic base to adult proportions and function; and (3) the dynamic relationships between cortical processing and cortical representation in the perceptual as well as the motor sphere of memory. This book attempts to cover these three subjects within its conceptual framework. Having discussed the first item in the previous chapter, albeit in sketchy fashion, I shall proceed with the second item. To introduce it, let us first go back to the thinking of one of Hebb's contemporaries, who had a much broader view than Hebb did of the cortical network and who conceived the manner of its development well beyond that of the cell assembly.

GROWTH OF THE NETWORK

Caminante, no hay camino,
Se hace camino al andar.
(Traveler, there is no path,
By walking the paths are made.)
—Antonio Machado, 1912

The first proponent of cortical memory networks on a major scale was neither a neuroscientist nor a computer scientist but, curiously, a Viennese economist: Friedrich von Hayek (1899–1992). A man of exceptionally broad knowledge and profound insight into the operation of complex systems, Hayek applied such insight with remarkable success to economics (Nobel Prize, 1974), sociology, political science, jurisprudence, evolution theory, psychology, and brain science (Hayek, 1967). In the 1920s, he wrote a theoretical essay entitled *The Sensory Order* which, for personal and historical reasons, would not appear published until much later (Hayek, 1952). Considering the neurobiological knowledge available even at the time of its publication, there is nothing dilettantish about that scholarly work. It is there that Hayek presents his concept of a cortical memory network in the context of the main topic, which is not memory itself but, significantly, perception, perception as the *source* of memory and as the *product* of memory. By postulating that *all* perception—and not just a part—is a product of memory, Hayek carries to the extreme one of Helmholtz's (1925) central notions, indeed one of the basic tenets of modern psychophysics.

According to Hayek [1952], perception is an *act of* classification performed by nets of interconnected cortical cells on the qualities of objects and events. Those qualities are not inherent in physical objects or events but are a set of relations previously established in a neural net by simultaneously occurring experiences. All perception is categorical in that it is an interpretation of an object or event made in the light of past experience by the network, which acts as a preformed classifying apparatus of cortical connections.

How is that apparatus formed? Here Hayek invokes a principle very similar to that of Hebb. In essence, it coincides with what we have called *Hebb's second principle* (sensorisensory association) transposed to the level of cell groups. As Hayek [1952] puts it, sensory impulses from different sources arriving simultaneously in two or more neurons will, possibly by circulating activity modify the synapses between them, such that subsequent arrival of one impulse will activate all the neurons that were originally activated together.

The result of all this will be that a system of connexions will be formed which will record the relative frequency with which in the history of the organism the different groups of internal and external stimuli have acted together. Each individual impulse or group of impulses will on its occurrence evoke other impulses which correspond to the other stimuli which in the past have usually accompanied its occurrence (Hayek, 1952, p. 64).

It is the total or partial identity of those "other impulses" with those evoked by the initial stimuli that makes them members of the same class. That system of connections for classifying stimuli is hierarchical. If two classes of objects or events are evoked simultaneously, their co-occurrence and coactivation will lead to connections representing a class of classes, and then there will be connections for classes of classes of classes, and so on. The order of cortical connectivity in that growing hierarchy of multiple classification will be isomorphous with (i.e., it will topologically correspond to) the order of sensory qualities previously established by the experience of the species and of the individual organism. In that order, topography (e.g., retinotopy) is simply a special case of topology.

That system, which constitutes the memory network or topological "map" (Hayek rarely calls it a network but rather a map), is also highly dynamic. With experience, it will not only grow upward to form ever higher hierarchies of classes but downward and sideways, to form new classes within previously existing ones, to reclassify objects, events, and their qualities.

It is not difficult to glean from such a system of connectivity the answer to several of the most pressing problems of cognitive neuroscience—namely, the neural base of stimulus constancy, generalization, discrimination, concept formation and, of course, perceptual memory. Although devoid of mathematical elaboration, Hayek's model clearly contains most of the elements of those later network models of associative memory that I have just singled out and that, with their algorithms, have not come any closer than it does to solving those problems in a neurally plausible manner. It is truly amazing that, with much less neuroscientific knowledge available, Hayek's model comes closer, in some respects, to being neurophysiologically verifiable than those models developed 50 to 60 years after his. It is no less amazing that virtually none of their developers ever cites him.

The main reasons for dwelling here on Hayek's model is simply that it has certain properties, absent from most others, that conform exceptionally well to recent neurobiological evidence on memory and that make it particularly suited to the current discourse. Those cardinal properties and their implications are summarized here:

• The *relational character* of all sensory perception and the denial of an "absolute core of sensation", in opposition to Mach (1885) and Von Helmholtz (1925); with it, the stage is set for phyletic memory and for the application of connective principles to the evolution of the sensory apparatus and primary sensory areas.

• The *categorical and hierarchical character* of all perception and memory, which provides a logical explanation for the hierarchical organization of connective systems in cortical areas of association.

• The *wide-ranging scope* of the principle of categorization, in perception and memory, which substantiates the need for a system of interconnections at least as rich and wide-ranging as that which has been discovered in the primate neocortex.

• The constant *dynamic interaction* between perception and memory, which explains the almost complete overlap, indeed identity, of processing and representational networks of the cortex that modern evidence indicates.

Hayek's model has problems, however. In the first place, it is incomplete; it could not be otherwise, considering its scope and the many gaps, present when he conceived it and still present today, in our knowledge of neural processes. More than anything, Hayek's model is merely an example of what he calls "the explanation of the principle," to characterize a high-level class of central representation.

Then there is the problem of the definition of the basic representational element, in other words, what others have called the *feature detector*, the *module*, the *submodule*, or the *semantic symbol*. Hayek (1952) denies that any such thing is necessary and asserts that sensory qualities are defined strictly by relationship, at all levels. This may well be true at any phenomenal level, but it is hard to accept for the lowest neural levels of a representational hierarchy. By definition, an order involves elements, the ordered elements. It is certainly possible, in fact desirable, to construe an order between classes or suborders, and this is probably what goes on in association cortex. However, at some level down the organization, it seems necessary to postulate neural units or sets of units that stand for something very concrete in the physical world. Of course, in modern neurophysiology, that function can be ascribed to the columnar module of sensory cortex. Anyway, to postulate something of the kind, which Hayek never does, is a perfectly reasonable corollary of his own thinking: The columnar module has developed in evolution and ontogeny by the same principle of relational connectivity that accounts for all perception and for all memory.

Hayek's model successfully avoids the problem of the so-called grand-mother cell because, in it, categorical representation is dispersed in a wide network of interconnections. Nonetheless, its radical connectionism appears, at higher levels, as implausible in neural terms as it appears at lower levels. Without constraints, it could easily run into a "connective explosion" that would obliterate even the most discrete of perceptual categories. Besides, there is neuropsychological (Damasio, 1990a) and neurophysiological (Desimone et al., 1984) evidence of categorical representation in some discrete cortical domains. A way to solve the problem, and to avoid the explosion, is to take the position later defended here. Briefly, the overarching category or concept is represented by a network made of the common elements and connections of multiple lower-level networks. This position, however, does not invalidate Hayek's "explanation of the principle" at higher levels of the representational hierarchy any more than it does at lower levels.

Edelman (1987), in his model, envisions a different principle of network formation while preserving the basic role that cortical networks have, in Hayek's model, for perception and memory. (Incidentally, Edelman is one of the few theoreticians of the brain to acknowledge the importance of Hayek's contribution.) Edelman's theory of *neuronal group selection* starts by assuming a genetic endowment of neuronal groups, such as the columnar modules of the cortex, with an inherent degree of variability and plasticity in their connections. They constitute the units of selection of the primary repertoire. By exposure to external stimulation and a hebbian mechanism, certain groups of cells, which tend to fire together, will be selected by stimuli insofar as the groups respond to them, and thus their connections will be strengthened (figure 5.1). Some of those connections will make recurrent or reentrant circuits which are an essential feature of the model and of all its theoretical and computational elaborations (Tononi et al., 1992). Groups not selected will be crowded out by the competition, in good agreement with the pertinent data from Merzenich and colleagues (see chapter 4). In that manner, a second repertoire will be formed. In it, a group will be one of many that will recognize (i.e., will respond more or less well, but now much more quickly, to) a signal similar to the one that shaped it. I stress *similar*, not identical. Because of reduplicaton, many groups can respond more or less well to such a signal. That tolerance for

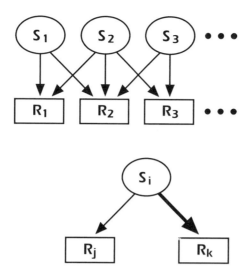

Figure 5.1 Edelman's principle of group selection. At birth, a primary repertoire of responses (R_1, R_2, R_3 . . .) by cortical neuron groups can be potentially elicited by any of a series of stimuli (S_1, S_2, S_3 . . .). After learning or repeated experience, a given stimulus, S_i, will elicit mainly or only one of those responses, R_K.

variations in the signal (degeneracy) is one of the strengths of the system. It ensures wide distribution of information and a degree of stimulus constancy—in other words, equivalence of response to variants of the same stimulus.

The system thus conceived is selective and adaptive, like evolution: hence the name of "neural Darwinism" which Edelman gave it. It shares with Hayek's model the merits of distribution of information, probabilistic response, and robustness. Nonetheless, in the computer simulations that Edelman (1989) and his colleagues devised to substantiate it, there is a lingering possibility of "grandmother groups."

The growth of the network in Edelman's model, as in Hayek's and Kohonen's models, is *unsupervised* and self-organized. It does not follow preestablished rules as in *supervised learning*. The latter, by contrast, is governed by rules inherent in the system, such as error correction, that act as an internal teacher. The best-known example of a supervised learning model is the *backpropagation model* of Rumelhart and colleagues (1986). This is a connectionist model that postulates feedforward processing in a network of three layers composed of, respectively, input units, hidden units, and output units (figure 5.2). As the response of the network to current input deviates from the input pattern, the weights of synaptic contacts from hidden to output units are changed to correct the discrepancy and, as a consequence, further retrograde adjustments are made in the contacts between input and hidden units. For these reasons, the error-correcting rule, which is based on a well-known algorithm first introduced by Werbos (1974), is designated back-

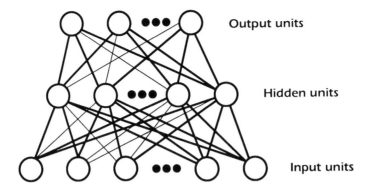

Figure 5.2 A neural network constituted by three layers of fully connected units. Learning consists in a process of error correction by backpropagation, leading to a system of stable synaptic weights, such that the output will reflect the input closely.

propagation. The rule is, in essence, what mathematicians commonly call a *delta rule*, here used as an optimization procedure to diminish incrementally discrepancies between input and output.

The backpropagation algorithm is biologically implausible. Other models of supervised learning have been reported to account better for the behavior of cerebral networks (e.g., the model by Mazzoni et al., 1991, based on reinforcement learning). Nonetheless, backpropagation has enjoyed enormous popularity as a tool to produce models of learning by machines and, despite its implausibility as a brain mechanism, it has served us well to develop a computer model whose hidden units simulate with remarkable fidelity the dynamics of active memory (see chapter 9).

Shaw and his colleagues (Shaw et al., 1985; Shenoy et al., 1993) have developed a learning model that reconciles several of the differences between the models thus far described. Their *trion model* is not dependent on reentry, which is not one of its assumptions. It is an unsupervised model obeying the selection principle much as Edelman's model, yet it is compatible with supervised learning for certain tasks. The trion model is inspired by Mountcastle's (1978) concept of the cortical columns and, as such, close to one of the basic principles of cortical organization. Thus, if the trion model proves tenable, the column may be not only the elementary functional unit but also the elementary network of cortex.

The trion is envisioned as the essential component of the column—in other words, as the minicolumn—a highly structured and interconnected conglomerate of some 100 neurons, approximately 60 μm in cross-section, that can fire at one of three levels—above average, average, and below average (figure 5.3). Thus, a column with a small number of trions has, built-in, a large repertoire of potential quasi-stable, spatiotemporal firing patterns. Those patterns change in rapid succes-

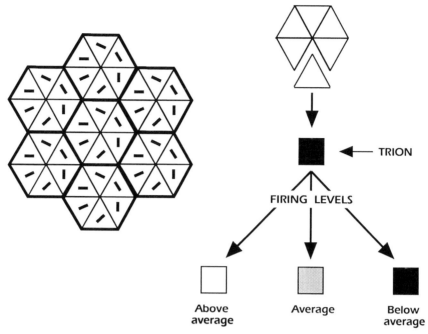

Figure 5.3 Schematic representation of Mountcastle's (1978) principle of cortical organization, as the basis for the trion model. Columns of cortical cells, here represented by hexagons, encode variations of a given sensory parameter, such as line orientation in the visual cortex. The columns are composed of minicolumns (triangles), each encoding a particular orientation. The trion, coinciding with the minicolumn, is the basic functional unit of cortex, which can fire at three frequency levels with respect to average. (From Shenoy et al., 1993, with permission.)

sion, spontaneously and according to full probabilistic (Monte Carlo) rules. Those rules can be overcome at any time by a hebbian rule: On arrival of a stimulus or combination of associated stimuli, a given pattern prevailing at the time is forced to persist by only the slightest change in the connective structure of the trion. Thus, the pattern becomes fixated, so to speak, such that subsequent encounters with one of those same stimuli will reelicit it. The power of the model resides in its large repertoire of responses, which is open to selection and to very fast learning (one-trial learning, in fact). Whereas in the Edelman model the object of "Darwinian" selection is the group, here it is the pattern of cell response, one among a great variety of them, already present before learning and ready to be selected.

The trion model may be a microcosm of the process of formation of larger networks. It seems well suited for fast learning on a relatively small scale, spatially and temporally. On the other hand, more global models such as those mentioned previously seem better suited for cortical networks, as we envision them, that span large territories of associative neocortex. Only further research on the neurobiology of the cortex can tell us which of these models explains best the growth of memory networks. It seems certain, however, that the growth of any such network is predicated on the presence of considerable plasticity, even in the adult organism. That means the capacity not only to strengthen preexisting synapses but to form new ones. It also probably means the capacity to develop new axon terminals and new dendrites and dendritic spines. In any event, it is function and usage that ultimately will determine the direction of connectivity and the expansion of the network. Conversely, lack of function and usage is bound to lead to regression and competitive loss. The adage, "Use it or lose it," probably expresses the very essence of what happens.

Based on the discussions in the previous two chapters, it seems reasonable to postulate that cortical memory networks grow in the general direction of ontogeny—that is, away from primary areas and into the areas of association. In other words, it seems logical that memory networks expand toward ever higher levels of the processing hierarchies for perception and for action. Note, however, that the connectivity up those hierarchies includes convergence as well as divergence every step of the way and, in addition, there is ample recurrence and backflow. What is most unclear is precisely how much of that wiring is genetically or epigenetically layed out and how much of it has developed during, and as a product of, individual life and experience (i.e., by learning).

If our presumption of network expansion into association areas is correct, networks can be envisioned to grow from phyletic memory into individual memory, at least as a general trend. That alone leads to an important corollary and prediction—namely, that variability in connectivity and in function should increase in the direction of network growth. This prediction is borne out by anatomical as well as physiological data.

Before concluding this section, I will summarize the principles of network formation that seem most reasonable in light of the previous discussion. At the root of the process there is a hebbian or quasi-hebbian mechanism of strengthening, and perhaps also formation, of synapses. Synaptic strengthening would involve the local depolarization of the membrane on arrival of simultaneous inputs—in other words, simultaneous conjunction at the presynaptic level. Groups of cells would be synaptically linked more strongly by simultaneous arrival of inputs to them.

At the lowest level of a cortical sensory hierarchy (for the moment, the reference is to perceptual networks, though similar processes could apply to motor networks), synaptic enhancements will take place in primary sensory cortex by coincidence of inputs on neurons from the same receptors and excited by similar stimuli. In phylogeny as well as ontogeny, this coincidence forms the lowest networks of a hierarchy, the basis of phyletic memory and the rudiments of individual memory. The process continues throughout life by expansion of networks into ever higher levels of integration within association cortex. Ever more complex co-occurring inputs will be associated and classed as similar or belonging together in some way. If the co-occurring stimuli are of the same modality, the associations will be circumscribed to unimodal association cortex. If they are not of the same modality, they will involve polymodal areas. Figure 5.4 illustrates in highly schematic manner the principles of memory network formation just proposed.

A group or class of stimuli that have been associated into a network can, by subsequent encounters, become associated with other stimuli that did not belong originally to the network and, by co-occurrence, become members of it. For that to happen, it is required only that a member stimulus or feature of the original class co-occur with any given new stimulus. The first will evoke the class (i.e., it will activate its network) and, by coactivation, will incorporate the second. This implies that an associative network in higher cortex, an entire class in memory, rapidly can establish new connections with incoming stimuli.

By a similar process, stimuli of two different classes can, by co-occurrence, link the two classes together to form a new supraordinate class, and this one, in turn, can associate with others at the same or lower levels. An important point is that a memory network can accrue associations in different levels of the representational hierarchy, up and down.

Certainly a connectionist process such as the one outlined is fully compatible with Hayek's assertion that all perception, and consequently all memory, is abstract and categorical at some level. At the highest levels, however, it is to be expected that convergence will lead to more general and abstract associations than at lower levels. Nonetheless, I believe it is erroneous to think of concepts, categories and names merely as representations made by convergence of associations at the top. This is the error that leads to the grandmother cell and its infinite regress. The reasonable alternative is to view the abstract concept as based on the entire network or networks that support it in their connections, and therefore, as widely distributed. This is not incompatible with some concentration of conceptual and semantic representation in certain areas of confluent association, such as Wernicke's area in posterior association cortex.

Ultimately it is function and usage that create the system of multiple interconnected networks for representation and classification of sensory information. In that system, experience opens new connections that will serve to interpret and accommodate even newer experience, which in turn will open newer connections, and so on: hence, the intimate and mutual relationships between experience and representation, be-

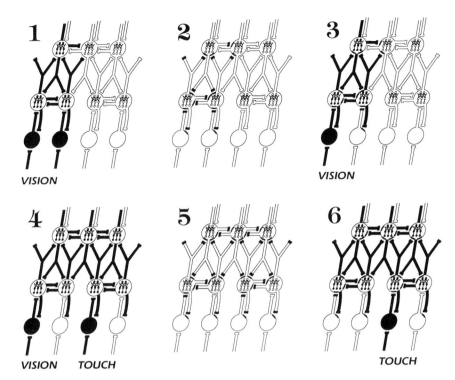

Figure 5.4 Scheme of memory network formation and activation. Each of the six network diagrams shows eleven interconnected units or groups of units (secondary nets or nodes). All major patterns of anatomically demonstrated connectivity are represented: parallel straight-through, convergent, divergent, and recurrent. Active units are represented in black, inactive in white. (*Diagram 1*) Two incoming visual inputs coincide in time; synaptic efficiency is enhanced at points of convergent and recurrent activation. (*Diagram 2*) Shown in black are enhanced synapses (latent memory) that are now excitable by either input. (*Diagram 3*) One input only activates the new network, which now incorporates some of the units formerly activated only by the other input. (*Diagram 4*) Coincidence of a visual and a tactile input. (*Diagram 5*) Enhanced synapses, some of which constitute the new bimodal net. (*Diagram 6*) A tactile stimulus activates the whole net, including units in territories of visual representation; the touch of the object evokes its visual memory.

tween perception and memory. Both use the very same networks to categorize information and to retain it.

PROPERTIES OF THE NETWORK

The paths are open and the network has been formed. Now the question we must ponder is how does it work? The remainder of this book attempts to answer this question. Before proceeding, however, it is necessary to define better the object of this study, at least in general terms, first structurally and then functionally. The following is a broad outline of the theoretical approach taken here to the structure and function of cortical networks.

Structure

My basic claim is that a memory is a cortical network, an array of connective links formed by experience between neurons of the neocortex, and that the function of cortical neurons in memory derives exclusively from their being part of such networks. The networks of phyletic memory and the lowest and most primitive components of individual memory networks (i.e., those in primary sensory and motor areas) can be viewed as topological feature maps, in that their neurons encode sensory and motor features. At higher levels of individual memory, however, the concept of *feature* becomes progressively more dependent on idiosyncratic connections and less on concrete physical parameters. Perhaps for this reason, the modular organization of primary sensory cortex disappears almost completely as we proceed into association cortex. At all levels and for all kinds of networks, the information networks contain is defined by the structure of each network—that is, by its neuronal elements and the connections that link them.

There are as many networks as there are memories and, in theory, their number is potentially infinite but, of course, many different networks share, to a greater or lesser extent, their constituent elements, cells and connections. At low levels of processing and representational hierarchies, all networks share one aspect or another of phyletic memory, a part of the apparatus of primary sensory or motor cortex. On the sensory side, the lowest-level constituents of a perceptual network are the columnar modules of sensory cortex or some other suitable group of functionally homogeneous neurons. They are the "feature detectors," which encode primitive attributes of the sensory environment. On the motor side, the lowest constituents of a network are the groups of cells in motor cortex (area 4 in the primate) that, by their concerted action, determine a vector of movement in a given part of the body, a motor feature.

Perceptual and motor networks permeate upward through the sensory and motor hierarchies and, as they do, they become generally more complex. As their pathways diverge, some networks or their parts become progressively more independent and idiosyncratic; they share less in common with others. At the same time, as pathways converge, networks also converge and share with others their more abstract and categorical aspects. High up in the hierarchies, the nodes of networks are simply other, more discrete, networks that are subcomponents of associative memory representing its relatively concrete aspects. Essentially, at higher levels of a hierarchy, those subordinate networks take the place that tightly interconnected clusters of cells occupy at lower levels (see figure 5.4).

Incalculable numbers of cells, linked by connections within and between levels of a hierarchy, contribute to the many parts of a given network. Conversely, because many networks overlap one another and share, in part, the same connections and cells, it follows that any connection and any neuron can be a member of many different networks, of many different memories. How big is a network? What shape does it have? The answer to these questions, of course, must differ enormously depending on the content of the network and on the memory it represents. Both questions naturally bear on the much-debated question of the localization of memory, which will be discussed in subsequent parts of this book in many different contexts.

For several reasons, a distributed perceptual or motor cortical network should be *two-dimensional,* at least coarsely. In the first place, the cortical processing hierarchies are laid out on the cortical plane; the most reasonable models of associative memory are laminar (e.g., that of Kohonen, 1984). All associational connectivity between areas is horizontal. Besides, in primary cortex and perhaps also association cortex, functional differentiation is greater on the horizontal than on the vertical plane. In fact, from a functional point of view, the neocortex of primary areas is strikingly homogeneous across cortex (because of its columnar organization) and heterogeneous in horizontal directions. It is on the horizontal plane—assuming, of course, a flattened cortex without sulci—that cortical connectivity displays the combinatorial power by which it can make practically infinite networks and practically infinite memories.

In any event, it is reasonable to suppose that the size and shape of a given network, literally of a given memory, should depend on its content and the directions in which it has grown; in other words, they should depend on the spread of its connectivity. Thus, simple sensory memories of one modality, for example, would take up relatively small sectors of sensory and parasensory association cortex, whereas a more complex perceptual memory, such as an episodic memory, would extend into higher-order association areas.

A *conceptual network* would be a large network involving broad areas of unimodal and polymodal association cortex. Because it would include parts of many networks with common connections, it would be not only widely distributed but also robust. As we shall see, there is considerable evidence indicating that conceptual networks have such properties. Only by assuming the wide distribution of, and multiple access to, the substrate of abstract memory (including what has been termed *semantic* and *nondeclarative memory*) is it possible to understand that extensive cortical damage is required for patients to manifest what Kurt Goldstein (1959) called the "loss of abstract attitude"—that is, the marked tendency to concrete thinking and expression. Also in this manner, we can understand why amnesic patients preserve abstract and procedural memory, which is robustly anchored in extensive cortical networks with multiple access. On the other hand, as noted previously, multiple access and wide distribution are compatible with concentration of conceptual and semantic representation in areas of convergent association. This would explain the loss of ability to recognize and name certain categories of objects that some patients exhibit after discrete cortical lesions (Damasio, 1990a).

Finally, an important structural property of networks is their heavy endowment of recurrent feedback connections, which flow downstream in the processing hierarchies of which they are a part. These recurrent or reentrant connections are a prominent feature of several of the computational models of cortical network (Kohonen, 1977; Palm, 1982; Edelman, 1987; Sporns et al., 1989). For the time being, let us just say that they provide the network with the capacity to turn on itself and to reach down into lower levels. Of course, reentry allows the network to maintain reverberating activity within it, a feature probably of the utmost importance for short-term memory (in accord with Hebb, 1949). In addition, however, this access of the network to lower levels can be important in acquisition of new memory, discrimination, and selective attention.

From Structure to Function

Now that we have considered how function makes structure, let us consider how structure makes function. Here the focus is on the cardinal properties a network should have for acquisition and retrieval of memory. In subsequent chapters, in the context of specific types of memory, additional properties and functions shall be discussed.

A memory network is a highly dynamic structure, meaning that it is constantly open to change and, under certain circumstances, it does change. This also means that, when activated, the network can play a decisive role in behavior. To discuss a memory network's changes and its behavioral role, and to simplify this discussion, we can assume that the established network can be in only one of two states: the *inactive* or latent state (see figure 5.4, diagrams 2 and 5), in which its neurons, without external input, maintain a relatively low and steady level of discharge that can be characterized as spontaneous background discharge; and the *active* state (see figure 5.4, diagrams 3 and 6), in which the discharge of the network's neurons, for whatever reason, is substantially above that level.

The assumption of a spontaneous background level of discharge presents certain difficulties, yet it seems necessary for accommodating a large body of empirical evidence. Spontaneous neuronal firing could be determined by factors that have little to do with the memory function of the network; it may reflect, for example, nonspecific activity arriving to the network through neurotransmitter systems of subcortical or limbic origin. Then again, that spontaneous discharge actually may reflect an underlying process of memory consolidation resulting from experience and, in fact, subcortical or limbic influences may have much to do with it. Nonetheless, background firing is a reasonable baseline to assess relative changes of network activity as a result of stimulation leading to memory retrieval or acquisition. A certain level of spontaneous discharge may be a precondition for effective activation or inhibition of a network. As Sejnowski (1981) has pointed out, it may be regarded as a bias that places neurons near threshold for excitation or inhibition.

The activation, or rather reactivation, of a network in perception and memory retrieval is a very fast process. It is much faster than any hebbian process of network formation as we understand it and as has been previously discussed. The slow and iterant mechanism of synaptic facilitation on which much neural plasticity is based is no longer applicable. Here we must postulate a process by which any of the set of stimuli that originally formed the network is capable of reactivating it and thus recreating the pattern of neuronal activity that defines the memory.

In the act of perception, a content-addressed memory network is reactivated quickly and in its entirety. It is unlikely that this occurs by a process of serial activation, one part of the network after the other and from one node to the next. Rather, what is needed (and has indeed been postulated) is a fast process of synaptic modulation in which the neurons of the network act as coincidence detectors and are extremely sensitive to correlated signals (Gerstein, 1970; Abeles, 1982; Aertsen et al., 1989). The neurons are activated and are induced to fire by temporal correlation of action potentials arriving to them through the connective links that incorporated them into the network originally. These impulses arrive by way of convergent, divergent, and, above all, parallel channels. The reactivation of a network most likely involves massive parallel conduction.

Although speed of conduction and activation have been stressed, we are not advocating here any mechanism of signal transmission other than by action potentials. Bear in mind, though, that neural transmission can take place by other means, such as fast-conducting surface potentials of dendritic origin or derivatives of postsynaptic potentials other than the action potential itself. Indeed, correlations of such surface potentials can also activate the coincidence detectors that are the neurons of the network. It is difficult to imagine, however, how activation by these other means would achieve the prompt and selective activation of any one among many overlapping cortical networks.

Reactivation is fast but not instantaneous. In the upper reaches of cortical hierarchies and networks, impulses evoked by sensory perception take a long time to arrive. As will be seen in the next chapter, we commonly encounter neuronal latencies of 100 to 300 msec in the association cortex (inferotemporal, parietal, or prefrontal) of the monkey.

This certainly denotes a much slower process of transmission than that of any digital machine. The point to emphasize, however, is that within that time all the elements of a huge cortical network can be activated. Considering synaptic delay and refractory periods, this only can happen by parallel conduction and a tightly connected array of coincidence detectors.

Von der Malsburg (1985) argues that the recognition resulting from an activated representational system depends exclusively on its profuse connectivity and the power of correlation, taking issue with proponents of conventional networks that are spatially fixed and work on a frequency code. His is a probabilistic and dynamic connectionist system in which correlations are processed in their own right, thus making the network flexible in the spatial and temporal domains. By their high sensitivity and fast response to correlations (in a few milliseconds), subsets of tightly interconnected neurons rapidly can encode sensory features, elementary symbols, despite considerable variations in physical appearance of the stimulus (the discussion is centered on vision). This would create a topological order within those neuronal subsets that would provide generalization and stimulus constancy to sensory representations in a way that rigid and static networks cannot.

Malsburg's model is attractive because of its probabilistic, correlational, topological, and dynamic features. All of them are assumed also in my model, which qualitatively does not differ too much from his. Indeed the nodes of the network I propose, the subordinate networks mentioned in the previous section, could be the subsets of neurons that Malsburg postulates, although the operational properties of ours, unlike his, are not submitted to computational treatment. However, it is unclear why it is necessary to assume such velocity of response or to dispense with a frequency code as he does. In fact, latency data indicate that cortical neuronal responses on recognition of a stimulus are much longer than those he envisions, and a frequency code, after the network is activated, is fully compatible with both his model and my views.

Electrophysiological data suggest the importance of temporal correlation for encoding information in the visual system of the cat (Eckhorn et al., 1988; Gray and Singer, 1989; Engel et al., 1991; Jagadeesh et al., 1992). Widely separated groups of neurons in primary visual (striate) cortex respond to a visual stimulus with highly correlated trains of oscillations (30–80 Hz, approximately 40 Hz as a rule). Such correlated synchrony suggests the cooperative role of the neurons in encoding the various aspects of the stimulus within a network of visual cortex. The value of this inference in terms of perception is diminished, however, by the fact that the data generally are obtained from the anesthetized animal and from relatively peripheral levels of the visual system. The transmission of a synchronous stimulus along separate channels is inherently correlated from its origin and bound to induce close temporal correlations centrally. Furthermore, oscillatory activity within the same range of frequencies just noted has been observed in the lateral geniculate body and traced to the retina, where it appears to be an inherent property of ganglion cells firing spontaneously and without stimulation (Ghose and Freeman, 1992).

Oscillatory activity has also been observed in the awake and behaving monkey's somatosensory cortex (Ahissar and Vaadia, 1990), temporal pole (Nakamura et al., 1992b), frontal cortex (Abeles et al., 1993) and, synchronously, in somatosensory and motor areas (Murthy and Fetz, 1991). From such observations, and others, the idea has emerged that synchronous oscillation is a manifestation of a temporal sensory code at the root of *perceptual binding*—in other words, the encoding of the identical or associated sensory qualities of objects (Engel et al., 1992). Naturally, reentry and lateral inhibition are assumed to be important features of encoding and binding networks (Horn et al., 1991; Tononi et al., 1992). Still, to uphold the principle of oscillatory perceptual binding, more experimental evidence is needed of the neural distribution and frequency specificity of the oscillations.

As noted in the previous chapter, lateral and recurrent inhibition is one of the common features of functional connectivity in the cerebral cortex. Its role is obscure but could well be that of deactivating networks that overlap or are near the one presently activated, thus enhancing the contrast of the active representation with respect to all others. In that way, its specific spatiotemporal pattern of activation (i.e., increased firing of pyramidal cells) would stand out above the rest. If this supposition is correct, there ought to be significant anticorrelations between the firing of the units of that network and the firing of those in other networks.

Let us now return to the activated network and concentrate on its more general characteristics with regard to perception and memory. As previously noted, that activation involves all levels of the network, from the lowest to the highest. The present model predicts that, up the hierarchy of representations, the activation of network elements is progressively less dependent on current stimulation and more dependent on past history and experience. Thus, by rapid conduction and correlation, vast networks can be reactivated by simple stimuli to recreate elaborate memories. Because of it, we need only see a small part of an object to conjure the whole object in our mind. From what we can see, however little, we make up the rest, or rather, the network does it for us.

That presumptive and a priori interpretive classing of the world is the essence of perception and goes on unconsciously most of the time. It is the essence of the categorizing process that neocortical neuronal networks most likely perform on sensory input (Marr, 1970). It is what prompted Hayek (1952, p. 143), expressing K. Popper's thinking, to say that "*all* we know about the world is of the nature of theories and all 'experience' can do is to change those theories." To change those theories, which we constantly and unwittingly test in our daily life, is to change the networks.

The recall of a categorical memory—what, in the previous section, we have characterized as a conceptual network—must involve the activation of vast areas of neocortex that may be anatomically discontiguous because of the multimodal and heterogeneous nature of its contents. I tend to agree with Damasio (1989, 1990b) that the memory of objects and categories cannot simply be allocated to one of the polymodal areas just because that memory is anchored in several sense modalities. Rather, as Damasio postulates, the memory is probably dispersed. Its recall may require the concomitant activation of such dispersed areas. In his scheme, this is achieved by impulses from a "convergence zone" (e.g., hippocampus) to those outlying neocortical areas (figure 5.5). In my scheme, that convergence zone is not indispensable—though the hippocampus most probably participates in the process of recall (see chapter 8)—because excitation easily can spread between distant areas via corticocortical connections. In either case, we have binding on a grand scale, supported by reentry and, as Damasio

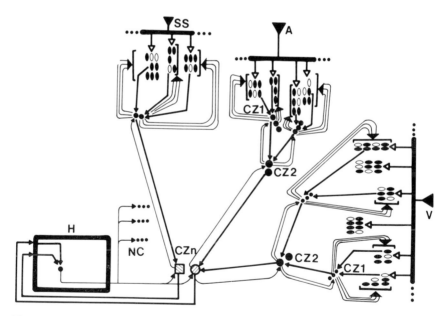

Figure 5.5 Damasio's scheme of activation of the neural architecture for perception and recall. Cortical areas for sensory analysis (A, auditory; SS, somatosensory; V, visual) feed into cortical and subcortical convergence zones (CZ). Feedback from these zones keeps the areas of representation activated. The hippocampus (H) is a cardinal convergence zone involved in the binding—in part, through noncortical (NC) neural stations—of widely dispersed representations. (From Damasio, 1990b, with permission.)

also postulates, effected by synchronous activation (again, according to him, possibly manifest in the form of oscillatory rhythms).

We have come full circle in our discussion, for now we are about to consider again, briefly, how the network changes and grows. To do so, we have to reinvoke Hebb and his principles. First, however, we must discuss another facet of network dynamics—the sustained activation of a network—along with its purpose and circumstances.

By a process of rapidly spreading excitation through correlated inputs, a sensory impression has reactivated a cortical memory network in the act of perception. After that, and under certain conditions, the network may stay active—that is, its neurons may continue to fire above spontaneous background level. The conditions under which this can happen are numerous. Three appear most likely: (1) Sensory inputs related, by experience, to the network keep arriving. (2) A new stimulus, although largely in accord with the network (falling within its class), is in some way discordant (it "disproves the theory") or else contains ambiguities that need to be resolved; this may call for a reclassification, the splitting of the network and of the class it represents. (3) Still another possible reason for sustained activation is that the network calls for later behavioral action. When we deal with motor memory, we will see that a motor network may be simply an extension of a perceptual one and not separable from it except by time, which is why, after the activating stimulus is gone, the perceptual network has to remain active until the action congruent with it is consummated. This temporary activation is the kind of short-term memory that is commonly understood as working memory (Baddeley, 1983). It is the short-term memory that I include under the broader category of active memory.

These eventualities require a mechanism to keep the network active, especially if it is to be modified, expanded, split, or utilized by the organism to perform an action in the short term. Such a mechanism of sustained activation is not known. A reasonable working hypothesis is that it involves reentry loops and recycling activity within the network itself. In chapter 9, I present a spiking model of short-term active memory that my colleagues and I have developed based on this principle (Zipser et al., 1993). Regardless of the mechanisms by which a network is and remains activated, it seems indispensable to postulate the concept of a threshold of excitability beyond which the cells of the network stay active. As Braitenberg (1978) proposes, a network "holds at a threshold θ" when at that threshold all its neurons, once excited, stay that way because of their reciprocal connections. Further he states that the threshold should be controlled by feedback from the activity of the network itself, to prevent its excessive excitation and, at the same time, to keep it above a certain minimum (figure 5.6).

Braitenberg (1978) derives an interesting corollary from the idea of threshold control: A network maintained at a certain threshold would

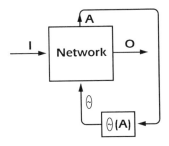

Figure 5.6 Reentrant activation (A) of a network at a given threshold (θ) according to Braitenberg (1978). I, input; O, output.

be a suitable substrate to accommodate the binary character of the recognition of objects—in other words, the classification of objects. An object "is" or "is not," in phenomenal terms, depending on whether or not that threshold is reached. Before reaching that threshold, however, the excitation of a part of the network would be sufficient to *ignite* the network at large, thus satisfying the requirement for completion of the representation of the object by perception of only one of its parts.

In more concrete neurostructural terms, the recycling of excitation that keeps a network active may extend beyond any conceivable and discrete portion of cortex. It may involve nuclei of the thalamus. Later, I will discuss experimental evidence for reentrant activation, in short-term memory, between dorsolateral prefrontal cortex and the nucleus medialis dorsalis (Alexander and Fuster, 1973) or between different cortical areas of association (Fuster et al., 1981; Quintana et al., 1989) (see chapter 9). Also involved in the sustained activation of the cortical network may be the amygdala and the hippocampus which, having played an important role in the formation of the network, play it now also in its expansion or modification. This brings us back to the acquisition of memory, the subject of chapter 3 and of the previous section (Growth of the Network).

An activated network can accrue new associations by co-occurrence and a quasi-hebbian mechanism, much as the network was generated and shaped by previous experience. Thus, the network in its active state acquires new connections; it expands. Note here that the activation of the network is the precondition for the acquisition of new memory as well as for the short-term retention of reactivated memory, new or old. Network activation is the common ground of both forms of short-term memory. As noted in chapter 2, much confusion about nomenclature could be avoided if the commonality of cortical substrate and state were recognized and accepted for both kinds of short-term memory. One important difference is worth noting, however. Whereas new memory involves the opening of new synapses, the short-term activation of old memory per se probably does not.

The formation of new memory on an old network may, as has repeatedly been mentioned, consist in the splitting of that old network to reclassify its information—in other words, to form a discrimination. For that, the network, by way of its recurrent connections, must reach down into its lower levels, must turn on itself, and establish new contacts that will dichotomize the information it originally contained. To use a human analogy akin to animal discrimination paradigms, what started as the class or network to represent, for example, traffic light splits into two; one for red and the other for green.

The traffic-light analogy, with its connotation of alternative actions, is a convenient lead-in to a brief discussion of motor networks. It will restate some of the concepts already presented in chapter 4. My position in this book is that motor networks develop and function according to the same principles as perceptual networks. At the lowest level of the cortical motor hierarchy—namely, the primary motor cortex (MI)—the co-occurring and convergent inputs that form the network come, through lateral thalamus and somesthetic cortex, from kinesthetic proprioceptors and possibly from the cerebellum. The simultaneous hebbian conjunction is, at those levels, of signals encoding movement primitives. These signals often are called *efferent copies* and constitute a form of feedback from movement. The networks, at this stage, are relatively small and represent relatively concrete vectors of striate muscle movement. At higher stages, in premotor and prefrontal cortex, the signals associated are more diverse and more general; they include sensory inputs from telereceptors coming through association areas of posterior cortex. Premotor and prefrontal networks represent more global movements, higher classes of action, than motor cortex networks. As the networks reach into dorsolateral prefrontal cortex, they represent action in the most general and conceptual sense (see chapter 7); they represent something close to what has been called *schemata* of action (Arbib, 1981). Somehow implicit, they have a substantial temporal dimension that is not realized until the network ceases to be merely representational and becomes operational.

It is there, in prefrontal cortex, that the more general aspects of perceptual networks and memory meet the more general aspects of motor networks and memory. Closing the highest links of the perception-action cycle (see chapter 9) are the long fiber tracts from posterior association cortex that converge on prefrontal cortex (see chapter 4). Through those long connections, perceptual networks reach frontal cortex and acquire motor associations. Likewise, motor networks acquire sensory associations reaching back into posterior cortex.

After being activated in an act of perception and recognition (perception is largely re-cognition), a network, whether perceptual or motor, may not stay more than fleetingly active. In normal behavior and phenomenology, there is a constant turnover of activated networks and memories. However, a network activated for any of the reasons stated earlier, including short-term or working memory, does not necessarily stay equally active in its entirety. For one thing, different parts of the network may have different thresholds, and these may change. Here we have to bring in a new concept which, as we will see in subsequent chapters, has considerable empirical support: The part of the network that stays most active at a given time is the part that controls or comes under the control of behavior at that time. That portion of active network is what I call the *focus of representation,* which is a concept identical to that of focus of attention but extensible to the motor sphere and not limited, as it usually is, to the perceptual sphere. The evidence for this concept will be discussed in later chapters (especially chapters 8 and 9). Suffice it here to say that shifts of neuroelectrical activity in a representational network during behavior indicate that different components of the network are involved in different aspects of behavior. Alternatively, the shifts may occur between networks, in which case different networks are involved in different behavioral functions. In any case, there seems to be a kind of sequential distribution of labor among components of a network, or among networks, in the behavior that follows the perception and recognition of a stimulus demanding attention, discrimination, short-term memory, and motor action. When perception leads to motor action, the activation of the cortical network and, with it, the focus of representation can be presumed to propagate over the cortical surface, generally following the scheme of figure 5.7.

In conclusion, the implications of the current theory are threefold: (1) In temporally extended behavior, there is a shifting focus of representation within or between cortical networks; (2) representational networks become *operational networks* (just as the opposite can also be true, in memory acquisition); and (3) in the processing of information from perception to action, *serial processes* are more prevalent than in perception and recognition, where parallel processes dominate.

Finally, a question seems to be the product of these considerations: Is what I call *focus of representation* the equivalent of consciousness? For the moment, let us just say that the shifts in that focus may correspond to the vicissitudes of what has been called the *stream of consciousness.* We will discuss this question again later (see chapter 10).

NEUROSCIENCE OF THE NETWORK

Despite the abstract and tautological nature of some of the argument thus far, the place and purpose of the present chapter should by now be clear to the reader. It is near the center of the book because it bridges, by inductive and deductive reasoning, the empirical base of the previous three chapters with that of the next four. Here I have presented only

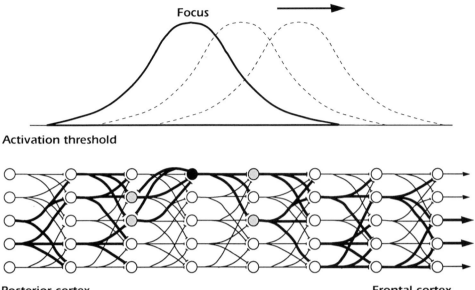

Focus

Activation threshold

Posterior cortex   Frontal cortex

Figure 5.7 General progression of a wave of network activation from the perceptual to the motor sector of the cortex. The focus of representation is where, at a given time, activation of the network is maximal above a certain threshold. Both serial and parallel processing are assumed. Reentry (schematized by two backflowing connections) allows the persistence of the focus of representation, as in active memory.

the principles of a model that I believe to be neurally plausible in light of chapters 2 through 4 and testable in chapters 6 through 9.

Next is a précis of methodology for the study of cortical memory at the level of analysis at which we have set it. The ideal scenario for the future is, of course, a full description of the cortical substrate of memory and of the computational algorithms that explain neural transactions in memory acquisition and retrieval. It seems unlikely that this scenario will ever be realized. It is of the nature of complex dynamic systems that no one can ever achieve complete knowledge and control of all the relevant variables that interact in them at any given time. This is true for social systems, economic systems, ecological systems and, of course, for the brain, which is the most complex system of all.

Nonetheless, progress has been and will continue to be made by successive approximations to the essence of cortical memory and the mechanisms of its acquisition and retrieval. At the basic level, the most promising advances should now come in the area of molecular neurobiology of the cortex and the hippocampus, especially with regard to the development of axons, dendritic processes, and synaptic contacts in both these structures. Particularly helpful will be new knowledge on the development of N-methyl-D-aspartate (NMDA) receptors and the changes in membrane biophysics they mediate.

Investigations of limbic and cortical connectivity will lead to better understanding of the makeup of memory networks. Of special interest is the neurobiology of cortical connections. Developmental connective correlates of cognitive functions should be closely examined. Individual morphological differences should be explored in association cortex, with keen regard to individual differences in memory function. This should be done in normal development, in adulthood, and in aging, as well as after injury and during recovery.

In the next four chapters, we will examine what has been done and what should be done to elucidate cortical memory. The study of the cortical network in memory requires a methodology that is adequate for a dynamic system whose functions are the product of complex neural associations and are irreducible to its elements; it should be a methodology appropriate to the level of discourse established in this chapter. It should approach the network as the memory itself, interrelated with many others, widely distributed and, above all, as a dynamic entity, subject to changes of state and content. This requires that the organism under study be aware and behaving.

Obviously, it is in its active state that the functions of the network can best be investigated. In fact, it would be futile to try to investigate those functions by focusing on single static elements of potentially multiple networks, and especially futile to try to do so when neither the network nor its elements are engaged in active representation. Instead, for the study to be fruitful, the system must be put in behavioral situations in which memory is being acquired, temporarily retained, or retrieved. The experimental paradigms in which this can be done will be discussed in later chapters, along with the research rationale and the data.

Questions regarding the role of cortical areas as the seat of memory networks can be approached by examining memory acquisition or retrieval after there has been a cortical lesion, either experimental or clinical, as has been done for more than a century. Studies of this kind are useful in that they give us approximate ideas about the location and extent of networks or, at least, of their most critical components for the type of memory and behavior under study. They do not tell us anything, however, about how a memory network works. In addition, the methods of brain injury and ablation are beset with difficulties deriving from secondary and compensatory changes that the brain undergoes after lesion and that have uncontrollable effects on memory function.

The use of reversible cortical lesions—by cooling, for example—circumvents some of these difficulties. Moreover, reversibility of lesion offers the advantage of allowing the repeated use of one animal as its own control. This is important when fine functional differences are to be examined between the normal condition and the inactivation of a cortical area. Reversible lesion methods, such as cooling, also have limitations, however. Among the most troublesome is the difficulty in producing with them a sharply defined and homogeneous inactivation of cortex.

The neurophysiology of the cortical network presents special challenges and opportunities. Again, the most informative studies are those conducted in the unanesthetized and behaving organism. Regardless of the level of analysis (single-unit, multiple-unit, or field-potential recording), the critical behavioral variables—namely, those that control behavior or change with behavior—should be carefully defined. Here some emphasis is necessary on the value of discrimination behavior as an important tool for memory study.

Because, as we assume, a cortical memory network is extensive and has many components, it is impractical to record the totality of its neural potentials at any given time. What is needed is a precise adjustment of behavioral variables to the level of physiological analysis, so that restricted parts of the network can be electrically investigated and meaningful inferences drawn from that about the functions of the network. That analysis can be taken down to the single-unit level if the area explored includes neurons of the network and if those neurons are activated by a discriminant stimulus that controls behavior. These conditions can be met in microelectrode explorations of certain cortical areas during discriminant behavior. Of course, a cell or group of cells may be part of many networks. If it is selectively activated by the discriminant stimulus, it can be assumed to belong to the perceptual network activated by that stimulus; if activated in relation to a particular motor response, it can be assumed to be part of the motor network.

By separating in time the discriminant stimulus from the corresponding motor response—that is to say, by introducing a delay between them—we force the animal to retain the discriminant stimulus in short-term memory before it performs the response to it. This procedure ensures that the perceptual network will remain activated during that delay, and the motor network may also remain activated in anticipation of movement. Here I should repeat that both the perceptual and the motor network may be part of the same general network activated by the stimulus, although the two components are activated at different times. This difference in time of activation may simply reflect the temporal shift of processing within the network and, with it, the shift in focus of representation. Latency, frequency, and time-series analyses of unit discharge throughout the discriminant trial can thus reveal the participation of the units under study in the structure and functions of that network. Of special interest is the unit's participation in short-term working memory, or more precisely, in the temporarily activated memory network.

Such is the methodology employed by this author in a number of microelectrode studies of association cortex of the monkey, which will be discussed in coming chapters. The principal obstacle for such studies is that they require exacting and lengthy procedures of animal training, testing, and data analysis. Some of the additional obstacles and limitations are presently being overcome by simultaneous recording with multiple microelectrodes. This approach provides the added advantage of allowing cross-correlations of unit firing, from which interesting inferences may be drawn regarding the spatiotemporal activation patterns of cortical networks and, above all, the mechanisms of short-term memory.

Modern methods of functional brain imaging, such as positron emission tomography, show much promise for the study of cortical memory. Particularly attractive for studies of memory are those methods that have high temporal resolution, such as PET with $H_2^{15}O$ and functional magnetic resonance imaging. They yield rather precise dynamic pictures of the distribution of cortical metabolism and blood flow and are, therefore, of great potential value for studying the activation of networks in memory acquisition and retrieval. Recent versions of the technology are applicable to animal study. Combined with microelectrode methods, they may be helpful in studies of learning and memory acquisition.

Computer modeling and simulation will remain valuable for the study of cortical memory. The most promising models will continue to be those that are based on processing along parallel but interactive channels and that incorporate self-organized and content-addressable memory. Efforts should be made to develop physiologically testable and open models—that is, models that can generate physiologically testable hypotheses and that are amenable to change as the data dictate.

6 Organization of Perceptual Memory

In previous chapters, the theoretical framework for cortical memory has been laid out and pertinent hypotheses have been advanced. It has been proposed that individual memories are self-organized neuronal networks of potentially infinite variety that extend beyond primary sensory and motor cortex into the so-called cortex of association. In the recognition and retrieval of a memory, one such neocortical net of certain proportions is activated; its neuronal elements, mainly pyramidal cells, are induced to fire at frequencies above their "spontaneous" baseline. While the net is active, new memory can be added to it through the creation of new associations in accord with the principle of synchronous convergence. It is also in its active state that a memory network controls behavior and presumably gains access to consciousness.

In this and subsequent chapters, the validity of those ideas will be assessed with regard to perceptual and motor memory, at least to the extent that available empirical methods allow it. The attempt will be made to delineate the topographical distribution and the dynamics of memory networks in the primate cortex. The focus of this chapter is the topography of perceptual memory; its dynamics will be dealt with in chapters 8 and 9.

One of the basic assumptions of this work is that memory and perception are practically and even theoretically inseparable. Perception makes memory and memory makes perception in a continuous interplay that renders the experimental dissection of these two cognitive functions extremely difficult with the traditional approach of keeping one of them constant while varying the other. As psychophysical data demonstrate (to wit, a rich collection of well-publicized visual illusions and the phenomenon of blindsight), not only do we remember what we see but we see what we remember, imposing on reality the assumptions, expectations, hypotheses, and preconceptions from prior experience. This would be the so-called top-down control of perception. In this sense, perception is a form of doing and far from the passive taking of mere sensation. In neural terms, this means that in the conscious organism, the network activated by a sensory stimulus has been, in all likelihood, shaped by previous experience with that stimulus and with others similar to or associated with it; it also means that the preestablished network shapes the quality of the perceived experience. Thus, it seems reasonable to assume that beyond primary sensory cortex (phyletic memory), the cortical networks of perception and memory coincide. They are the networks of what we call *perceptual memory*.

In the ensuing discussion and throughout this chapter, much value is placed on discrimination as a measure of perception. This emphasis on discrimination is based on the assumption enunciated in the previous chapter that perception is essentially a series of acts of classifying the sensory world from memory. Methodologically, the experimental discrimination is nothing but a forced act of perceiving (i.e., of classifying or categorizing two or more sensory stimuli). Thus, the ability of an animal to discriminate stimuli gives an indication of how well it perceives them. Its ability to learn the discrimination measures the formation of perceptual memory, and its ability to retain one of the stimuli in a short-term memory task measures the efficacy of active perceptual memory.

For reasons of methodology, including the necessity to control sensory stimuli and their prior associations, perceptual memory can best be investigated separately within each sensory modality. This is also the most useful approach for reviewing the available evidence. From the separate study of modalities, general principles may be expected to emerge that are applicable to polymodal memories, which are based on temporal coincidence or near-coincidence of inputs of several modalities.

For each sensory modality, the available data concerning the cortical distribution of perceptual memory of that modality will be reviewed. In chapters 8 and 9, the activation of perceptual networks and their dynamics in memory retrieval, attention, and active short-term memory will be discussed. In discussing these processes, special emphasis will be placed on microelectrode records of neuronal discharge and tomographic data from behaving and conscious subjects.

VISUAL MEMORY

Primates are eminently visual animals and, consequently, much of their cortex of association appears involved in visual functions. In fact, it has been stated that more than two-thirds of the macaque's neocortex is devoted to vision. This may be an overstatement, for the reckoning is based on neuropsychological evidence that parietal and frontal areas, in addition to occipital and temporal areas, are involved in visually guided behavior. Indeed, posterior parietal cortex seems essential for encoding visuospatial information, whereas prefrontal cortex subserves the temporal organization of visuomotor behavior. Visual behavior shares both those functions, as well as their supporting parietal and frontal cortices, with behaviors that are guided by auditory and somesthetic stimuli. Be that as it may, the most intensively explored perceptual representations in the primate cortex are, by far, those of the visual modality. Interestingly, some of that research was prompted by clinical observations.

The term *agnosia* was coined around 1890 by Freud (1953) to characterize the inability of certain patients to recognize objects and persons in the absence of visual sensory dysfunction. For many years, especially in the neurological literature of the early part of this century, numerous reports appeared on cases of visual agnosia resulting from lesions of posterior cortex (e.g., Kleist, 1934). At all times, however, the term and subject of agnosia, of which there are many kinds, have been controversial, and the exact nature of the lesions causing it remains obscure in most cases. Nonetheless, there is little doubt that in cases of so-called agnosia, what is critically impaired is precisely perceptual memory. It is not surprising that reports of agnosia should have influenced the design and discussion of systematic studies of visual cognition in non-human primates.

In their landmark study, Klüver and Bucy (1938) noted that monkeys with bilateral resections of the temporal lobe, including inferotemporal cortex and limbic structures, exhibited (among other things) a peculiar inability to recognize familiar objects and their biological significance. A similar syndrome was observed in the human (Terzian and Dalle Ore, 1954). It is apparent that what those investigators described as "psychic blindness" was tantamount to visual agnosia from inferotemporal (IT) cortical injury. Indeed, more selective lesions of extrastriate cortex subsequently were shown to cause severe deficits in higher visual functions. Ablations of IT cortex (area 21, TE), in particular, induce deficits in the learning and performance of a variety of visual discrimination tasks (Chow, 1951; Iwai and Mishkin, 1969; Cowey and Gross, 1970; Mishkin, 1972; Gross, 1973; Horel et al., 1984). It is clear from the bulk of this evidence that the integrity of that large cortical region is critical for cognitive visual functions, including visual memory. This is in keeping with the anatomical and physiological evidence that IT cortex is the last and highest stage of visual information processing, where the aggregate of serial and parallel processing channels terminate that originate in the retina (see chapter 4).

What is not clear, however, from neuropsychological data alone, is precisely which cognitive functions the various parts of the IT cortex subserve in the visual domain. Lesion studies are inconclusive on this issue. Let us briefly consider one of the best such studies to illustrate the difficulties they encounter. To uncover functional specialization within IT cortex, Iwai and Mishkin (Mishkin, 1972) produced strip lesions of this cortex at various anteroposterior planes in monkeys to be trained, or already fully trained, in visual discrimination tasks. Animals with posterior IT lesions were, with some difficulty, capable of learning several discriminations concurrently, that is, discriminations of several pairs of objects, each pair presented every day—along with other pairs—in a series of consecutive days. These animals had much trouble, however, relearning a single discrimination between two visual patterns (figure 6.1). Conversely, animals with anterior IT lesions (near the temporal pole) relearned with relative ease the single-pattern discrimination but only with great difficulty the concurrent discriminations. From this apparent double dissociation of tasks and lesions, the researchers concluded that posterior IT cortex is essential for visual discrimination, whereas anterior IT cortex is needed for visual memory. One problem with this interpretation, aside from the evidence that the task impairments were only relatively and quantitatively different, is that it does not take fully into account that both tasks required both memory and discrimination, albeit perhaps to different degrees. It can be argued that both lesions affected visual memory and their results were all basically variations of a memory defect: Posterior IT lesion affected the more concrete aspects of visual representations and anterior IT lesion their

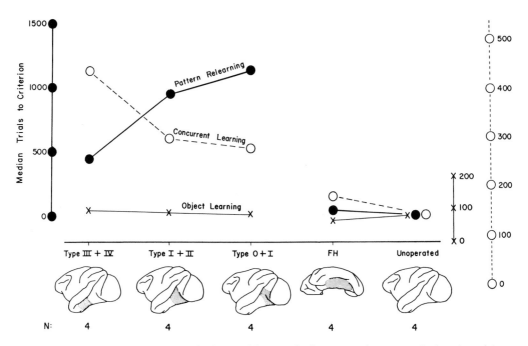

Figure 6.1 Results of selective ablations of inferotemporal cortex on the learning of three visual discrimination tasks: object learning, pattern learning, and pattern relearning. Five groups of animals are tested, with lesion area shown in gray. The numbers of trials to criterion are represented with different scales for the three tasks. (From Mishkin, 1972, with permission.)

more complex and categorical aspects (where interference from other concurrent information would perhaps be most deleterious). This would be in accord with our hierarchical view of perceptual memory organization, which is supported, in the case of vision, by the hierarchical connective organization of extrastriate cortex and which later will be substantiated further with single-cell data.

There is now a considerable body of human neuropsychological evidence implicating the temporal cortex in visual memory, although with regard to localization this evidence is no more conclusive than the animal data, despite the methodological advantage of verbal communication in the human. As is often the case in human neuropsychology, there are problems largely related to the variability and arbitrariness of lesions that do not adjust to scientific rationale. Nonetheless, the human evidence is revealing and fully in accord with the suspected importance of IT cortex for visual memory. Milner (1958) first demonstrated that patients with right temporal lobe lesions had difficulties recognizing familiar objects from partial views of them. Kimura (1963) reported, in such patients, deficits in tachistoscopic recognition of images. Other studies (Milner, 1968; McCarthy and Warrington, 1986) confirmed the visual-memory deficits from temporal lesions, whether on recognition or free recall. More recently, patients with temporal lobe lesions have been shown to have deficits in performance of paired-associate tasks that test visual short-term memory (Petrides, 1985). In none of the studies mentioned, however, were the lesions circumscribed to IT cortex. Most, if not all, cases investigated were in patients who had undergone temporal lobectomies, which included at least partial amygdalectomy and hippocampectomy. Given the well-known importance of limbic structures in memory, including possibly the retrieval of old memories, it is somewhat risky to attribute the reported visual-memory deficits exclusively to IT cortex removal, although such an interpretation is certainly in harmony with the monkey data.

Fragments of visual memory can be recorded with microelectrodes from the monkey's temporal cortex. At first, this was done almost inadvertently in the context of physiological investigations of IT cortex. In recent years, the issue has been more formally approached by some investigators, and their studies will be reviewed next. It should be noted, however, that most of them leave unresolved what to some is a crucial distinction—namely, the distinction between the sensory response of any given IT neuron to the physical properties of a stimulus and the associative activation of that neuron as a member of an assembly that encodes, by virtue of prior history, the mnemonic experience to which the stimulus belongs. In my view, and in light of our discussions in chapters 4 and 5, the distinction may be a nonissue because, in the association cortex of the conscious organism, physical quality is inextricably tied to perceptual (i.e., mnemonic) quality. Only the rather impractical study of the natural history of every stimulus, from the neuron's perspective, might help resolve the matter to everyone's satisfaction.

Even in the anesthetized monkey, Gross and his colleagues (1972), who were the first to study systematically the visual properties of IT cells, found units that reacted selectively to unusually complex and more or less natural stimuli, such as the images of hands and faces. Subsequent investigations in the awake animal have not only confirmed but expanded those findings. Particularly intense has been the search for cells that respond to faces of monkeys or humans (Perrett et al., 1982; Desimone et al., 1984, Baylis et al., 1987; Rolls et al., 1989a; Young and Yamane, 1992). These units characteristically react with increased firing frequency to a wide range of visual stimuli but especially to images of one or several faces (figure 6.2). Often, the response of one such cell to a face is relatively independent of the position, size, color, and degree of exposure of the image. Otherwise, a "face cell" may respond in particular to frontal or profile views or to individual features of the "preferred" face; its responses to visual stimuli with emotional connotations are reported to be minor (e.g., Perrett et al., 1982), as are its

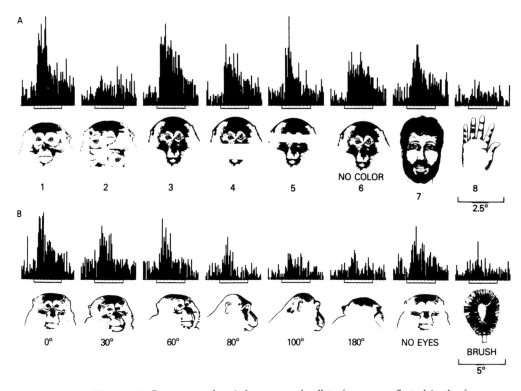

Figure 6.2 Responses of an inferotemporal cell to faces, as reflected in the frequency histogram of the cell during stimulus presentation. Monkey faces are presented complete, in fragments, or with jumbled features. (From Desimone et al., 1984, with permission.)

responses to the jumbled features of the face into a meaningless geometrical pattern. Some IT cells are responsive to the sight of moving objects and subjects (Perrett et al., 1985).

Ever since Gross observed those unusual IT cells, the quest was on, in the classical tradition of sensory neurophysiology, to find exactly the physical parameters, or combinations thereof, that accounted for unit responses to complex visual stimuli. Interestingly, the responses appeared, in some cases, sharply and remarkably tuned to the stimulus across retinal translations (regardless of the retinal domain in which it fell). Thus, the quest promised to solve what some (e.g., Klüver, 1933) have called one of the most important riddles of physiological psychology—namely, the problem of stimulus equivalence. Indeed we know that, up to striate cortex (V1), the characteristics of the visual world can be found encoded in a spatial (retinotopic) order of neural elements that respond to discrete features of that world, but we also know that visual perception clearly transcends that order. A behaviorally and phenomenologically meaningful stimulus remains effective and just as meaningful even if its size, position, or perspective changes drastically in the real world and in the retina. Is that not, in fact, an essential property of perception—and of memory? It was only logical to look for its physiological explanation in IT cortex, especially after finding there the presence of such neural elements as face cells.

However, the search for the selective physical constants that activate IT cells independently of retinal coverage has met with only moderate success. Mathematical functions have been found that explain relatively well the invariant responses of certain cells to certain stimuli across retinal translation, in terms of either spike counts or spike pattern (Schwartz et al., 1983; Richmond and Optican, 1987; Eskandar et al., 1992). Some of those responses (e.g., responses to contour regardless of size) can be related to a single complex parameter, such as relative spatial frequency (e.g., the number of points of a star). Nonetheless, the results of such research address only a relatively narrow range of natural forms. Tanaka (1993) and his colleagues have expanded that range by identifying cells that respond to a long series of simple *object primitives* (my term) and seem to be arranged in columnar fashion.

In any case, it seems that with its parametric reductionism, the research just summarized misses the essence of visual perception and memory, both of which are based on categorical, classificatory, and binary decisions that the higher visual system makes with its many cells, despite noise and enormous variance, in both real-world and single-unit activity. Furthermore, this research ignores the possibility, indeed probability, that what drives IT cells is not merely the physical characteristics of any given stimulus but a combination of the stimulus and its history. It would be the confluence of external (sensory) and internal (memory) factors that would activate the net in which the cell is immersed. *Internal factors* here means the prior associations of the stimulus, engraved in the network, which include its emotional and biological connotations (see chapter 5).

In sum, visual binding is probably the product of the interplay of exogenous and endogenous factors on cells of IT cortex. Thus, for optimal response, IT neurons may require both the appropriate visual input and the associated descending input from past history and from the neural substrate of motivation (limbic input?). Significantly, face cells have also been found in the amygdala (Leonard et al., 1985; Nakamura et al., 1992a), a limbic structure supposed to be critically involved in the evaluation of the motivational significance of sensory stimuli (Fuster and Uyeda, 1971; Sarter and Markowitsch, 1985). Amygdala units, in the monkey, have been seen to respond selectively to socially significant visual scenes as well (Brothers and Ring, 1993).

If only because they are activated by ethological stimuli of presumably acquired meaning, face cells are most probably an integral part of memory networks. Rolls and coworkers (1989a) have shown that such cells have a degree of plasticity; by successive exposure to different faces, the cells modify their responses to them. This evidence can be adduced in support of the notion that face cells are part of long-term memory networks subject to learning changes. It has been suspected that these cells and their networks are damaged in cases of prosopagnosia—that is, agnosia for faces (Bodamer, 1948; Whiteley and Warrington, 1977; Walsh, 1978; Tranel et al., 1988). These are patients with certain cortical lesions who are incapable of recognizing faces, even of familiar persons. They appear to suffer from a discrete and categorical visual memory defect for faces (Damasio, 1990a; Damasio et al., 1990). However, the lesions of these patients, in the relatively few cases reported for which there is thorough neuropathological description, appear to have been located primarily in more posterior regions (e.g., fusiform gyrus) than the regions of the monkey where face cells have been found. Face cells have been reported in the middle and superior temporal gyri of the human (Ojemann et al., 1992).

In monkeys, as noted earlier, face cells have thus far been encountered mainly in discrete locations of anterior IT cortex, especially in the depth of the superior temporal sulcus and in the amygdala. Some have been found in area TPO (Bruce et al., 1981; Perrett et al., 1982), a transitional area between IT and superior temporal cortex in the depth of that sulcus (Seltzer and Pandya, 1984), which has been supposed to be important for cross-modal integration. Because of its polysensory properties the area has been physiologically characterized as the superior temporal polysensory (STP) area (Bruce et al., 1981).

Face cells are not the only cells that appear to participate in visual memory networks. Evidently, other IT cells do too, even though they seem attuned to much simpler stimuli than faces and, for this reason, there has been a tendency to consider them merely as sensory feature analyzers. Our research indicates that at least one important class of IT neurons, the color-responsive neurons, can be part of memory networks. After appropriate behavioral training of the animal, a proportion of these cells behave as if they have been incorporated in such networks. Let us briefly review the evidence.

In a study designed to examine the activity of IT units in short-term memory, we (Fuster and Jervey, 1981, 1982) trained monkeys to perform a delayed matching task with colors. Because the task was somewhat difficult and we required from the animal high levels of performance, the training procedure was lengthy, of the order of months. It can be assumed a priori that, by the time a monkey had been fully trained, the colored stimuli that he had to use in the task had become thoroughly consolidated in long-term memory and, therefore, in well-established memory networks. Here is what the animal was supposed to do (figure 6.3). He faced a panel with five translucent stimulus-response buttons, one on top and the other four in a row below. Trials of short-term memory were presented every minute or so. A trial began with presentation of one of four colors by transillumination of the top button (approximately 2.5 cm in diameter, 8 degrees of visual angle). This was the sample color for the trial; the animal had to acknowledge having seen it by pressing the button (top) on which it appeared, thus turning it off. After that, there ensued a forced delay of some 15 to 20 seconds, during which time the animal had to remember that particular color. At the end of the delay, four colors appeared on the lower buttons, one of them the sample. The monkey had to then press the button with the sample color and, if he did, he received automatically a squirt of fruit juice to the mouth as reward. Both the sample color for each trial and its position in the choice buttons were changed in random order from one trial to the next. The trained monkey performed the test with remarkable proficiency and committed few errors.

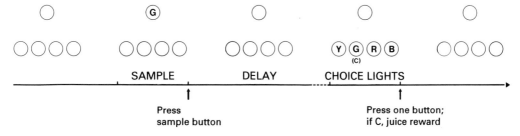

Figure 6.3 A trial in a delayed matching-to-sample task with colored stimuli (time *from left to right*). C, correct response; B, blue; G, green; R, red; Y, yellow.

After the animals were trained, microelectrodes were driven through IT cortex during performance of the task. Thus, extracellular unit records were obtained from extensive areas of posterior and anterior IT cortex (figure 6.4). A number of cells in the cortex of the IT convexity and the lower bank of the superior temporal sulcus showed responses to the sample color when it appeared at the beginning of each trial. In some of the cells, those responses were color-differential—that is, they were significantly greater for one or two colors than for the others. Those color preferences continued to be manifest in the activity of some cells during the delay, after the sample color had been extinguished but while the animal had to memorize it.

Consider the unit in figures 6.5 and 6.6. Although activated by all four color samples, the cell prefers yellow. That preference persists in the form of sustained and selectively elevated discharge during the retention period (delay) after the yellow sample (see figure 6.6). This becomes evident by averaging the discharge of the cell for all trials of each color sample. The resulting four frequency curves can be seen to remain orderly and almost perfectly stacked (yellow>red>green>blue) throughout the three trial periods—sample, delay, and match—with some inhibition during blue-sample delays. Clearly, the preferential and sustained activation after yellow through the 17-second retention period is not simply a sensory afterdischarge. If the delay is shortened, the activation is commensurately shortened. The cell returns to baseline (approximately 10 spikes/sec) promptly after the match, regardless of sample color (yellow included), even though the monkey has had to look at the sample color for a second time at the time of choice, when all four are presented simultaneously. It is reasonable to conclude that the cell, which prefers the yellow sample, remains activated above baseline after that sample because it has to be remembered. The activity of the cell returns to baseline after yellow has been seen again and properly matched; activity presumably reverts to baseline because now the trial is over and it is no longer necessary to retain the color.

The point to be stressed here about IT units such as the one just described is not simply that they participate in working memory (as they apparently do and will be further discussed in chapter 9) but rather that their participation in this kind of memory is a consequence and a clear indication of their belonging to long-term memory. Their color responses per se are unremarkable and generally less selective than those observed in occipital area V4, for example, where cells engage in color analysis. What is remarkable is that IT responses outlast a stimulus if, and only if, that stimulus needs to be remembered for the short term to perform the task. That can mean only that the cells are part of an internal order established with the task and for the task, embedded in the array of neural associations that connect a particular visual stimulus

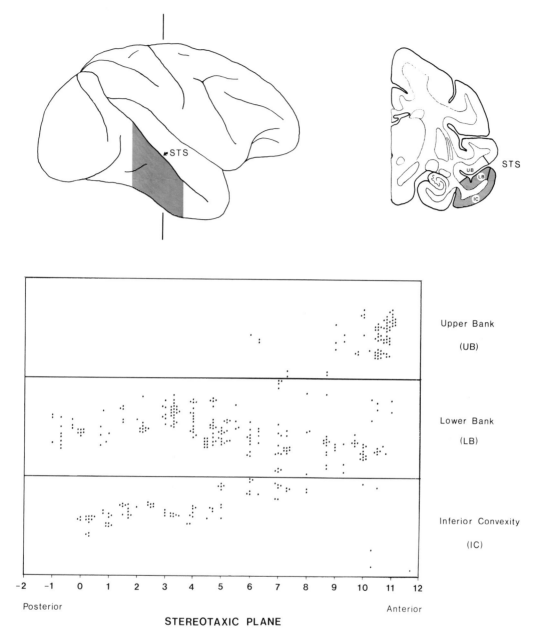

Figure 6.4 Inferotemporal (IT) area explored with microelectrodes during performance of the task in figure 6.3. (*Top*) The IT area is shaded in lateral view and in coronal section. (*Bottom*) Schematic distribution of the units recorded in the upper bank (UB) and lower bank (LB) of the superior temporal sulcus (STS) and in the inferior convexity (IC) of the temporal lobe. (From Fuster and Jervey, 1982, with permission.)

Organization of Perceptual Memory

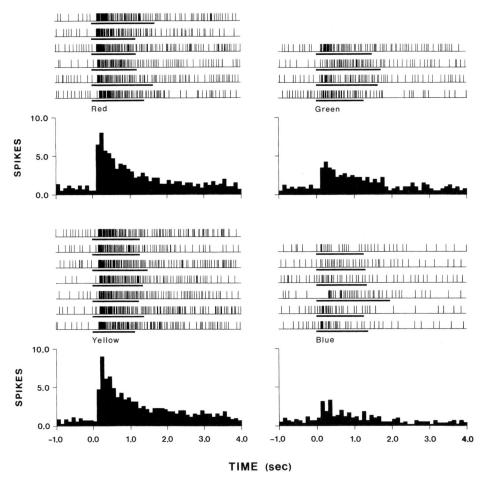

SPIKES

10.0

5.0

0.0

Red

Green

SPIKES

10.0

5.0

0.0

Yellow

Blue

-1.0   0.0   1.0   2.0   3.0   4.0   -1.0   0.0   1.0   2.0   3.0   4.0

TIME (sec)

Figure 6.5 Responses of an inferotemporal cell to the four sample colors (all of equal luminance). Cell responses are represented in spike rasters and average frequency histograms. Note that the unit is especially activated by yellow or red sample.

to the context in which it appears, to the reward, and to the motor act that leads to the reward. It means, in other words, that the cells are part of well-established memory networks that are activated by the stimulus and remain activated for as long as necessary to reach the behavioral goal. The fact that many other IT cells are activated during the delay in a nondifferential manner (i.e., without regard to color) does not exclude them from either short-term or long-term memory. They may simply be part of networks that encode the properties of the stimulus common to all trials and samples (brightness, position, reward association, motor associations, etc.). What is different about these IT cells is that they do not encode a particular property (color) whose relevance changes from trial to trial. Thus, their relation to memory is less evident in the experiment.

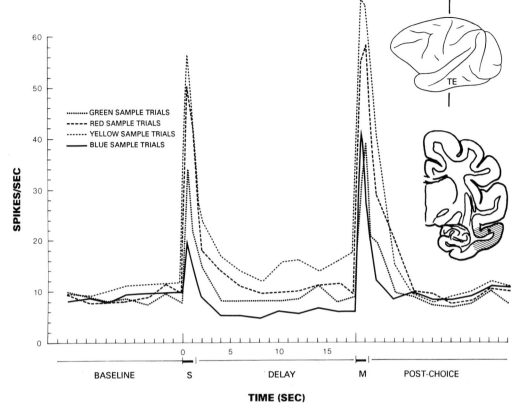

Figure 6.6 Average firing frequency of the cell in figure 6.5 through delayed matching trials with the four sample colors. Cell location, in area TE, is marked by dot in brain section at right. Note that the cell is sharply activated by yellow at the time of sample presentation (S) and at the time of matching (M). Note also that the cell's discharge is higher than baseline during memorization (delay) of yellow and reverts to baseline after trial termination. (From Fuster and Jervey, 1982, with permission.)

Miyashita (1988) attempted to determine more directly to what extent the protracted responses of IT cells to sample stimuli in a delayed matching task such as ours were learned. More specifically, he tried to establish that those cells were indeed part of a long-term memory substrate. He trained monkeys to perform delayed matching with a large variety of stimuli, not just four as we did. His stimuli were colored, computer-generated fractal patterns on a video screen. On each trial, the monkey was presented with one such stimulus and, after a delay, with a second one. If the two stimuli were identical, the monkey had to do nothing; if they were not, he had to touch the screen. The animals were first overtrained to perform the task with 97 sample stimuli, designated *learned stimuli*. In the course of unit recording from anterior IT cortex, the monkey had to perform the task with two sets of stimuli

Organization of Perceptual Memory

intermixed: the learned stimuli and a new set of stimuli. Some units, as ours, showed elevated and sample-dependent discharge during the retention period (delay). However, in Miyashita's experiment, the delay discharge of those units after a learned stimulus was always larger than after a new stimulus. Miyashita (1988) inferred that this was so because the units had stronger associations with the old stimuli than with the new ones. If that inference is correct, as it appears to be, this is another indication that IT units respond to visual stimuli and retain their features because they are part of permanent memory nets that represent the stimuli.

The single-unit study just reported is, like ours, a direct challenge to the concept of separate short-term and long-term stores for visual information. Instead, these studies suggest one permanent visual memory store in IT cortex that has within it innumerable representational networks. Under certain circumstances and with appropriate visual stimulation, the networks can be activated for a short time to serve as the substrate of so-called working memory. Thus, the neuronal data support the idea of one memory store, active or inactive, for the short and the long term (see chapter 5), which is in agreement with neuropsychological data. There is no convincing evidence from cortical lesion studies, in either human or monkey, to support the concept of two memory stores, for vision or any other modality.

Visual memory networks, however, are not restricted to IT cortex. There is abundant evidence from nonhuman primates indicating that those networks extend into other areas of association cortex, especially when the visual information contained in them has spatial or temporal attributes that are important for behavior. Ungerleider and Mishkin (1982) proposed two cortical extrastriate systems for vision, one for *what* and the other for *where*. The first would consist of the interconnected areas of occipital and temporal regions that process visual information beyond striate cortex, including peristriate and IT areas (see chapter 4, figure 4.13); this would be the system for object vision. The second system would consist of areas of prestriate and posterior parietal cortex, especially area PG; it would constitute the system for spatial vision. Although there is considerable neuropsychological evidence (discussed later) for involvement of posterior parietal cortex in the codification of spatial relationships in the visual world, the idea that this cortex is visual is questionable, and the concept of a spatial vision system has been effectively challenged by Ettlinger (1990). His argument is based on the fact that spatial features are inextricably part of object vision and the evidence that visual-spatial relationships are also analyzed in areas outside the occipitoparietal system. In support of this argument, the evidence may be adduced that cells in IT cortex are responsive to movement (Perrett et al., 1985). Furthermore, posterior parietal cortex is involved in the encoding of spatial relationships perceived by touch and, possibly, by hearing.

In any event, this discussion is largely semantic and vitiated by excessive compartmentalization of perceptual and mnemonic qualities in sensory domains. It seems easily resolved by postulating, instead of a visuospatial system, a supramodal system of cortical networks for the analysis and representation of spatial relationships, although different components of the system would have different frames of reference, depending on such factors as sensory modality (Soechting and Flanders, 1992). The posterior parietal cortex, as we will see later in the context of tactile memory, would be a crucial node of these networks. Because vision and touch are fundamentally spatial modalities, their networks would encroach into that system and interact cross-modally within it. A beautiful example of multimodal integration toward the encoding of space can be found in the superior colliculus (Stein and Meredith, 1993), a mesencephalic structure with certain properties very similar to those of cerebral cortex.

Similar comments can be made for representations with temporal dimensions. It seems now well established that the perception of temporal "gestalts" requires the functional integrity of the prefrontal cortex, especially for the temporal organization of behavior (Fuster, 1989) (see next chapter). To the extent that visual objects and memories are part of those gestalts, neurons of the prefrontal cortex are part of visual networks that control behavior.

The preceding discussion has defined some of the neuropsychological and electrophysiological evidence implicating the cortex of the inferior portions of the temporal lobe in visual discrimination and memory. The focus has been on data from the monkey because it is in the monkey that the most systematic research on the subject has been conducted. Besides, the cortical connectivity of the visual system is better known in the rhesus monkey than in any other animal species (see chapter 4). It can be reasonably supposed, however, that these concepts concerning visual memory networks in the monkey apply also to the human. The pertinent neuropsychological evidence from the human is fully consistent with this inference. The last portion of this section is devoted to a brief discussion of the involvement of temporal cortex in semantic visual memory, which represents a somewhat more abstract form of visual memory than that to which we have been mostly referring.

Earlier it was noted that some human neuropsychological data implicate the IT cortex in memory networks for at least one category of visual objects, faces. Some of those data, however, implicate IT cortex in memory of other visual categories as well. Patients with temporal lesions, especially on the left side and involving the IT convexity, have been reported to exhibit difficulties in naming or recognizing certain grammatical classes of words, such as verbs (Miceli et al., 1984); others cannot name objects of certain categories, such as fruits or animals (Goodglass et al., 1966; Basso et al., 1988; Hillis and Caramazza, 1991). Rarely is it the case, however, that the defect is circumscribed to one specific category of objects. Close scrutiny often reveals that categorical differences may be attributable to spurious factors, such as the familiarity or perceptual complexity of supposedly differentiated categories, as is the case, for example, for the differences between living and nonliving things in visual agnosia (Gaffan and Heywood, 1993). Double dissociations, by lesion and category, have not been demonstrated persuasively. Deficits frequently cover more than one category, and the differences in categorical deficit are generally merely of degree. For example, a patient may have considerable trouble naming fruits, body parts, and articles of clothing, but little trouble with animals of various phyla, whereas another patient may show the opposite (Hillis and Caramazza, 1991).

Especially in view of the relative discreteness of some of the lesions responsible for the deficits observed, these findings do suggest a degree of topographical localization of certain semantic categories of visual memory in temporal cortex. At the same time, however, the findings speak for the widespread distribution of categorical visual representations and for the profuse interactions, in certain common nodal regions of temporal cortex, between the associative neuronal networks that support those representations. Again, we are forced to adopt an intermediate position (see chapter 5) between that of assuming universal connectivity, which precludes knowledge of stable neural architecture (Fodor, 1983), and any reductionist position that would pretend to localize categorical memory in discrete cell assemblies or representational modules of microscopic proportions (Tanaka, 1993). We may, however, plausibly argue for extensive modules of association cortex in charge of categorical representation, something akin to the "central modules" of Shallice (1988, 1991). Widespread IT networks, with multiple nodes of convergence, would serve the role of such modules for semantic and categorical visual memory.

TACTILE MEMORY

Now let us explore tactile memory and its representational substrate in the parietal association cortex. We will again begin with human findings, but this time referring first to some disorders of spatial cognition that may or may not be restricted to touch and that commonly result from parietal lesions. This will make for a good transition between modalities because the spatial disorders of touch and vision are closely related and frequently coexist.

Astereognosia (or *astereognosis*) is the inability to recognize objects by touch (Critchley, 1953; Corkin et al., 1970; Roland, 1976). This symptom is commonly observed in patients with parietal lesion, which is one reason for attributing to parietal cortex cognitive functions related to tactile perception and memory. It is questionable, however, that astereognosia is reducible to a disorder of the tactile modality, especially because astereognosic patients, in addition to their object-recognition problems, commonly have problems with orientation in space—evident, for example in map-reading tests. On this basis, Semmes (1965) proposed that astereognosia is the consequence of a general disorder in spatial representation that transcends whatever disorder the affected individuals may have in the somesthetic sphere. Thus, a distinction would seem necessary between astereognosia and tactile agnosia (Lhermitte and Ajuriaguerra, 1938).

The attribution of a general spatial function to parietal cortex appears justified also by other troubles commonly present in parietal cases. One of them is *autotopagnosia*, difficulty in pointing to one's own body parts despite one's ability to name those parts when pointed to by the examiner (Hécaen and Ajuriaguerra, 1952; De Renzi and Scotti, 1970; Ogden, 1985). This has been grounds for hypothesizing a body image in parietal cortex. Parietal patients also commonly manifest disorders of recognition of spatial relationships in vision (Butters and Barton, 1970; Faglioni et al., 1971; Villa et al., 1990).

Related to these spatial disorders is the phenomenon of *neglect*, which is most apparent after unilateral parietal lesions (De Renzi, 1982; Heilman et al., 1985). The symptom is characterized by a failure to perceive or respond to stimuli on the side contralateral to that of the cortical lesion. When asked to draw a clock, for example, the patient will leave blank and without numbers the half of the clock's face contralateral to the lesion. A patient of Caramazza and Hillis (1990) with a parietal lesion on the left side made a high number of reading and spelling errors on the right side of presented words (figure 6.7).

Unilateral neglect, however, can be conceived of primarily as a disorder of spatial attention, including internal attention (i.e., the focus of representation) and, consequently, a role can be ascribed to parietal cortex in this form of attention from the clinical evidence just described. This interpretation is in accord with results of lesion studies in animals. Parietal ablations in the monkey have been shown to induce a semblance of neglect for spatial location of stimuli of three modalities—vision, audition, and touch (Heilman et al., 1970). Disorders of visual attention have also been induced by parietal lesions in other monkey studies (Latto, 1986; Lawler and Cowey, 1987). Pohl (1973) showed, and others (Ungerleider and Mishkin, 1982) later confirmed, that monkeys with posterior parietal lesions have trouble learning the so-called land-

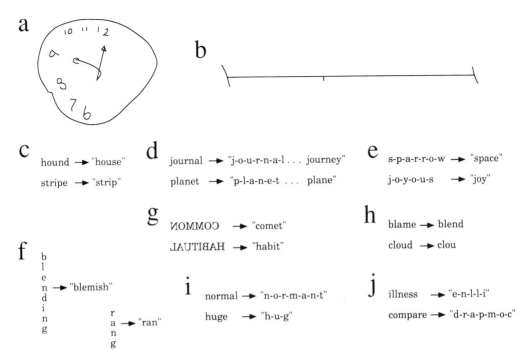

Figure 6.7 Performance of a patient with left parietal lesion in various tasks: (*a*) drawing a clock; (*b*) bisection of a line after demarcation of extremities; (*c*) reading horizontal words; (*d*) reading horizontal words after loudly spelling them; (*e*) naming words after hearing them spelled; (*f*) reading vertical words; (*g*) reading mirror-reversed words; (*h*) written spelling; (*i*), oral spelling; (*j*) backward spelling. In all cases, the patient makes errors of omission or commission in the right half of a canonical internal representation. (From Caramazza and Hillis, 1990, with permission.)

mark task (figure 6.8). In this test, the animal is presented with two identical and widely separated rectangular objects covering two food wells; a third object (the landmark), placed between the two but near one of them, indicates that the latter is the correct one to choose for it conceals the food. The deficit of posterior parietal monkeys in this test was used to support the argument for a "visuospatial" system (see the previous section) including posterior parietal cortex, area PG in particular (Ungerleider and Mishkin, 1982). However, even the landmark deficit can be interpreted as a spatial attention deficit (Lawler and Cowey, 1987; Ettlinger, 1990). In summary, human as well as monkey lesion results have led to the idea that the posterior parietal cortex is an essential component of a cortical system for spatial attention (Mesulam, 1981). Consistent with this view is the finding of increased blood flow in posterior parietal cortex of humans performing visual tasks that required attention to spatial location (Haxby et al., 1991; McIntosh et al., 1994). Shortly, we will discuss unit data from area 7, including PG, that further support the conclusion just emphasized, but before doing

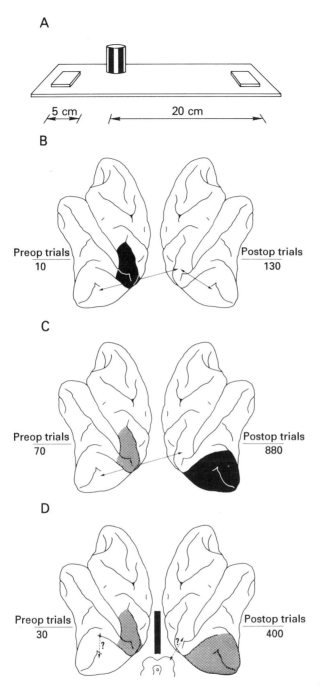

A

5 cm 20 cm

B

Preop trials
10

Postop trials
130

C

Preop trials
70

Postop trials
880

D

Preop trials
30

Postop trials
400

Figure 6.8 (*A*) Landmark task: The monkey must choose the food well closest to the striped cylinder, which is positioned on the left or right at random from one trial to the next. (*B*) Number of trials necessary to perform the task at criterion level before (10 trials) and after (130 trials) the left parietal ablation marked in black. (*C*) Number of trials to criterion (respectively, 70 and 880) before and after the subsequent lesion of the right visual cortex. (*D*) Number of trials to criterion (respectively, 30 and 400) before and after the subsequent section of the corpus callosum. Arrows indicate connections presumably left intact after each lesion. (From Ungerleider and Mishkin, 1982, with permission.)

so we must consider neuropsychological and unit studies in the monkey that directly address the question of parietal tactile memory.

In a manner similar to that in which IT lesions produce visual discrimination deficits, lesions of posterior parietal cortex (areas 5 and 7) produce deficits in tactile discrimination of objects and their features, such as roughness, shape, and size (Blum, 1951; Wilson et al., 1960; Ettlinger and Kalsbeck, 1962; Murray and Mishkin, 1984). Two important caveats are necessary here, however. The first is that it is relatively difficult to ablate posterior parietal cortex without injuring portions of SI cortex that are essential for tactile somesthesis but not necessary for the cognitive aspects of tactile discrimination. It is possible that a posterior parietal ablation induces secondary degeneration in neural elements of SI projecting to posterior parietal cortex. Therefore, the results of experimental parietal lesions must be viewed with caution, for in those results a sensory deficit may contaminate the cognitive deficit.

The other caveat is that, at ieast as much as by lesions of posterior parietal cortex, tactile discriminations may be impaired by lesions of SII, the cortex in the parietal operculum of the lateral (sylvian) fissure which, as mentioned in chapter 4, also receives projections from SI (Ridley and Ettlinger, 1978; Garcha et al., 1982; Murray and Mishkin, 1984). This is supported by recent single-cell data (Pons et al., 1992). Hence, the question of functional analogy between posterior parietal and IT cortex remains open. Some investigators (Ridley and Ettlinger, 1978; Mishkin, 1979; Murray and Mishkin, 1984) have argued that SII, rather than posterior parietal cortex, is the equivalent of IT cortex for touch and, therefore, the substrate for tactile discrimination and memory. Because both posterior parietal and SII cortex receive direct projections from SI, it is possible that the two work in parallel (Ettlinger, 1990) and constitute the highest stage of tactile cognitive processing. Deoxyglucose labeling indicates that both are more or less involved in roughness discrimination (Hörster et al., 1989).

Since the pioneer work of Mountcastle and Powell (1959; Powell and Mountcastle, 1959) on the monkey, the role of SI cells in the sensory aspects of touch has been well recognized and extensively investigated (see the review by Kaas, 1983). Four striplike areas of cortex constitute the physiological cortical substrate for primary sensory analysis of tactile features: 3a, 3b, 1, and 2 (figure 6.9). In the macaque, the first three are located in the depth and posterior wall of the central sulcus, the fourth (area 2) in the crown of the postcentral gyrus and anterior wall of the lateral extremity of the intraparietal sulcus (figure 6.10). All four areas contain neurons that respond to stimulation of skin receptors and deep-tissue receptors (e.g., from joints). The hand is represented in all four areas (Whitsel et al., 1971; Iwamura et al., 1980; Kaas, 1983; Chapman and Ageranioti-Bélanger, 1991; Ageranioti-Bélanger and Chapman,

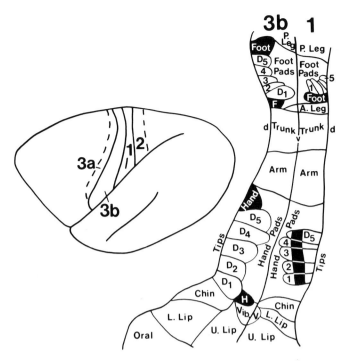

Figure 6.9 Cytoarchitectonic fields for somesthesia (touch) in the owl monkey, in which—for lack of a central sulcus—tactile fields and representations are in superficial cortical convexity. A, P, anterior, posterior (leg surface); D, digit; d, v, dorsal, ventral (trunk); F, foot; H, hand; L, U, lower, upper (lip); Vib, V, vibrissae. (From Kaas, 1983, with permission.)

1992), which receive inputs from ventral thalamic nuclei (figure 6.11). As noted in chapter 4, there is an orderly flow of projections from areas 3 to 1, 1 to 2, and 2 to 5 and 7. All projections are reciprocal. Areas 5 and 7 exchange projections as well.

Duffy and Burchfiel (1971) were the first to propose a processing hierarchy of somatic areas in parietal cortex comparable to that of visual areas in the occipitotemporal region. They did so based on the observation of units in area 5 that, unlike those of SI, responded to stimulation of several joints or of both skin and joints. Some units even responded to stimulation in parts of all four limbs. They interpreted these observations as evidence that the neurons of area 5, in the upper reaches of a hypothetical tactile processing hierarchy, were capable of integrating somatic information over wide areas of the skin and body. The existence of such a somatic hierarchy later was substantiated by other studies that revealed progessively higher levels of tactile integration from area 3 to area 5, especially evident with regard to the hand (Iwamura et al., 1980, 1983, 1985, 1993; Pons et al., 1985). As we progress upward in that hierarchy, we find that units integrate information

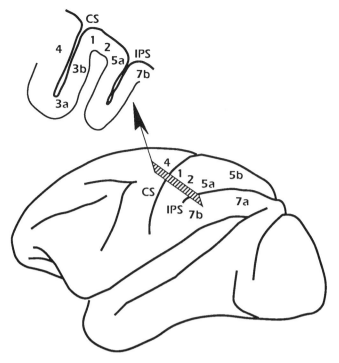

Figure 6.10 Parietal areas (Brodmann) in the rhesus monkey (cross-section *above*). CS, central sulcus; IPS, intraparietal sulcus.

from wider regions of the hand, and their receptive fields become larger. At all stages of the hierarchy, integration probably is accomplished not only between corticocortical inputs but between cortical and thalamic inputs. Unit studies have made it increasingly apparent that area 5 is the highest stage of representation of object qualities and spatial relationships within manipulated objects. Early on, Sakata and colleagues (1973), from observations comparable to those of Duffy and Burchfiel (1971), had accordingly concluded that area 5 contains a neural code for position and form in three-dimensional space.

Across the intraparietal sulcus, in the inferior parietal lobule, Hyvärinen and Poranen (1974) were the first to note the role of area 7 cells in integrative behavior that involves the hand as well as the eye. They discovered units that were activated by looking at, and reaching with the hand, a given target in space. It seemed that those cells occupied the highest stage of a different hierarchy from that for touch, this one apparently dedicated to the representation of extracorporeal spatial relationships.

In a classic and comprehensive study, Mountcastle and coworkers (1975) systematically investigated and described the properties of cells in the two areas of posterior parietal cortex, 5 and 7, that appeared to sit on top of parietal processing hierarchies. In area 5 they found, in

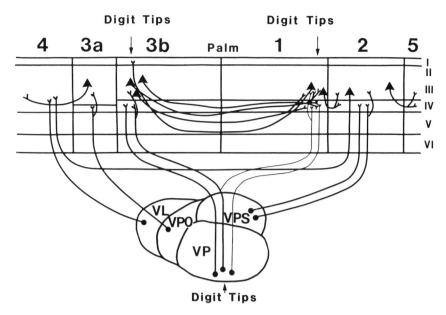

Figure 6.11 Connectivity of somatosensory areas in the monkey. For thalamic nuclei: VL, ventrolateral; VP, ventroposterior; VPO, ventroposterior oral; VPS, ventroposterior superior. (From Kaas, 1983, with permission.)

addition to skin and joint units, units that were activated in forward arm projection and manipulation. In area 7, they also found arm projection and manipulation cells and, in addition, cells that were activated in eye tracking and fixation. They characterized the projection and eye movement cells as *command neurons*. Especially in area 5, they noted units that are excited in active touch, even though they may fail to show receptive fields on passive touch. This phenomenon has since been observed by others also in area 2, an area that only with difficulty can be distinguished anatomically or physiologically from area 5 (Iwamura and Tanaka, 1978):

The latter phenomenon is a clear indication of the participation of areas 2 and 5 in haptics (from the Greek *haptein*, meaning "to feel actively")—in other words, in the sensorimotor functions that underlie the exploration of the world with the hand (Gibson, 1966). These functions are essential for stereognosis (i.e., the recognition of objects by manipulation). In the monkey, the activation of area 5 units in certain forms of arm movement and manipulation has been substantiated by a number of studies (Kalaska et al., 1983; Chapman et al., 1984; Seal and Commenges, 1985; Koch and Fuster, 1989).

Thus, to repeat and sum up, with regard to haptics and stereognosis, there is abundant evidence from single-unit studies for the notion of a processing and integrating hierarchy in parietal cortical areas, beginning with areas 3a and 3b and proceeding through 1 and 2 up to 5. Thalamic input is maximal in early stages and diminishes in higher stages. Another tactile hierarchy can be assumed to proceed from SI to SII, where the cells have somatic properties in some ways similar to those of area 5 but without the strong motor components (Robinson and Burton, 1980; Pons et al., 1987).

Microelectrode evidence implicating parietal neurons in tactile memory, as neuropsychological studies seem to suggest, is beginning to emerge. Koch and Fuster (1989) explored the units of areas 2 and 5 during a haptic short-term memory task, much as Fuster and Jervey (1981, 1982) had explored IT units during a visual short-term memory task. Remarkable similarities were encountered, along with some differences, all of which will be discussed in the context of memory dynamics (see chapter 9). At this time, what is important to note is that during a task in which the monkey had to memorize a shape (cube or sphere) perceived by touch, units were found, especially in area 5a (PEm), showing sustained elevation of discharge during the memorizing period. In some of them, the elevations were differential and related to the object being memorized (figure 6.12). The units apparently were involved in haptic short-term memory, whereby the same argument can be used here with these parietal cells that was made with IT cells regarding visual memory. The activation (stimulus-differential or not)

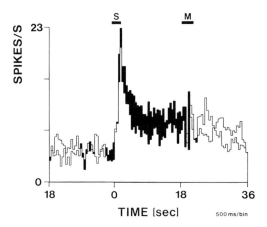

Figure 6.12 Frequency histograms from a cell in area 5a of a monkey performing a haptic delayed matching-to-sample task with two stereometric objects, a cube and a sphere (approximately 2.5 in maximal diagonal length or diameter, respectively). In the sample period (*S*, beginning at time 0), the animal has to feel one of the two objects and then memorize it during an 18-second delay for choice at matching time (M), when both objects are presented simultaneously. The animal performs the entire task without sight of the objects, which are presented in random order and choice position. Note that the cell is sharply activated by sampling (palpating) either object and stays activated throughout memorization. (The sphere-sample histogram, in white, is superimposed on the cube-sample histogram, in black.) The cell shows preferential activation during memorization of the cube.

of parietal neurons in working tactile memory is an indication that these neurons are part of haptic memory networks that have developed with the learning of the task. Those are long-term memory networks (i.e., tactile engrams) that are activated periodically and remain activated whenever, and for as long as, the engrams need to be retained in active memory for performance of a tactile task. More support for these ideas will be presented in chapter 9, where active memory is discussed along with haptic memory tasks using more discrete tactile stimuli than the stereometric objects utilized in the experiment just mentioned.

Now let us turn briefly to area 7, the other sector of posterior parietal cortex, and to its neurons with apparent spatial integrative functions. As already mentioned, with the observations of Hyvärinen and Poranen (1974) as well as those of Mountcastle's group (1975), it became clear that many area 7 units are attuned to movements of eyes and arm toward specific positions in surrounding space. Some are activated by ocular fixation and others by the tracking of visual targets (figure 6.13). Their activation is conditional on the motivational value and attraction of the target. For this reason, the cells have been assumed to play a critical role in the attention of the animal to objects and events in surrounding space (Lynch et al., 1977; Sakata et al., 1980; Bushnell et al., 1981; Motter and Mountcastle, 1981). Some units have been observed that have the peculiar property of becoming activated by passive touch of certain skin location (e.g., a small patch on the surface of one arm) *and* by sight of the investigator's hand moving toward that particular location (Leinonen et al., 1979).

A controversy arose with regard to the sensory or motor properties of cells in area 7. The concept of command neurons was challenged by the finding of cells in that area that responded to discrete visual stimuli and apparently had well-defined receptive fields (Robinson et al., 1978). This seemed to support the notion that those cells were sensory rather than motor, a notion that was challenged, in turn, by evidence that some units of area 7 discharged in correlation with direction of gaze and eye movement, even in the dark (Sakata et al., 1980). The argument seems unimportant and simply based on different methodological perspectives. Both the motor (command) concept and the sensory concept miss the essentially integrative nature of the job of the cells and their networks in these areas of association cortex. (The same reductionistic argument has been heard in regard to prefrontal cortex, especially the frontal eye fields.) As shall be discussed in chapters 7 through 9, neurons in associative areas are thoroughly enmeshed in various aspects of the perception-action cycle—that is, in the cybernetic cycle that governs behavior in the temporal domain, where percept leads to action, action leads to change, change leads to new percept, and so on. If, in our experiments, we concentrate only on the sensory or motor prop-

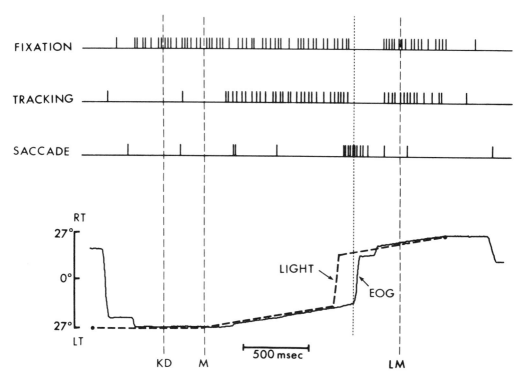

Figure 6.13 Three types of cells in area 7 of the monkey during an oculomotor task. Fixation cells are active during periods of steady gaze and smooth pursuit of a visual target but are suppressed during saccades. Tracking cells are active during smooth pursuit movements (to the right in the example) but not during fixation or saccades. Saccade cells are active only before and during saccades. Below, records of electrooculogram (EOG) and movements of target light (both in degrees to right [RT] or left [LT] of center of gaze). KD, key depression; M, start of target movement; LM, light dimming. (From Lynch et al., 1977, with permission.)

erties of the cells, we may be led to attribute to them a fictitious role in isolation of the circuitry and connections that give them their true role.

That role, for the cells of area 7, seems to be to integrate signals from sensory receptors with motor actions of eyes and limbs that relate the organism to relevant objects in environmental space. Those are the relationships that break down in the patient and in the monkey with posterior parietal lesion, and thus their symptoms of inattention and neglect toward objects and events in outside space become understandable.

There is some experimental evidence also of the participation of area 7 neurons in memory networks. In the posterior bank of the intraparietal sulcus, there is a subarea of 7 (LIP) in which cells are attuned exquisitely to the direction of gaze. Andersen and his colleagues (1990) trained monkeys to perform eye saccades toward certain visual targets. They observed that, when the animal was forced briefly to withhold a saccade and "remember" its target for subsequent action, LIP units maintained elevation of discharge congruent with target position and gaze direction. Despite the much shorter time scale (less than 0.5 seconds) of these activations, they seem to have the same functional significance as those of area 5 units in a different (tactile) memory task. Thus, in area 7, instead of tactile information, some cells appear to represent the relative position of targets in space or the direction of gaze to foveate them. They also appear capable of retaining that information for a short term.

In conclusion, both major areas of posterior parietal cortex, areas 5 and 7, may be regarded as the highest neural stages for processing information about tactile features and spatial relationships within and between objects with respect to the self. Area 5, possibly together with the collateral cortex of SII in the parietal operculum of the lateral fissure, seems to represent percepts mainly acquired by manipulation (haptically) through skin and deep-tissue receptors; those percepts concern the tactile characteristics of objects (texture, shape, size, etc.). Area 7, on the other hand, seems to represent information acquired by touch as well as vision and concerning the spatial relationships between the subject and external objects. The concept of stereognosis may be extended to encompass those relationships across space as well as the more discrete spatial relationships within objects that define their texture, shape, and size. Consequently, the posterior parietal cortex, and SII, may be considered, in a broad sense, the substrate for stereognostic memory—that is, for perceptual memory of the spatial features of objects and events. Obviously, such a broad purview of representation can be understood only if the networks in which parietal neurons participate extend beyond parietal cortex and interact with networks in other areas of unimodal and polymodal association cortex.

AUDITORY MEMORY

The cortical substrate of auditory memory is better understood in the human than in nonhuman primates. There are several reasons for this, but two stand out above all others. One is language, a rich form and carrier of auditory information unique to humans which, for the most part, is lateralized in the cortex of one hemisphere. The other reason, which may appear trivial yet is methodologically crucial, is the notorious and paradoxical difficulty that such an intelligent animal as the rhesus monkey has for learning fine auditory discriminations.

Language as the means for studying auditory memory presents distinct opportunities but also difficult challenges. On the one hand, the lateralization of auditory cognition, with language in the dominant hemisphere and nonverbal material in the other, minimizes the common problem of distinguishing cognitive neuropsychological deficits from primary sensory ones. This is partly true because input from both ears is almost equally distributed in the primary acoustic cortex of both sides—Heschl's transverse gyrus in the upper temporal plane, most of it hidden in the sylvian fissure (figure 6.14). That bilaterality of auditory input is also the reason why cortical deafness is so rare. On the other hand, the memory for words and sentences is inextricably tied to all human memories. Language is learned in the context of other experience and recalled, implicitly or explicitly, as part of that context. Words, and the concepts for which they stand, are associated by experience with a vast variety of nonauditory material, as Freud (1953) first pointed out in 1891 (figure 6.15). It is because of this that the large sector of individual long-term memory that we call *semantic memory* is so widely distributed in the cortex. For the same reason, long-term semantic memory can be accessed through a multiplicity of perceptual channels (Warrington and McCarthy, 1987). Consequently, in the dominant hemisphere, the representations of words and language appear idiosyncratically localized and tied to individual experience, as the studies by Ojemann and his colleagues suggest (Ojemann, 1983; Ojemann et al., 1990). That is also why semantic aphasia is so difficult to differentiate from acoustic agnosia.

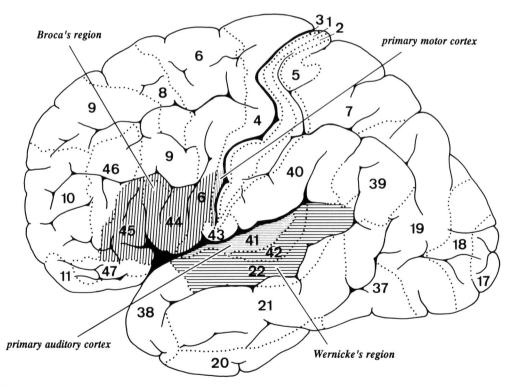

Figure 6.14 Auditory and language areas on the left hemisphere. (From Pulvermüller and Preissl, 1991, with permission.)

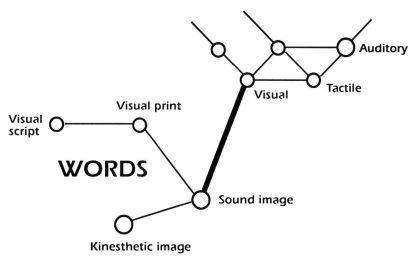

Figure 6.15 In schematic diagram, word-object associations as envisioned by Freud (1953).

Receptive or semantic aphasia is the agnosia for words and sentences. Patients with this disorder have difficulty understanding what is being said to them, even though their audition is unimpaired on audiometric testing (Penfield and Roberts, 1966; Geschwind, 1970). Semantic amnesia is the perceptual amnesia of language. The amnesia for particular names is called *anomia*. *Acoustic agnosia* is the perceptual amnesia of nonverbal auditory material, such as music (amusia) and sounds. The two categories of auditory memory, verbal and nonverbal, have been extensively investigated in patients with lesions of the cortex of the temporal lobe and, more generally, lesions of the large conglomerate of cortical association areas of parietal, temporal, and occipital cortex that has come to be named, for short, *PTO cortex*. The PTO region includes unimodal association cortex for the three modalities—auditory, visual, and tactile—as well as the polymodal association cortex of the supra-marginal gyrus, the angular gyrus, and the posterior third of the superior temporal gyrus (Wernicke's area). A problem with clinical studies of either form of auditory memory is, again, the ill-defined nature of most pathological lesions, which limits their localizing value. However, modern imaging methods are beginning to provide valuable help in this respect. For example, musical sight-reading and keyboard performance have been noted to activate metabolically cortical areas that are adjacent to, though not identical with, Wernicke's area and Broca's area, respectively (Sergent et al., 1992). Thus, the sensory and motor aspects of musical memory, to judge by the topography of their activation, have different cortical distribution from those of verbal semantic memory.

From the studies of auditory agnosias and aphasias, both of which reflect disorders of long-term memory, as well as the studies of auditory short-term memory, some indirect evidence emerges for our contention that the cortical substrates for short- and long-term memories are identical. At the very least it is fair to conclude that none of these studies produces evidence to the contrary. It has been established that semantic aphasias and amnesias are largely the result of injury to PTO cortex of the left or dominant hemisphere, usually including, but not circumscribed to, Wernicke's area (Luria, 1966; Barbizet, 1970; Walsh, 1978; Mayes, 1988). Some of those syndromes are clearly the result of interruption of associations between the visual and auditory modalities. Thus, lesions between left occipital and temporal lobes can cause disconnection syndromes in which the patient cannot use in the domain of one modality information from the other (Walsh, 1978); he or she cannot, for example, draw a clock on verbal request, although capable of copying its visual image. Disconnection syndromes (Geschwind, 1965b), in general, illustrate how the different components of one memory network interact with one another. They also provide much suggestive evidence that one and the same engram can be accessed from multiple sensory sources, the same sources through which presumably, the polymodal information was gathered that originally shaped the network.

Auditory short-term memory commonly is tested by audioverbal tests. The subject is given auditory cues (e.g., lists of words or digits) and is asked to repeat them immediately or shortly afterward. The same information may be provided to both ears or different information to each ear (dichotic listening). By use of such tests, it was determined long ago that left temporal lesions, unlike right temporal ones, cause auditory memory deficits if the material to be retained is verbal (Milner, 1958; Kimura, 1961; Sparks et al., 1970). Conversely, tonal memory is impaired by right temporal but not left temporal lesions (Kimura, 1964; Schulhoff and Goodglass, 1969; Zatorre and Samson, 1991). In reported cases of either type, long-term memory is not systematically tested the way short-term memory is. Therefore, it is difficult to ascertain to what extent the auditory short-term memory deficit is simply a manifestation of a broader deficit in the substrate of visual memory for words or for the visual image they conjure, which is presumably diminished by a commonly coexisting lesion of IT cortex. Furthermore, many of the cases reported in the relevant literature are cases of temporal lobectomy. Therefore, the same caveat is appropriate here as was appropriate with regard to visual memory deficits from temporal lobectomy: The possible importance of damaged limbic formations in those cases cannot be easily discounted.

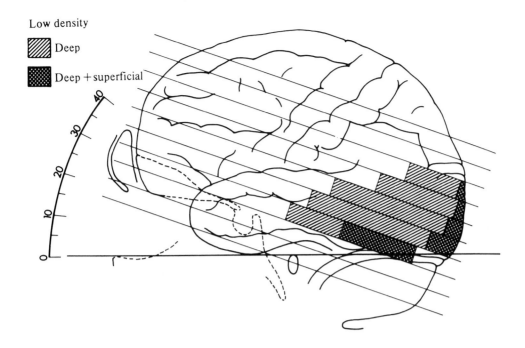

Low density

Deep

Deep + superficial

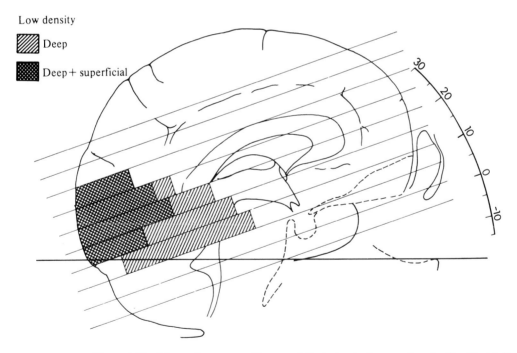

Low density

Deep

Deep + superficial

Figure 6.16 Schematic tomographic map of the lesion in the case described by Davidoff and Ostergaard. (*Top*) lateral view. (*Bottom*) medial view. (From Davidoff and Ostergaard, 1984, with permission.)

Organization of Perceptual Memory

The interactions between modalities in memory networks, the apparent identity of stores (for short-term and long-term), and related methodological problems are illustrated by the case reported by Davidoff and Ostergaard (1984). The patient was a man who, at age 47, suffered a vascular lesion encroaching on occipital and temporal lobes of the left side (figure 6.16). After the lesion, he exhibited color anomia—that is, he was unable to name colors correctly when they were presented to him. He was, however, capable of discriminating them, as could be ascertained by asking him to sort them in a color-matching task. When requested to remember shapes that could not be verbally encoded, he was able to recognize them without fail after periods of up to 8 seconds but, when requested, he was unable to do the same with colors, even with much shorter retention delays. From these findings, the authors argued that the patient had a short-term memory deficit restricted to color, thus arguing for a short-term store for color. Because the patient was not tested for long-term memory, a general deficit in this function cannot be excluded, however. In fact, the color anomia of the patient suggests that he did indeed suffer from a long-term perceptual memory deficit for color. It also suggests that, instead of or in addition to that perceptual trouble, he suffered from a visual-auditory disconnection that prevented the visual input from gaining access to a verbal code. Incidentally, Geschwind (1965a) reported in considerable detail a case of disconnection in which color anomia was associated with *alexia*, the incapacity to read and understand written material. In any event, the argument for separate memory stores could be validated only with clinical cases that showed the opposite of what the patient of Davidoff and Ostergaard (1984) purportedly showed: good short-term memory and bad long-term memory. No such results of neocortical lesion have been reported with regard to color, words, or any other kind of sensory information.

Two Canadian investigators, Penfield and Perot (1963), electrically stimulated the brain of conscious neurosurgical patients treated for epilepsy. By stimulating a number of points on the surface of the temporal cortex, they were able to elicit in some 8 percent of the cases what they called "experiential responses." For the most part, those responses appeared to consist of hallucinatory perceptions and were reported by the patient as having a certain compelling quality. The evoked pseudoperceptions varied widely, ranging from fragments of poorly defined sensory experience to complete private memories or unfamiliar scenes. Most were auditory, some visual. Both kinds were more commonly elicited by right- than by left-hemisphere stimulation. Music was a common experiential response, mainly from right-sided stimulation. Whereas auditory responses were evoked mostly by stimulation of the superior temporal gyrus (T1), the fewer visual responses appeared scattered but mainly in prestriate, IT, and polar regions. These intriguing results suggested that normal memories and perceptions could be elicited by direct stimulation of their representational substrate in temporal cortex. The value of the results is diminished, however, by the presumably abnormal excitability of the responsive tissue stimulated, which was invariably in the vicinity of an epileptic focus. At most it may be said that, even in pathological brains, artificial stimulation can induce perceptions and memories within physiologically plausible boundaries of association cortex. This was most apparent for audition, because the effective points for evocation of auditory experiences were largely circumscribed to the auditory association cortex of the superior temporal gyrus (T1).

Electrical stimulation can be used not only to elicit memory but also to suppress it if the stimulus surpasses certain intensity. Again, in the course of neurosurgical operations for treatment of epilepsy, Ojemann and his colleagues (Ojemann, 1983, 1991; Ojemann et al., 1990) endeavored to explore the effects of brief faradizations of the cortex of conscious patients on their ability to name objects and to remember words for a short term. In the testing of short-term memory, the subject was given a word or series of words and asked to repeat it after a delay. Stimulation under these conditions was found to have remarkably specific blocking effects on both object naming and retention of words (figure 6.17). Depending on the location stimulated, naming of certain objects could be blocked but not that of others, all within small portions of the cortical surface. Stimulation had also a suppressor effect on verbal memory, and that effect was most marked when the stimulation was applied during presentation of the verbal cue or the ensuing delay, not during retrieval. As could be predicted from the nature of the tests and the mnemonic material utilized, the effects could be obtained only by stimulation of points in left or dominant hemisphere. A high incidence of errors was observed by stimulus block in Wernicke's and Broca's areas.

Remarkably, stimulation could block the naming of a given object in one language but not in another (Ojemann and Whitaker, 1978), an indication that different languages, in the same individual, have different cortical distribution. Another of Ojemann's findings was the cortical scatter and individual variability of the points from which blockage could be induced. Some of those points were far away from language areas. There was no consistent pattern of effective locations within the parietotemporal region. The suppression appeared to act prominently on the short-term engrams of words, but it may be argued that what was interfered with by the electrical block was the activation of long-term engrams (i.e., networks) mobilized by the experimenter for the short term. How else, but by postulating the selective blockage of long-term memories could the individual variability of the effects be understood? Indeed, the idiosyncrasy of stimulation effects can best be inter-

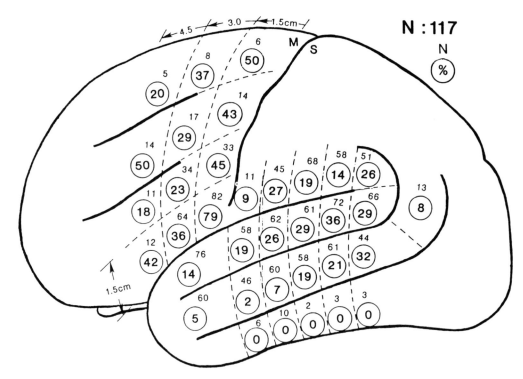

Figure 6.17 Lateral view of left hemisphere with mapping of the incidence of naming errors on direct cortical stimulation in 117 subjects. The upper number in each zone represents the number of subjects in whom a site was tested in that zone; the lower, circled, number indicates the percentage of subjects in whom naming errors were elicited by electrical stimuli within that zone. (From Ojemann, 1991, with permission.)

preted as the expression of the individuality of associative connections that characterizes cortical memory beyond sensory cortex. The evidence for verbal activation of extensive long-term memory networks is strengthened by unit data acquired also by Ojemann and his colleagues (1990). Neuronal populations in widespread temporal areas were seen to be activated by listening to or by repeating specific words. In my view, Ojemann's results are one more argument for the commonality of short- and long-term memory stores. These results also argue for the broad cortical distribution of language and semantic memory. Here, reasons could be given for distributed categorical representation of auditory memory that are similar to those given for representation of visual memory.

The hemispheric lateralization of oral representation and communication is not limited to the human brain. It has been observed in birds (Konishi, 1985) and nonhuman primates (Dewson, 1977; Petersen et al., 1978), although analogies with human language should be viewed with great caution. Heffner and Heffner (1984) explored by the cortical ablation method the laterality of discrimination of species-specific vocalizations in Japanese macaques. With a combination of aversive (shock) and appetitive (water) reinforcement, they trained such monkeys to produce different instrumental responses to different "cooing" sounds of conspecifics. After being trained, the animals were submitted to ablations of temporal cortex and then retested on the discrimination. Unilateral ablation of the left but not the right superior temporal gyrus, including auditory cortex, impaired the discrimination, although only temporarily. Bilateral ablations of the same cortex permanently abolished the discrimination. The conclusion is that perception of species-specific vocalizations is mediated by the aditory association cortex of the superior temporal gyrus, especially that of the left hemisphere. By lesions of that cortex, deficits in auditory sequence discriminations of nonvocal sounds have also been observed (Dewson et al., 1970), though without evidence of hemispheric lateralization. Bilateral, but not unilateral, lesions of the same cortex induce a marked deficit in auditory short-term memory, as measured with a delayed tone-matching task (Colombo et al., 1990).

The activity of neurons in auditory association cortex of monkeys in discrimination and memory tasks has not yet been investigated in detail. It is known from microelectrode studies, however, that certain areas in the superior temporal gyrus and the anterior bank of the superior temporal sulcus, as well as areas more remote from the auditory system, have associative qualities and receive auditory input. One is Tpt, a small area in the posterior portion of the superior temporal gyrus (figure 6.18) where most cells seem to have mainly auditory functions because they respond primarily to auditory stimuli (Leinonen et al., 1980; Hikosaka et al., 1988); some of them respond also to somesthetic stimuli and a few to visual stimuli. Other areas with multimodal input, including auditory, are STP and TPO in the depth and anterior wall of the superior temporal sulcus (Bruce et al., 1981), and PGa, in the anterior wall of the medial extremity of the lateral fissure (Hikosaka et al., 1988). More remote areas with auditory input as well as input of other modalities are situated in medial, basal, and prefrontal regions of the cerebral hemisphere (see chapter 4). No one knows for sure the physiological role of any of these polymodal areas. Two general possibilities appear plausible and are not mutually exclusive. One is that those areas represent supramodal or categorical information acquired through several sensory modalities. The other is that they serve as transitional bridges for cross-modal activation of networks that cover associative territories for several modalities. Interestingly, the polymodal areas in the upper reaches of the monkey's lateral fissure and superior temporal sulcus are in a region that, in the human, would correspond approximately to Wernicke's area or related areas of the angular and supramarginal gyri (see figure 6.14). The role of these areas in the semantic

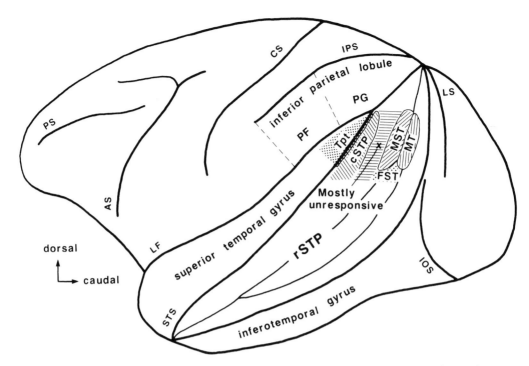

Figure 6.18 Polysensory association areas of parietotemporal cortex in the monkey, as revealed by microelectrode studies. (The superior temporal sulcus [STS] has been opened for better visualization.) CS, central sulcus; IPS, intraparietal sulcus; LS, lunate sulcus; AS, arcuate sulcus; IOS, inferooccipital sulcus; LF, lateral fissure; PS, principal sulcus. Cells in the following areas respond to stimuli of more than one modality, including auditory: cSTP, rSTP, PF, PG, Tpt, and TPO (not shown). (From Hikosaka et al., 1988, with permission.)

aspects of language, which is an eminently polymodal function, is well substantiated by neuropsychology.

Whatever the role of polymodal areas may be, there is evidence that unimodal association areas are themselves part of broad networks of perceptual memory that transcend their respective modalities. Some such evidence has been found in area 5, which is, as we have seen, one of the higher stages of the representational hierarchy for haptic information. Seal and Commenges (1985) found that some cells in area 5 responded to an auditory cue (a tone of 400 or 1000 Hz) *if* that cue was used by the animal to perform an arm movement. The cells were not responsive to the tone alone. In our haptic memory task (Koch and Fuster, 1989), where the animal used a click as a signal to advance the arm toward a stereometric object to be palpated in the dark, we found cells responsive to that auditory signal. Such cells were present not only in area 5a but also in area 2, which is hierarchically lower, and in 5b, which is higher (figure 6.19). Two findings were most remarkable about those cells. One was the short latency of their auditory response,

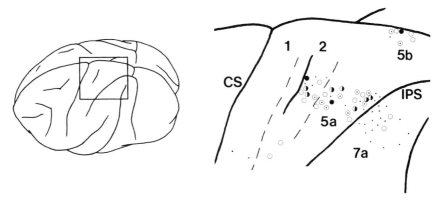

Figure 6.19 Auditory cells in haptic cortex. Circular symbols indicate where microelectrode penetrations revealed units responding to an auditory signal associated with palpation of a stereometric object. CS, central sulcus; IPS, intraparietal sulcus. (From Koch and Fuster, 1989, with permission.)

in some instances less than 20 msec. The other was that they usually showed, in addition to a reaction to the click, activation with arm movement. The anatomical pathway by which auditory input reaches neurons of area 5 as quickly as it seems to do is not clear. Possibly, that pathway transits through the thalamus. Also unclear is the kind of input those neurons receive from movement. Conceivably, the latter is proprioceptive input from the arm or else an efferent copy or corollary discharge from motor cortex, as some have speculated (Mountcastle et al., 1975). It seems reasonable to conclude, nonetheless, that both the auditory signal and the input from movement probably have shaped, in the training process, the network in which the cells are embedded, and thus the network is accessible to both thereafter. When the auditory signal arrives, the network is activated and perhaps somehow readied or primed to receive the somesthetic input. More evidence for such cross-modal interactions will be discussed in the next section and in chapter 9.

GUSTATORY AND OLFACTORY MEMORY

On account of their relative simplicity, the gustatory and olfactory systems lend themselves relatively well to empirical and theoretical treatment of perception and memory issues. Thus, the last part of this chapter will deal briefly with these issues as they pertain to taste and olfaction. The two systems are closely related to each other, and the problems concerning the neural substrate of their cognitive functions epitomize the general problems we have encountered with regard to the other modalities.

Agnosias for taste (*ageusias*) were described by Bornstein long ago (1940) in patients with bullet lesions of the orbitofrontal region. Experimental lesions of the same region in the monkey were noted to induce deficits in discriminations of taste (Bagshaw and Pribram, 1953; Patton, 1960). More recently, single-unit research of the monkey's orbital prefrontal cortex has contributed further evidence of the involvement of this cortex in taste functions. In the course of studies of prefrontal neuron discharge in instrumental behavior, my colleagues and I (Rosenkilde et al., 1981; Fuster et al., 1982) as well as others (Niki et al., 1972; Thorpe et al., 1983; Inoue et al., 1985) have observed in orbitofrontal cortex the presence of numerous cells excited (and some inhibited) by delivery to the animal of the liquid or solid food reward to reinforce its behavior. Those observations are now understandable in light of subsequent research on the central processing of gustatory information.

As already noted in chapter 4, a discrete taste area has been identified in caudolateral orbitofrontal cortex (Rolls et al., 1989b). From studies of the connectivity and the behavior of its cells, it is evident that this is the association cortex for taste, where gustatory information is processed further beyond the sensory cortex of the insula and frontal operculum. Rolls and his colleagues (1989b) have apparently been able to establish two fundamental facts about the physiology of this area: First, unlike the cells in earlier stages of the taste system, the orbitofrontal cells are adaptable and susceptible to motivational needs. Second, these cells associate gustatory input with input of other modalities. Let us briefly review their work.

The investigators analyzed the responses of single units in several structures along the gustatory pathway to different taste stimuli (glucose, HCL, NaCl, quinine, and others) in cynomolgus macaques (Scott et al., 1986a,b; Rolls, 1989; Yaxley et al., 1990). They explored the nucleus of the solitary tract, the frontal operculum, the insula, and the orbitofrontal cortex. Most cells in all locations were responsive to more than one stimulus. However, as the investigators proceeded upward in the system, they found that cells became progressively more sharply tuned. Sharpest tuning was observed in orbitofrontal units. Units at all stages below orbitofrontal cortex appeared insensitive to motivational need; they continued to respond to their preferred taste stimulus even after the animal had been satiated with food of that particular taste. Orbitofrontal units, on the other hand, responded less or not at all to their preferred stimulus (e.g., glucose) after the monkey had been satiated with food of the corresponding taste (figure 6.20). The cells seemed to reflect sensory-specific satiety. Furthermore, the investigators encountered considerable polysensory convergence in orbitofrontal cortex. Whereas a large proportion of units in this cortex responded to taste, others responded to olfactory and still others to visual stimuli.

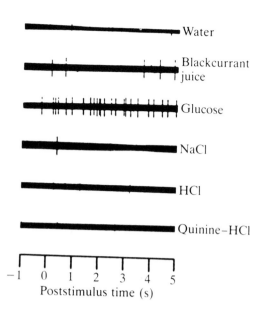

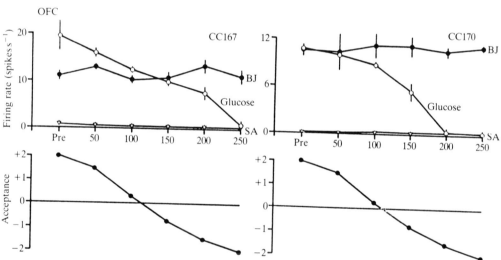

Figure 6.20 (*Top*) Responses of a neuron in orbitofrontal cortex (OFC) to six taste stimuli. (*Bottom*) The two upper graphs show the responses of two cells to black currant juice (BJ) and to glucose in the course of satiation with the latter (*abscissa*, milliliters of solution; SA, spontaneous discharge). The two lower graphs show the degree of acceptance of glucose by the monkey. (From Rolls, 1989, with permission.)

Organization of Perceptual Memory

Some units responded to stimuli of more than one modality. What is more, some cells responded selectively to a given taste *and* to a visual stimulus that, by discrimination training, had become associated with that taste. This cross-modal property illustrates the associative character of orbitofrontal cortex and the polymodal nature of the cortical memory networks to which some of its neurons belong.

Rolls (1989) speculates that tuning becomes sharper up the taste system so that associations can be formed without interference, and satiety can work selectively. He also proposes gustatory encoding by cellular ensemble (i.e., network) to allow for generalization, completion of partial representations, and graceful degradation (a concept akin to that of Edelman's "degeneracy"; see chapter 5). In doing so, he adopts Kohonen's (1984) basic concept of the associative memory network. Recall that I adopted essentially the same general posture but emphasizing, more than Kohonen and Rolls do, the role of synchronous presynaptic convergence. Finally, Rolls points out the importance of limbic feedback on orbitofrontal cortex for storage of taste memory as well as for its retrieval and top-down processing, including attention. The role of limbic structures in attention and memory retrieval will be further discussed in chapter 8.

The olfactory system and its relations to behavior have been investigated much more in lower species, especially rodents, than in primates. Consequently, this system's cortical organization and its cognitive functions in the primate are not yet well understood. However, because this system appears to have evolved less than other sensory systems, it is possible that some of the more general principles of olfaction discovered in those species apply also to the primate. Here the focus will be on what we know, however limited, about the role of cortical areas of primates in olfactory memory. I will conclude with discussion of a model of olfactory perceptual memory that, although inspired largely by data from lower species, is relevant to primate cognition.

Tanabe and colleagues (1974, 1975a, b) identified in the orbital prefrontal cortex of the monkey an area for olfactory discrimination. The area is somewhat medial to the orbitofrontal area for taste. When that medial orbital area was ablated, the animal was unable to learn or perform discriminations of odors. Microelectrode recording during olfactory discrimination tasks revealed neurons within that area that were selectively activated by the stimuli used by the animal in the task. These findings are in agreement with the clinical observation of olfactory discrimination deficits in patients with orbitofrontal lesions (Zatorre and Jones-Gotman, 1991). The human olfactory area has now been identified by positron emission tomography as a part of the junction of the inferior frontal and anterior temporal cortices (piriform cortex, bilaterally) and of the orbitofrontal cortex of the right side (Zatorre et al., 1992).

The close proximity to each other of two orbitofrontal areas, one for taste and the other for smell, suggests that the two are associative areas at roughly equivalent hierarchical rank. That proximity also indicates the probability of cross-modal interaction between the two. As noted earlier, units in the caudolateral (taste) area are receptive to olfactory stimuli. The same may be true, in reverse, for cells in the medial area with respect to gustatory stimuli. Obviously, the interactions between the two areas may be important for such an associative cross-modal quality as flavor.

In the rat, the reciprocal interactions of olfactory system with limbic structures have been substantiated in the behavioral context. Hippocampal or fornix lesions have been found to impede the formation (Eichenbaum et al., 1988) and utilization (Staubli et al., 1986) of olfactory memory. As in other sensory systems, the anatomical connections between olfactory system (olfactory bulb and piriform cortex) and hippocampus appear to run through the entorhinal cortex (Otto et al., 1991). Reciprocal connections between olfactory structures and amygdala have been established (Leonard and Scott, 1971). This behavioral and anatomical evidence suggests the possible role of hippocampus and amygdala in acquisition and retrieval of olfactory memory, which agrees with what appears to be true in the primate with regard to other modalities.

In this section, as in the previous ones of this chapter, the emphasis has been on the organization and topography of perceptual memory, even though functional data have been used for the purpose. Now I will present a functional model of olfaction that may have heuristic value for making the transition from the review of formation and structure of perceptual memory to the discussion of its dynamics in a subsequent chapter (8). As has been pointed out by others (Haberly and Bower, 1989), the olfactory cortex has a particularly suitable circuitry for the study of associative memory.

Based on what is known about that circuitry, Ambros-Ingerson and coworkers (1990) have developed a computational model of the neural architecture subserving olfactory memory. The model is based on simulation of the structural and functional properties of the olfactory bulb and the piriform cortex as now understood mainly from work with small mammals, the rat in particular. Essentially, the simulated system, which is composed of neurons in olfactory bulb and superficial layers of piriform cortex, can learn to discriminate and to recognize olfactory cues by hierarchically clustering the cortical cells that represent them (figure 6.21).

The model assumes and incorporates structure and operations that are biologically established or plausible: Through parallel sets of receptors in the bulb and by a mechanism of long-term potentiation, the statistical frequency of occurrence and the degree of similarity of external cues determine hebbian synaptic changes in the cortex that lead to

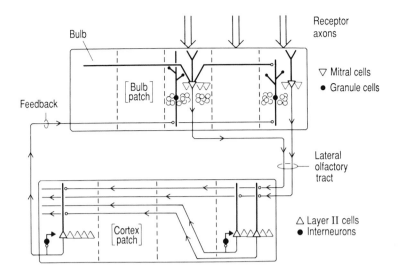

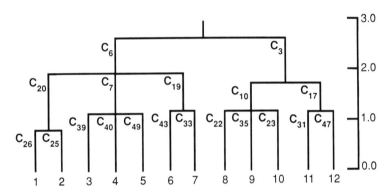

Figure 6.21 A hierarchical model of olfactory learning and recognition. (*Top*) The architecture of the model, simulating that of the olfactory system. Receptor input to the olfactory bulb is processed there by mitral and granule cells and then transmitted through the lateral olfactory tract to the olfactory cortex for further processing. The cortical network is trained by repeated exposure to a set of 120 cues in random order (10 instances each of 12 categories of olfactory stimuli or odors). After training, the units of the network recognize and discriminate the 12 categories more or less well. The analysis of the responses of the model's units to test stimuli reveals that, in the training process, the units have arranged themselves in hierarchical fashion, reflecting a hierarchy of the stimulus categories. (*Bottom*) The dendrogram depicts the hierarchical organization of the model's units after training. Unit C_6, for example, responds readily to stimuli of categories 1 through 7, whereas unit C19 responds less readily, but more selectively, to stimuli 6 and 7. (From Ambros-Ingerson et al., 1990, with permission.)

the progressive functional differentiation of the cortical neurons representing the cues. Feedback inhibition from cortex to bulb helps normalize the total firing in the bulb and thus allows for successive sampling and discrimination of cues by internal proliferation of the cortical networks. As a consequence of this process of unsupervised learning, cell groups will learn to fire to groups of cues according to the similarity of those cues. The end result will be a cortical hierarchy of cell clusters representing a comparable hierarchy of olfactory cues and covering a wide gamut of smells. The upper elements of the neural hierarchy will represent groups of more or less similar (i.e., categorical) smells; the lower elements will represent the more distinct and idiosyncratic smells. Thus, by a structure and an algorithm that need not be discussed here, the olfactory cortex would do precisely what we postulated in the previous chapter as the essence of memory formation: It would create a classificatory cortical apparatus of hierarchically organized cell networks based on the relative frequency and similarity of stimuli. The difference between the two approaches is that, whereas Ambrose-Ingerson and colleagues (1990) espouse top-down clustering of the representational hierarchy, I have adopted bottom-up clustering for categorization and perceptual constancy, as well as top-down clustering (the network turning on itself) for fine discrimination. Other than that, their model assumes learning and recognition in pre-piriform (primary) cortex, whereas mine displaces them upward to associaton cortex which, for olfaction, would be orbitofrontal cortex.

To form the olfactory hierarchy, as to recognize the stimuli it represents, the model of Ambros-Ingerson and colleagues makes use of a cyclical mechanism of environmental scanning for which they also find a biological foundation. This foundation is sniffing behavior and the accompanying electrical oscillation of the olfactory apparatus to which Freeman (1975, 1990) has attributed crucial information-processing importance. The cycling ("passes") of the computational model would provide the stimuli with statistical exposure to the system and thus with increased discriminability and clustering, both in learning and recognition. Their model recognizes objects first at categorical (high) level and then at successively lower levels, just as humans do according to psychophysical data they adduce. However, this is far from clear. It seems that only in highly selective attention do we perceive the world with temporally descending categorization of its objects.

Parallel processing, one of the assumptions of the Ambrose-Ingerson model, seems to be a necessary feature of any plausible system of olfaction (Kauer, 1991). However, neither the oscillatory feature nor the top-down clustering seem essential to the model except in computational terms. It is unclear why the continued neural exposure to sensation, without periodic sampling, could not accomplish the same objective of hierarchical clustering as does cycling or oscillation. As for the temporal clustering order, both bottom-up and top-down seem important and necessary. It may be true that in the making of a perceptual memory hierarchy, as well as in the recognition of objects, a certain degree of global categorization precedes fine discrimination, a point that Fair (1992) also makes. However, in the process of perceptual learning, concrete instance precedes both abstraction and categorical stimulus constancy. Only in the focusing of attention, it seems, is that top-down categorization (or recategorization) essential (see chapter 8).

POLYMODAL AND HIGH-LEVEL PERCEPTUAL MEMORY

The foregoing discussion of the organization of perceptual memory in posterior neocortex may be useful heuristically but is highly contrived. To establish the principles of that organization, which has been my primary intent in this chapter, it seems reasonable to separate memories by sensory modality. After all, this is the way our experimental methodology is arranged ordinarily for neatness and good control. In real life, however, the situation is very different and much more complex. All or most all our memories are perceptually mixed. Though their origin and recall may be—in proustian manner—anchored solidly in one of our senses, they are made of associations with experiences acquired through other senses as well. All our conceptual and semantic knowledge is much the same way. There is hardly an item of it that we have not acquired or firmed up by vision *and* audition *and* some other order of sensory qualities, to say nothing of affect and value. In any case, the higher we go in the hierarchy of knowledge and memory, the more detached these become from individual senses, places, and dates.

Our guide and justification for the parcelling of the discussion by sensory modality has been the assumption that we will be able to apply to higher levels of cortex and memory what we learn at lower levels. Within any given modality, we may have made some progress, for with our strategy we have been able to venture into the organization of categorical sensory perception and even into related semantic areas, such as language. Once we venture into polymodal, episodic, or conceptual memory, however, extrapolation falls quickly short of its goal. The reason is, of course, that we lose our empirical support. Curiously, our empirical failure is here a measure of our theoretical success, or at least of the viability of the conceptual model I have proposed in chapter 5, for my model predicts that, as we go up the hierarchy of a system of layered cortical memories, these become progressively overdetermined, better anchored in multiple associations and, hence, more accessible to recall. The higher the layer and the more widely distributed is a memory network, the less localizable it is and the less vulnerable to cortical damage. Thus, when we reach the level of individual declarative memories, let alone the level of factual knowledge and concepts, all our localizing methods, from the microelectrode to the field potential, from the selective lesion to the best tomographic imaging, are bound to fail us. The reasons can be gleaned in the simple diagram of figure 6.22.

To this day, the neuropsychological study of the effects of human brain injury has been the source of nearly all the descriptions of memory types and systems currently brandished in the literature (see chapter 2). When it comes to the cortex, however, the localization of any of those types or systems of memory appears futile. It has to fail if the model proposed here has any credence and memories are as spread out over the cortical surface as the model postulates. To illustrate the limitations of the neuropsychological method for defining the layer of perceptual memory affected by cortical lesion, as well as its gradient of decreasing vulnerability from the particular to the abstract, consider a hypothetical clinical example. (The choice of memories is meant to perk up the interest of those who enjoy the grandmother cell debate): Our subject, K, has never met his maternal grandmother, for she died before he was born, and his knowledge of her derives exclusively from family portraits and accounts. He did get to know his paternal grandmother,

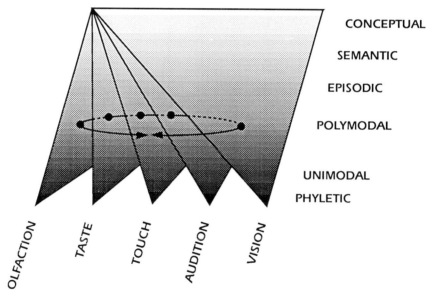

Figure 6.22 Schematic interplay and hierarchical organization of perceptual memories of five sensory modalities. The territory of representation for each modality fans out from primary sensory areas toward the highest areas of cortical association. As it does, it progressively overlaps larger territories of other modalities and progressively interacts more with them (interaction at one level is symbolized by the interconnecting ring). The result of that upward expansion of sensory representations and interactions is a hierarchy of perceptual memory networks that is increasingly anchored in more modalities, more diffusely distributed (therefore less localizable), and more resistant to damage.

however, who was an affable and witty lady who did her best to make the young K a happy child. She died when K was an adolescent. It is reasonable to suppose that, because of the multiple contacts and associations with her, her memory is better established in K's adult cortex than the memory of the other grandmother, whom he did not meet. Therefore, if K incurs posterior cortical injury, he is more likely to have amnesia of his maternal grandmother than of his paternal one. The most resilient representation, presumably anchored in his cortex by innumerable associations and memories, will be the *concept* of grandmother. This bit of conceptual memory would probably endure all but the most extensive lesion of K's posterior cortex, one leading to a total loss of Goldstein's "abstract attitude" (1959).

The point I am trying to make with this example is that the vulnerability of any memory to brain injury is inversely proportional to the number and solidity of the associations on which it rests. When a network is widely distributed in many directions, as it is for semantic and conceptual memory, its localization becomes elusive and resistant to discrete cortical injury, wherever it may be: Mass action and the *extent of the injury* will then take the upper hand. If this is true, then it is no wonder that pure agnosias and semantic amnesias are rare, especially if the lesion is discrete, whereas episodic amnesias are common, especially as we age (as does our cortex). Categorical memory survives even in the presence of declarative amnesia (Knowlton and Squire, 1993).

Global retrograde amnesia, which is characterized by an extensive and permanent loss of the ability to recall personal experiences, along with semantic memory, dating all the way back to childhood, also is rare. Judging by the pathological findings in the cases in which it has been observed, global retrograde amnesia results only from very extensive lesion or functional inactivation of neocortex. The reported cases occur either from massive neocortical damage (Cermak and O'Connor, 1983; Damasio et al., 1985; Kapur et al., 1992) or from damage to subcortical or paleocortical regions implicated in the activation of widespread neocortical territories in arousal, attention, and recall (see chapter 8): the mesencephalic reticular formation (Goldberg et al., 1981a) or the hippocampus and parahippocampal cortex (Schnider et al., 1992; Warrington and Duchen, 1992; Schnider et al., in press).

The case of Schnider and colleagues (1992; subsequent report soon to appear) is particularly interesting because it illustrates the importance of midtemporal structures for memory recall, in addition to memory consolidation (see chapter 3). It upholds the activating role of those structures on presumably large expanses of neocortex. The patient is a 66-year-old man who suffered an embolic infarct of both medial temporal lobes and the inferior temporo-occipital area of the left hemisphere. After recovery from his initial confusional state, the patient

remained disoriented in time and space, while showing a severe anterograde and retrograde amnesia. On leaving the hospital room for just a
few seconds, he could not find his way back. He never recalled prior
medical examinations or the names of the examiners and recognized
only his wife and children. His language was generally normal, with
the exception of difficulties in naming certain visual, auditory, tactile,
and olfactory items and sensations. Reading and writing, as well as
calculation and praxis on command, were normal. The severe anterograde amnesia was well substantiated by formal testing.

The patient's retrograde amnesia was massive and extended to his
childhood. He was able to provide only a vague and fragmented personal history. Six months after the vascular accident, he could not yet
recognize his closest friends, nor could he find his way in his own
town. Only in the vaguest terms could he recount world events, such
as World War II, without any dates or other details. Significantly, he
could not remember anything about some such events except the affect
they connoted. For example, questions about the nuclear accident at
Chernobyl would elicit from him only one descriptive word: "bad."

Apparently, the case is at odds with most of the literature on amnesia
from limbic lesion. Certainly, the patient differs from those with temporal lobe lesion, who have been reported to suffer from anterograde
but not retrograde amnesia. Schnider and coworkers attempt to reconcile the discrepancy by attributing the retrograde amnesia of their patient to his lesion of the left IT cortex. I find this explanation
unsatisfactory because the patient's amnesia was not circumscribed to
events or experiences of the visual modality. A more plausible explanation, in my view, is that the most severely injured structures—
namely, the hippocampus and parahippocampal cortex—are important
not only for the fixation of new memories but for the retrieval of old
ones (see chapter 8). The case of bilateral hippocampal lesion with global
retrograde amnesia, described by Warrington and Duchen (1992), also
supports this view. The degree of retrograde perceptual amnesia of
hippocampal cases may have been generally underestimated.

In sum, the global amnesia of the two cases cited here may be attributed to the absence of hippocampal activation of neocortical memory
networks, which rendered the patients incapable of deposition as well
as retrieval of memories. It is curious, in any event, that, in the first
case, the most resilient associations of those networks appear to have
been the associations with affect. This observation is fully congruent
with our view of the role of the amygdala in memory (see chapters 3
and 8), for the patient's amygdalas were practically intact.

In more general terms, we can infer that extensive lesions of posterior
cortex or disruptions of the mechanisms that activate it interfere, to
some degree, with retrieval of a wide range of perceptual memories of
all modalities at all levels of categorization. The reactivation of their

supporting networks, widespread as they normally are over the cortical surface, is only fragmentary. The global nature of the deficit, and also its spotty character, bear witness to the broad and capricious distribution of perceptual memories that extend beyond the narrow confines of phyletic and unimodal sensory memory.

From our knowledge of connective anatomy (see chapter 4), the theoretical model in chapter 5, and the empirical evidence presented in this chapter, a few general conclusions emerge on the distribution of perceptual memory. These conclusions, at the very least, may serve as useful working hypotheses for future research.

In principle it is reasonable to conclude that all perceptual memory is based mainly in neuronal networks of posterior cortex—that is, in the vast region of neocortex that covers the parietal, temporal, and occipital lobes, from the rolandic fissure and the temporal pole to the occipital pole. Unimodal perceptual memory is based in primary and associative areas of sensory cortex; the latter include the IT cortex for vision, the superior temporal cortex for audition, and the posterior parietal cortex (superior and inferior parietal lobules), in addition to SII, for touch and somesthesis. Gustatory and olfactory memory is based in paralimbic areas of orbitofrontal and prepiriform cortex. Polymodal memory is based in those same unimodal associative cortical areas and, in addition, in intermediate polymodal areas (i.e., areas of multisensory convergence). All forms of declarative memory, including episodic and semantic memory, consist of wide networks intimately interlinked with those of unimodal and polymodal memory. At high levels of categorization, the networks of semantic memory, although still amply based, would have certain neuronal ensembles with high connective confluence that would serve as nuclei for representation of categories and names. Some of these semantic nodes seem especially common in lateral and inferior aspects of the parietotemporal region. Conceptual knowledge would be so broadly based in networks of posterior association cortex as to defy localization by any means now available.

7   Organization of Motor Memory

Motor memory is the neural representation of motor acts and behavioral sequences. In chapter 5, it was postulated that cortical networks of perceptual memory expand into the frontal lobe following the principles of self-organization mainly by synaptic convergence and there, by associations with action, contribute to forming the cortical networks of motor memory. In this chapter and the next two, I present evidence that frontal networks not only are representational but can become operational and participate directly in motor control and the enactment of behavior.

As in the previous chapter with regard to perceptual memory, here we must resort to functional data to gain insight into the structural organization of motor memory. In chapters 8 and 9, functional data will be used again to explore the dynamics of that organization. First, let us reconsider the basic concept of motor memory.

So ingrained in us is the idea that memory is acquired through the senses that we find motor memory difficult to comprehend. We have no trouble discussing operationally the learning of motor skills, motor tasks, or motor habits, but we are inclined to reject the idea that any of that could be called *memory*. Further obscuring the identity of motor memory is the phenomenal appearance that the memories of most actions are reducible to the memories of the kinesthetic, visual, or other sensory—ergo perceptual—traces that those actions may have engendered or been accompanied by.

Most psychologists and cognitive neuroscientists accept the notion of motor memory, although usually by another name, such as *procedural memory* or *habit* (see chapter 2), but the neurophysiologist often will deny the concept or dismiss it as an arcane and useless philosophical concept. Even to those who accept it as a viable concept, the neurophysiology of motor memory seems beyond the grasp of modern methods. One purpose of this chapter is to show that this is not the case and that motor memory has a neural organization that we can begin to delineate with current methods.

There are at least two major reasons to search for the neural substrate of motor memory. One is to clarify the foundation of motor learning; the other is to clarify the central representation of those schemes of complex behavior, commonly called *programs* or *plans*, that evidently are stored somewhere and somehow in the brain and control behavior with minimal or no sensory input. We do not know much about that substrate, but we do know enough to establish some of its general properties. Enough evidence is available for us to at least attempt to substantiate three principal ideas:

1. The neural circuitry of motor memory is, to a large degree, identical to, and inseparable from, that of motor action.

2. Motor actions and memories, as well as their neural substrate, are organized in hierarchical fashion, much as perceptions, their memories, and their substrate (see chapter 6).

3. With learning and practice, some motor memories shift their base away from the cortex, where they originate, and become relegated to subcortical structures.

NEURAL HIERARCHY OF MOTOR MEMORY

The skeletal motor apparatus of the primate supports an enormous range of adaptive behaviors. Taking the temporal dimension into account, it is correct to say that any muscle group, or any limb, has practically infinite degrees of freedom. In the human, so does the oropharyngeal musculature—that is, the apparatus for the spoken language. Clearly, however, the motor behavior that one observes in nature, or even in laboratory conditions, can be classified into discrete categories according to such factors as biological or social significance, innate or acquired origin, and the muscles involved.

Ever since Hughlings Jackson (1958) first proposed it within an evolutionary framework, the theory of a hierarchical organization of movement in the nerve axis has had widespread appeal (Bernstein, 1967; Paillard, 1982; Brooks, 1986). It is well supported by not only phylogenetic but also developmental and clinical evidence. One of its key elements is the concept that movements are represented in an orderly fashion at various levels in the central nervous system depending on such features as their complexity or the degree to which they are voluntary: In general, elaborate and deliberate actions are represented in the cerebral cortex, simple and automatic actions in subcortical structures, the cerebellum, the brain stem, and the spinal cord. Less widely accepted is the implication that movement is hierarchically controlled from the top down. (Later, I will touch several times on this dynamic issue.) Here, for the moment, I adopt only the topographical aspects of the hierarchical theory, inasmuch as they are helpful to outline a tax-onomy of motor memory and its representational substrate.

At the lowest levels of the neural hierarchy for movement, in the spinal cord and brain stem, are the *reflex arcs* that mediate some of the most primitive defensive motor reactions of the organism. These reactions, at the bottom of the hierarchy of adaptive behaviors, can rightfully be considered part of the innate memory of the species, and thus part of what I have termed *phyletic memory*. The defensive reflexes are normally under some degree of inhibitory control from higher stages; consequently, in certain cerebral injuries, they are characteristically released from that control and accentuated. Besides, some of them are conditionable. By repeated pairing of a stimulus innately eliciting a given reflex (unconditioned stimulus) with a stimulus of another kind (conditioned stimulus), the two stimuli become associated, so that eventually the conditioned stimulus alone will unleash the reflex motor response (conditioned response). The cerebral circuitry involved in the initial stage of formation of the new reflex is unclear. In their pioneering studies of the cortical unit discharge of conscious monkeys, Jasper and his colleagues (1958) observed that some neurons in motor cortex increased or decreased their firing in anticipation of a conditioned avoidance response to shock. Similarly, in the cat, the neurons of sensorimotor cortex appear to be involved in the establishment of a classic conditioned reflex (Woody, 1982). Pyramidal lesions, however, do not disturb well-established reflexes (Wiesendanger, 1981), an indication that once they are formed, those reflexes are only subcortically represented. In any case, what seems clear is that synchronous convergence, at whatever level and by whatever mechanism, is at the root of conditioned reflex formation. The conditioned reflex may be the most elementary example of the operation of the principle of synchronous synaptic convergence, which I have postulated as essential to the formation of cortical memory (see chapter 3). The conditioned reflex also epitomizes, albeit in rudimentary fashion, the accretion of individual memory on phyletic memory.

A particularly good example of synchronous convergence at work is the conditioning of the eye-blink reflex, which can be experimentally accomplished by pairing an air puff to the cornea with an auditory stimulus. Thompson and his colleagues (Thompson, 1986; Steinmetz et al., 1992) have meticulously investigated the circuitry and the mechanism of that reflex and, by so doing, have been able to localize the critical convergence in the nucleus interpositus of the cerebellum (figure 7.1). This nucleus plays a critical "binding" role even if the conditioned stimulus happens to be a burst of current to the auditory cortex (Knowlton and Thompson, 1992). The motor memory network (i.e., the motor trace), however, not only may reside there but may extend to the cerebellar cortex.

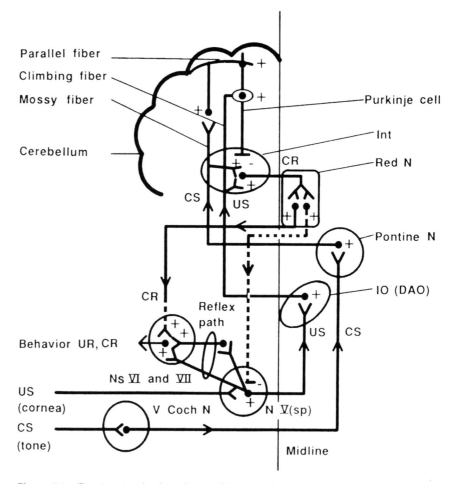

Figure 7.1 Circuitry involved in the conditioning of eye blink (conditioned response [CR]) by pairing an air puff to the cornea (unconditioned stimulus [US]) with a tone (conditioned stimulus [CS]). The critical convergence appears to take place in the nucleus interpositus (Int). IO (DAO), dorsal accessory portion of the inferior olive; N, nucleus; UR, unconditioned response; V Coch N, ventral cochlear nucleus. (From Thompson, 1986, with permission.)

The cerebellar cortex is well-known to take part in "downstream" motor coordination through control circuits that involve the motor cortex, the pontine nuclei, and the inferior olive (figure 7.2) (Kemp and Powell, 1971). This cerebellar participation in motor control seems not so critical for the structuring or initiation of behavior as for the fast regulation of movement in progress (Eccles, 1967). Nevertheless, some evidence suggests that, even there, time-locked events can induce lasting changes in synaptic efficiency (Thach, 1978). The increased synaptic efficacy from the synchronous convergence of inputs through climbing fibers is one of the essential features of Marr's (1969) cerebellar theory.

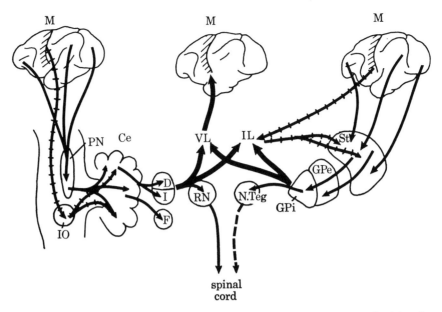

Figure 7.2 Schematic diagram of the circuitry of the motor system emphasizing the parallel organization of cerebellar and basal-ganglia pathways. Ce, cerebellar cortex; D, dentate nucleus; F, fastigial nucleus; GPe, globus pallidus, external segment; GPi, globus pallidus, internal segment; I, interpositus nucleus; IL, intralaminar nucleus of the thalamus; IO, inferior olive; M, motor cortex; N. Teg, tegmental nuclei; PN, pontine nuclei; RN, red nucleus; St, striatum; VL, ventrolateral nucleus of the thalamus. (From Kemp and Powell, 1971, with permission.)

Somewhat higher in the motor hierarchy, in the diencephalon, seems to lie the substrate for certain elaborate forms of phyletic motor memory. Since the experiments of W.R. Hess (1954), it has been known that the electrical stimulation of certain regions of the hypothalamus can unleash a variety of emotional reactions and instinctual behaviors. These behaviors tend to be brief and stereotypical and obviously are fragments of instinctual ("prewired") programs. This conclusion agrees with the physiological evidence that hypothalamic nuclei play a critical role in sexual, aggressive, and feeding behaviors.

The fact that in higher primates, especially the human, instinctual behavior with diencephalic representation is thoroughly enmeshed with culturally acquired and neocortically represented social behavior illustrates two important points: First, instinctual programs, part of phyletic motor memory, can be nested within broader behavioral programs of higher order—that is, within cognitive plans and strategies. Second, in the course of normal behavior, different levels of the neural motor hierarchy—some presumably representing innate and others acquired schemes of action—cooperate in continuous and reciprocal interaction for the pursuit of biological and social goals. The issue here is not whether an upper hierarchical layer drives a lower one, or vice versa, as psychoanalytical theory would have it. The issue is that different layers with innate and acquired representations can work intimately together in the integration of purposeful behavior. Obviously, under the circumstances, it makes no sense to speak of serial processing, either from the top down or from the bottom up. In motor control, profuse parallel processing and reentry undoubtedly take place between layers. One of the most pervasive errors of contemporary neuroscience is to equate the terms *serial* and *hierarchical*. Indeed, motor control is widely distributed in the central nervous system and implemented largely by parallel processing (Alexander et al., 1992). Still, neither wide distribution nor parallel processing is incompatible with a hierarchical organization of motor representations, the existence of which does not necessarily imply serial processing in behavior. To reemphasize what should be clear already from our previous discussion of perceptual memory (see chapter 6), parallel processing probably takes place on a massive scale between different layers of hierarchical representation.

Thus, to understand motor processing, we cannot adhere strictly to hierarchical concepts. These concepts are nonetheless useful to understand the distribution of motor representations, which is our present concern. Our next step up the hierarchy of motor representation is the basal ganglia though, judging from neural circuitry, it is debatable that, in that hierarchy, these nuclei are higher than the cerebellum (Kemp and Powell, 1971).

In the globus pallidus, as well as the caudate and putamen, neurons have been shown to encode either the direction of limb movement or the position of a manual target in spatial coordinates (Crutcher and DeLong, 1984; Mitchell et al., 1987; Crutcher and Alexander, 1990). In tasks with an instructed delay, some neurons (figure 7.3) also show increased discharge during preparation for movement (Liles, 1974; Crutcher and DeLong, 1984; Kimura, 1986; Alexander, 1987; Alexander and Crutcher, 1990b; Schultz and Romo, 1992), albeit for not as long a time before movement as do some cortical neurons (figure 7.4). On the basis of the apparent participation of units of any given striatal region in different phases of motor integration, as well as the somatotopic organization of the units within the region, Alexander and colleagues (1992) have argued persuasively against serial and for parallel processing of movement, as well as for the coexistence and coactivation of several levels of processing within regions. Neither the anatomical nor the physiological evidence they adduce, however, is incompatible with our notion of the basal ganglia as representational levels under the neocortex in the hierarchy of cerebral structures that represent a corresponding hierarchy of behavioral structures or programs. We have already indicated that in the implementation of those programs, during normal behavior, there must be continuous, parallel, and reciprocal transactions between levels. The evidence that there is reduplication of

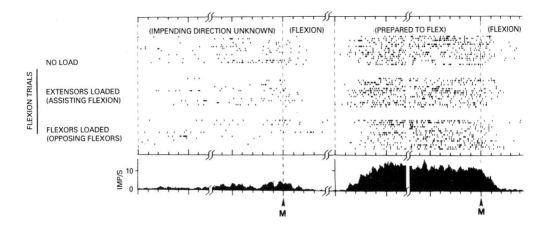

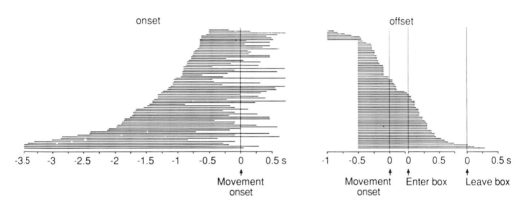

Figure 7.4 Temporal relationships of the activity of 74 neurons in caudate nucleus and putamen to several components of a self-initiated movement (monkey). Horizontal lines indicate the time of increased activity of the 74 cells, rank ordered according to onset (*left*) and offset (*right*) times. (From Schultz and Romo, 1992, with permission.)

somatotopy in the various levels is another argument for the hierarchical view, because different hierarchically organized motor programs share the same peripheral effectors.

To sum up, the basal ganglia in general, and the striatum in particular, may be viewed as harboring a stack of intermediate representational layers of the motor hierarchy that extends from the spinal cord to the cortex. Those nuclei, at the base of the cerebrum, would represent at least some of the programs for the execution of automatized actions and habits (Marsden, 1982).

Now let us summarize the general principles of hierarchical motor representation in the nerve axis that we have gleaned thus far and will develop further in forthcoming sections. These principles can be succinctly expressed by reference to coordinates or gradients in three principal dimensions.

Innate-Acquired Dimension

At the bottom of the motor memory hierarchy, represented in the circuitry of the spinal cord, pons, and cerebellum, lie the genetic representations of action, the inborn reflexes. Already there, we encounter the rudiments of acquired memory in the form of conditioned reflexes. The hypothalamus is the diencephalic base of instinctual programs representing, so to speak, the biological motor memory of the species. In the basal ganglia, we encounter programs and structures of acquired and temporally extended action that reach their culmination, in terms of complexity, in the prefrontal cortex.

Particular-General Dimension

There is, along the nerve axis, a gradient of progressive motor abstractness from the bottom to the top. At the lowest levels, the represented actions are discrete and well-defined, spatially and temporally. As we progress toward the cortex, the schemes of represented action become broader and have a larger span in space and time. They represent progressively more complex movements and longer behavioral sequences. Their overarching goals become temporally more distant and abstract, and they require that more interim goals be reached to attain them. The plans formed in and under the agency of the prefrontal cortex are presumably the most general and abstract. They are also the most idiosyncratic and creative of the organism.

Automatic-Voluntary Dimension

The most automatic acts of all are the spinal reflexes. At higher levels, in the cerebellum and basal ganglia, learned automatic acts are represented—acts that, by repetition and practice, have become habit. Still higher up, in neocortical levels, voluntary action is represented. A substantial body of neuropsychological and electrophysiological data, some of which will be reviewed later in this chapter, indicates that the cortex of the frontal lobe plays a critical role in voluntary behavior. The dorsolateral prefrontal cortex, at the top of the motor hierarchy, is essential for the planning (i.e., for cognitive representation) of future voluntary action (Fuster, 1989). However, neither this cortex nor any other part of the frontal lobe can be considered anything like the *center of will*, which is a useless concept of neural representation.

MOTOR PROGRAMS

Before proceeding with the discussion of motor representation in the cerebral cortex, it is appropriate to discuss briefly the concept of *motor program*, which becomes increasingly relevant as we ascend the representational hierarchy of movement. As motor representations get more complex, their temporal dimension expands and the question becomes increasingly pressing: Where and how is the syntax of the action (Lashley, 1951) represented? Indeed, to use the computer metaphor, this is a question of structural relationship between neural "hardware" and neural "software." Unfortunately, at this time, the question cannot be answered. One can merely speculate on possible answers, and this I shall do in the discussion of the prefrontal cortex, which my colleagues and I postulate is the supreme synthesizer of action. At present, we simply must assume that, beyond a certain level of the motor hierarchy, what is represented gains substantial temporal structure and thus becomes what has received, in the literature, such designation as *program, plan, strategy,* or *frame*. All these terms and the concepts behind them can be placed under the rubric of motor memory and treated alike, for at present there are no solid reasons to make distinctions between them, at least on neural grounds. I favor the term *program* (Brooks, 1986), even though it has computer connotations that may be misleading when applied to the nervous system.

Any sequence of normal behavior is defined by its goal and the sequence of movements to attain it. For the attainment of their goal, complex behavioral sequences usually require a series of intermediate steps that involve the reaching of interim or preliminary goals. Each of them may, in turn, require the reaching of ancillary subgoals, and so on. Thus, we can visualize a hierarchy of goals, with the ultimate goal of the sequence on top and the others nested at various layers underneath. The same can be done with the corresponding structures and substructures of motion in the sequence to reach the ultimate goal. The resulting hierarchy of behavioral structures resembles considerably the hierarchy of sensations that make up perception. Furthermore, in the same way that perception is an act of classifying the sensory world from prior experience (perceptual memory), motor behavior involves classifying and actively selecting motor acts from prior experience (motor memory) that are conducive to their respective goals. As there is a neural hierarchy for the representation of perception, there is a hierarchy of neural structures to represent the hierarchy of motor behaviors. The latter spans the entirety of the nerve axis, from the spinal cord to the cerebral cortex ("from coccyx to cortex"). Also, like the perceptual hierarchy, the motor hierarchy participates intimately in the processing of information. The programs of behavior represented in it control the very behavior they represent. Thus, as the neural foundation of perceptual memory guides perception, that of motor memory guides action. The guidance of the action, again like the perceptual process, undoubtedly involves the interplay of programs (memories) represented at different levels of the hierarchy.

The parallel between perception and goal-directed action extends to their sharing of cognitive constancy, a property that here is essential for understanding the latitude and flexibility of the motor programs we envision, especially in the cortex. Just as the perception—or identity—of an object is invariant across a multitude of changes in its physical parameters, so does a structure of behavior remain appropriate to its goal regardless of innumerable variations in the individual movements that lead to it. In this sense, and just as we spoke of perceptual constancy, we can now confidently speak of motor constancy. The program to govern the motor sequence must accommodate that fundamental feature of behavior. Obviously, this is one of the places where the analogy between the motor program and the computer program fails. The many degrees of freedom of the motility to reach a goal are unmanageable by any preprogrammed computer algorithm, as Alexander and coworkers (1992) have aptly remarked. Moreover, finding a wide range of solutions to one and the same problem is not a practical objective of computer programs, whether the processing is to be in series or in parallel. The biological motor program, in contrast to the computer program, must be flexible and ready to correct for unforeseen contingencies the organism may encounter. In other words, it must be ready to operate in ad hoc conditions. Such are probably the characteristics of the broad, novel, and schematic representations or motor engrams at the top of the motor hierarchy, supposedly in the neocortex. On the other hand, the programs representing and implementing old and well-practiced motor habits are undoubtedly much more rigid, precise, and of the nature of machine programs. They are probably based in subcortical structures.

However, for reasons to which I have already alluded, it is highly unlikely that any program is represented in its entirety in any one given layer of the hierarchy. Most behavioral structures are mixed. They contain segments that are novel and unrehearsed as well as segments that are old and thoroughly practiced. To illustrate the point, let us consider a simple example of human behavior with both extremes, such as finding one's way on foot in a town one is visiting for the first time. The visitor's goal is, say, the post office. He or she leaves the hotel with a plan in mind containing the essential information on how to reach it. The plan is, in some respects, vague and fragmentary, based on broad verbal instructions from someone and a glance at a map. Having never been to the place, the visitor lacks practical experience with such things as the length of city blocks, the presence and location of street signs, and so forth. On the way, the visitor clearly is using a mixed motor program. It contains a scheme of voluntary action that is in some ways open-ended, flexible, and ill-defined, and it also contains at least one thoroughly ingrained and automatic subroutine: walking. At intermediate levels as well, the program contains elements lying between the fully voluntary and the fully automatic, some of which are called into operation by unanticipated contingencies, such as traffic lights or public works. On reaching the objective, the previously schematic plan of motor memory has been fleshed out and transformed into a more complete program. Subsequently, with repeated trips to the same post office, the program undoubtedly will become more automatic, stereotyped, efficient, and economical (in that it will require less of a cognitive load to execute); in sum, it will become more like the program to reach the post office in one's hometown.

It is the mixture of new and old components, which is present in most behavioral structures and their programs (as in the preceding example), that leads us to suspect that any given program is represented across several levels of the motor hierarchy. On similar grounds, we are led to suspect that the enactment of behavior requires continuous interactions between those levels. In fact, it is inconceivable that any behavior of minimum complexity can be represented and integrated in its totality at any given neural level.

Two lines of neurobiological evidence indicate that, indeed, in normal behavior, there is a running interaction between programs or program components at different hierarchical levels. One is the anatomical evidence of cortical-subcortical loops of connectivity linking frontal areas to basal ganglia and lateral thalamus (DeLong and Georgopoulos, 1981; Alexander and Crutcher, 1990c; Hoover and Strick, 1993). The other is the previously mentioned evidence that different, interconnected layers of the motor hierarchy (premotor cortex, supplementary motor area, motor cortex, putamen, globus pallidus) contain topographically organized representations of movement (Crutcher and DeLong, 1984; Alexander and DeLong, 1985; Mitchell et al., 1987; Georgopoulos et al., 1989; Kalaska et al., 1989; Crutcher and Alexander, 1990). The argument will be further developed in the next two chapters, in which I deal with the dynamics of memory.

Complicating our search for the topography of motor programs is yet another line of evidence suggesting that, with experience and repeated enactment, the central representations of organized movement may change their location or be displaced by others from their controlling role. The principal evidence for this derives from studies of the effects of cortical lesions on performance of cognitive tasks.

Consider a delay task, such as delayed response, delayed alternation, or delayed matching to sample. Each of the trials in it constitutes a discretely defined behavioral structure within the larger structure of the task. The trial ordinarily requires from the animal first to observe a visual cue (in delayed alternation, the cue is kinesthetic), then to retain that cue in active short-term memory and, finally, on appearance of a second cue, to perform a manual act contingent on the first cue. It is important to note that, after the animal has learned the task, its performance requires the utilization of two kinds of memory. One is the general memory of the task, the rules that govern it and the basic procedure to perform it; indeed, that kind of memory is practically identical to what has been called *procedural memory* (see chapter 2). The other is the short-term perceptual memory of the first cue. Monkeys with bilateral ablations of dorsolateral prefrontal cortex (area FD) have great difficulty learning to perform the basics of the task, and even more difficulty performing it correctly; in other words, they have difficulty acquiring the memory of the procedure and even more difficulty retaining the memory of a stimulus through the period of delay (for review of the issue, see Fuster, 1989). Nevertheless, with time and repeated testing, the animals eventually learn to perform the task and even do so correctly, especially if the delay is short (1 or 2 seconds). It appears that, in the absence of dorsolateral prefrontal cortex, some other part of the motor hierarchy can play the role of accommodating the procedural memory of the task and even helping the animal bridge a short delay. We can only speculate about what that surrogate motor structure may be. It is reasonable to suppose it is the premotor cortex, possibly in conjunction with the striatum, for these constitute stages of the motor hierarchy immediately under the prefrontal cortex.

Even motor programs in primary areas seem to migrate to lower levels after acquisition and practice. Following lesion of the somatosensory cortex of one hemisphere, a monkey has a great deal of difficulty learning a new skill with the contralateral hand (Pavlides et al., 1993). However, after acquiring a skill in the hand contralateral to the intact hemisphere, the lesion of its somatosensory cortex does not abolish the skill. Thus, corticocortical projections from somatosensory to motor cortex play a critical role in the learning of new skills but not in the execution of existing ones. Presumably, this is the case because the latter have become automatized and relegated to lower structures of the motor hierarchy.

These findings in the monkey are in agreement with the neurological evidence that patients with cortical lesions preserve the ability to perform automatic movements while having lost that of performing the same movements intentionally on command (voluntarily). This phenomenon was first described by Jackson (1958) in 1866. Both kinds of observations suggest the migration of motor programs from higher cortex toward lower cortical or subcortical levels as their execution becomes established. Cortical lesions force or expose the shift. Further evidence of that shift, in natural circumstances, can be found in results of studying cerebral blood flow by positron emission tomography in human subjects acquiring a motor skill (Seitz et al., 1990); as a subject learns the skill, cerebellar and striatal circuits appear to become increasingly activated during its performance while, in relative terms, the activation of cortical structures diminishes.

CORTICAL MOTOR REPRESENTATION

Whereas it is simplistic and inappropriate to speak of a center of will anywhere in the central nervous system, there seems to be no question but that the cortex of the frontal lobe, as a whole, is critically involved in the planning, initiation, and execution of voluntary action (Passingham, 1993). The mechanisms of voluntary action, however, are a highly complex subject on which speculations are plentiful but conclusive data scarce. Here my objective is simply to gather whatever evidence can be found that may allow us to establish the essential properties of the representation of voluntary motor behavior in the cerebral cortex, especially the frontal cortex. Under the rubric of *motor representation* we imply, in addition to the central representation of motor acts, the motor programs discussed in the previous section and a wide range of theoretical constructs that are supposed to characterize the antecedent cognitive representations of voluntary action, from the idea (Allen and Tsukahara, 1974) to the concrete schema of movement (Arbib, 1981). Only better understanding of neurophysiology eventually will allow the sorting out and precise definition of those relatively abstract representations. For the time being, in the absence of that understanding, it is not productive to debate in neural context such concepts as plan, program, kinetic image, motor engram, motor schema, or strategy, to name only the most common. All are reasonably appropriate at some level of discourse. Most differ only quantitatively along a certain dimension, such as time. None has a well-understood neural basis.

For reasons that should become apparent as we proceed, here I invert the order in which frontal areas should be discussed if I were to follow the hierarchical order—from the bottom up—that I have been following so far in this chapter up to the basal ganglia. The inverted order does not prejudge the order of processing or assume that the latter is sequential. It merely reflects the order in which frontal areas apparently are recruited for implementation of voluntary action. Because the emphasis here is on the cognitive aspects of action, it makes sense to respect the order in which frontal representations are called into the making of that action. Therefore, the prefrontal cortex will be discussed first.

Prefrontal Cortex

Phylogenetically and ontogenetically, the prefrontal cortex is one of the last neocortical regions to develop. In the course of mammalian evolution, it undergoes enormous growth (figure 7.5), which reaches its maximum in the human brain, where the prefrontal cortex constitutes nearly one-third of the entire neocortex. Judging by myelination and other neuroontogenetic criteria, it is one of the last neocortical regions to reach full structural maturity.

The prefrontal cortex of the primate is far from functionally homogeneous, and there is considerable evidence for the functional specialization of distinct areas within it. However, there is also evidence, from the monkey as well as the human, that this vast cortical region plays an overarching role in the temporal organization of behavior, a role that is manifest in a wide range of behavioral activities, including speech (Fuster, 1989). Two specialized functions of dorsolateral prefrontal cortex subserve that supraordinate role of temporal integration. Those two functions are mutually complementary and temporally reciprocal: One is a retrospective function of short-term sensory memory and the other a prospective function of short-term motor set. These two functions allow the prefrontal cortex to mediate cross-temporal contingencies (Fuster, 1985a) and to play its prominent role in the formation of new, complex, and temporally extended structures (*temporal gestalts*) of behavior. Partly on account of this, the prefrontal cortex can reasonably be called the *organ of creativity*. Most likely, the capacity for new and complex behavior rests above all on that prefrontal function of prospective set and on the related capacity to form internal representations of prospective action (planning). Whereas in the previous chapter I have referred to the role of prefrontal cortex in sensory representation, here I shall deal with its representation of action

One of the most common and striking disorders from large lesions of prefrontal cortex in the human is the difficulty in initiating and carrying out new goal-directed behavior. The patient with prefrontal damage has difficulty spontaneously initiating new sequences of speech or motor behavior (Kleist, 1934; Luria, 1970; Damasio and Van Hoesen, 1983; Stuss and Benson, 1986). Closely related to, and usually accompanying, this lack of initiative is the difficulty in formulating new plans. Trouble with planning is present in the majority of syndromes from substantial lesion of prefrontal cortex (Ackerly and Benton, 1947; Luria, 1966; Lhermitte et al., 1972; Walsh, 1978; Milner, 1982; Shallice, 1982; Owen et al., 1990). Indeed, there is almost universal agreement among clinicians and neuropsychologists that the planning disorder is the most

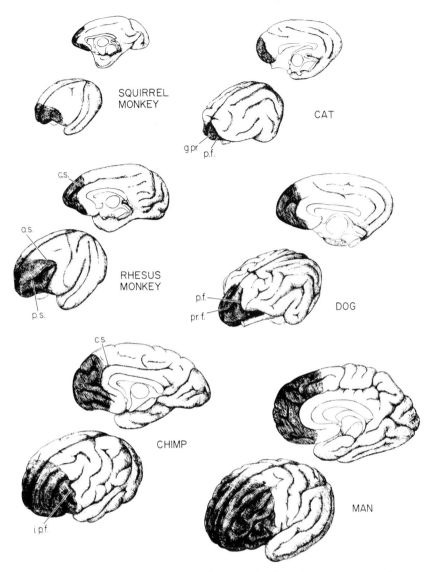

Figure 7.5 The prefrontal cortex (shaded) in six animal species. a.s., arcuate sulcus; c.s., cingulate sulcus; g.pr., gyrus proreus; i.p.f., inferior precentral fissure; p.f., presylvian fissure; p.s., principal sulcus; pr.f., proreal fissure.

characteristic and consistent cognitive disorder from prefrontal pathology (review in Fuster, 1989). Still, it should be noted that the prefrontal patient usually is capable of executing ordinary motor routines without trouble. In fact, ordinary routine seems to take the place of dwindling creativity in the life of the patient.

In addition to disturbing the planning and initiation of behavior, prefrontal lesions seem to disturb the short-term representation of specific movements as required for integration of temporally extended behavior. Frontal patients have trouble remembering the order and execution of externally or internally generated motor responses (McAndrews and Milner, 1991; Petrides, 1992).

In summary, it has been demonstrated that in the human the prefrontal cortex is essential for planning and initiation of action and, consequently, is essential for all manner of creative speech and behavior. There is evidence that it also is essential for the memory of recent actions. It is in the prefrontal cortex that we should look for the neural foundation of motor plans and for the neural evidence that "a plan of action is built up on the basis of the organism's goals and current perceptions" (Arbib, 1981, p. 1477), and that "the richest source of new plans is our old plans, transformed to meet new situations" (Miller and Chomsky, 1963, p. 486). It is probably also in prefrontal cortex where motor actions are temporarily represented as needed in the context of behavioral sequences.

The deficit of monkeys and humans with prefrontal lesion in delay task performance can be largely explained as a difficulty in forming and using internal representations. As noted earlier, the subject with prefrontal damage has trouble forming and using two kinds of such representations essential for bridging the delay and the cross-temporal contingency of the delay-task trial: the memory of the cue and the "future memory" of the appropriate motor response. Both must be formed and used anew for every trial.

That lesions of prefrontal cortex, in monkeys or humans, lead to deficits in the formulation or execution of plans and in the performance of delay tasks constitutes only indirect evidence that schemes of behavior are actually represented in the prefrontal cortex. Again, for more direct evidence of cortical representations, we must resort to functional data—that is, to physiological signs of the activation of those representations in operant conditions. We must resort to indices of neuronal activation while, we assume, the subject utilizes those schemes for the construction of motor acts—in other words, while the programs are mobilized that prepare the organism for motor action. Among other things we can assume that, if prefrontal neurons are part of motor memory networks that represent the action, their discharge should reflect activation before and during the action.

Notice, however, that this approach allows no clear distinction between the motor program as a representation and the motor program as the physiological operator (between hardware and software, in computer lingo). Thus, the approach cannot easily disambiguate the significance of neuronal activation preceding movement. Such activation may signify either the activation of the cognitive representation of movement or the preparation of motor networks for the movement itself (preparatory motor set). Alternatively, it may signify both, because representational and operational networks probably coincide: The same neuronal networks that represent the action may be in charge of mediating it. This interpretation derives from concepts of network dynamics discussed in chapter 5 (to be discussed further in coming chapters) and is supported by electrophysiological observations. Here, with regard to prefrontal networks, its validity is supported by neuropsychological data. For example, the neurons exhibiting the most pronounced activations in preparation for movement, during the delay of delay tasks, are found in the area that lesion studies have shown to be critical for learning the tasks (i.e., the area in and around the sulcus principalis) (figure 7.6). Cooling of the same area induces a reversible deficit in performance of a delay task, with variable probability or strength of contingency between the cue and the motor response after the delay (Quintana and Fuster, 1993). Judging by reaction time, the sensorimotor performance of human subjects with prefrontal lesions does not benefit, as it does in normals, from advanced knowledge (i.e., predictability) of the target of motor response (Alivisatos, 1992). These are neuropsychological indications that the prefrontal networks representing the memory of the task are those that mediate it.

Some of the possible neuronal mechanisms of task execution are discussed in chapter 9. In any case, there is no empirical evidence, in the prefrontal cortex or anywhere else, that the neuronal networks of perceptual or motor memory that are necessary for learning and thus for representing a delay task and its components are any different, or separate from, the neuronal networks that organize the action in performance of the task. There is no evidence here that, to use Bernstein's (1967) terminology, the motor engram is any different from the "ecphorator." Now let us examine some physiological evidence that they are indeed the same.

The earliest descriptions of prefrontal *memory cells*, as I have subsequently called them, were published in the early 1970s (Fuster and Alexander, 1971; Fuster, 1973). Such units are especially common in the region of the sulcus principalis, although they can be found practically anywhere in the prefrontal cortex (area FD of Bonin and Bailey, 1947; see figure 7.6C) of monkeys performing delay tasks. They are characterized by sustained elevated discharge (i.e., spike firing above spontaneous intertrial baseline) during the period of forced delay between the cue (memorandum) and the motor response. The magnitude of that activation of discharge (Fuster, 1973) is related to three factors: (1) the learning of the task (untrained animals do not show activation), (2) the level of correct performance, and (3) the need to mediate the cross-temporal contingency between the cue and the response. As we have seen in the previous chapter and will discuss further in the next two, memory cells have also been found in various areas of posterior association cortex; where they are found depends on the kind of cue utilized by the animal.

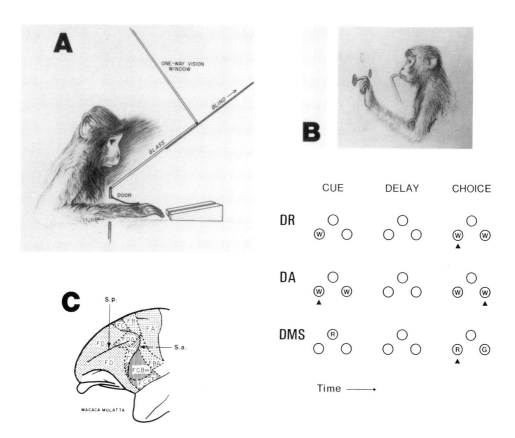

Figure 7.6 (*A*) Monkey performing the classical delayed response task. At the start of a trial, the animal observes the concealment of a food morsel under one of the two blocks. After a delay of a few seconds with a screen ("blind") blocking the view of the objects, the screen is raised and the animal is allowed the choice of one object. If the chosen object is the baited one, the animal retrieves the food, the position of which is changed at random from trial to trial. (*B*) Three delay tasks on a panel with three stimulus-response buttons: DR, delayed response; DA, delayed alternation; DMS, delayed matching to sample. W, white light; G, green light; R, red light. Correct responses (marked by black triangle) are rewarded with fruit juice. (*C*) Cytoarchitectonic map of frontal cortex (Bonin and Bailey, 1947). Bilateral lesions of area FD (prefrontal cortex) cause deficits in performance of all tasks in (*A*) and (*B*) without affecting visual or motor abilities. (From Fuster, 1989, with permission.)

Niki (1974a,b,c) was the first to observe that the sustained activation of some prefrontal cells during the delay was related to the impending motor response. Clearly, the discharge of these neurons was not related to the memorizing of the cue per se but to the movement that the animal was about to make (figure 7.7). Using delay tasks with long and constant delays (10 seconds or longer), it has subsequently been shown that some prefrontal units anticipate the motor response by several seconds and accelerate their firing as that response approaches (Fuster et al., 1982; Quintana and Fuster, 1992). In general, the use of tasks in

LEFT   RIGHT

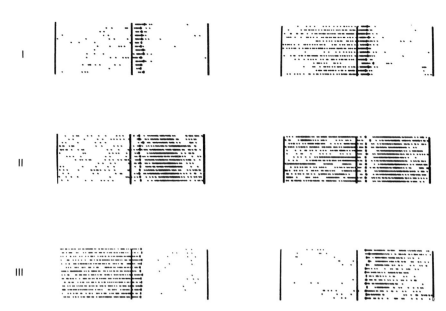

Figure 7.7 Firing rasters from three types of prefrontal cells (I, II, and III) in delayed alternation (see figure 7.6). Left-sided and right-sided response rasters are displayed separately. Vertical line in the middle of each raster marks the visual signal; animal's responses are marked by heavy dots. The period of 2 seconds of delay, before and after the signal, is delimited by two vertical lines on each side of the raster. During the delay preceding each response of the animal, all three cells show different firing levels, depending on response direction. (From Niki, 1974b, with permission.)

which the animal can predict the time to respond may reveal accelerating cell discharge in anticipation of motor response (Sakai, 1974; Komatsu, 1982; Funahashi et al., 1989, 1990) (figure 7.8).

Thus, delay tasks have revealed the coexistence within prefrontal cortex of two distinct types of cells. The first are attuned to the memorandum (cue) and the second to the consequent motor response (Niki and Watanabe, 1976; Fuster et al., 1982; Fuster, 1984; Quintana and Fuster, 1992). The two types of units, which are anatomically intermixed, tend to exhibit reciprocal trends of firing. The sensory-coupled (cue-coupled) cells decrease their firing as the delay progresses toward the response, whereas the motor-coupled (response-coupled) cells do the reverse (i.e., they accelerate firing as the response approaches), and they do it in proportion to the predictability of that response (see the next chapter; Quintana and Fuster, 1992). The evidence that the two types of neurons are intermingled and in close proximity (Fuster et al., 1982) suggests that the prefrontal networks representing the cue and those representing the response largely overlap. The two sets of prefrontal neurons and their respective networks would represent two

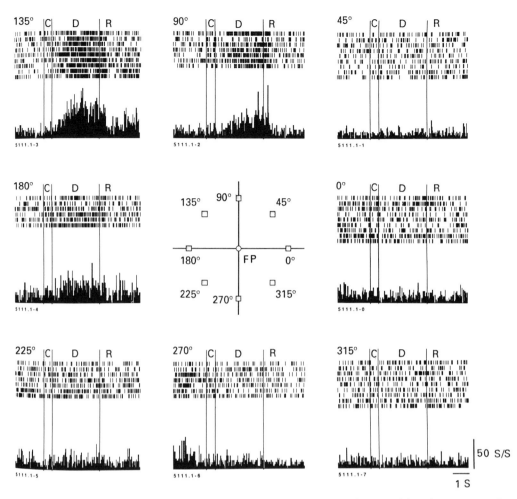

Figure 7.8 Activity of a prefrontal cell during an oculomotor delayed response task. Except for response, the monkey maintains eye fixation on a central location of the visual field (FP). Each trial begins with presentation of a point of light in one of the eight locations indicated in the middle diagram. A delay (D) of 3 seconds ensues, during which time the monkey must memorize the location of that cue (C). At the end of the delay, the animal must respond (R) by briefly directing the eyes to the location of the cue for reward. Note that the cell is activated during the delay of trials with cue in the left upper quadrant; note also that the activation tends to increase as the monkey prepares to respond to the site of the cue. (From Funahashi et al., 1989, with permission.)

mutually complementary and interactive representations—one *retrospective*, the short-term memory of the cue, and the other *prospective*, the short-term memory of the forthcoming response. The second would be what Ingvar (1985) has called a "memory of the future."

Neurochemical studies have indicated that the activation of prefrontal cortex during the delay of a delay task is mediated by dopamine receptors. The local injection of dopamine antagonists by iontophoresis has been noted to block that activation in manual delayed response (Sawaguchi et al., 1990). In an oculomotor delayed-response paradigm, it has been shown that those injections induce increased latency and errors of performance (Sawaguchi and Goldman-Rakic, 1991, 1994); the use of selective antagonists makes it appear that D1 receptors are those chiefly involved in the mnemonic properties of prefrontal cells. In general terms, the predominance of dopamine receptors in the dorsolateral prefrontal cortex points indirectly to the motor character of the structure (review and discussion in Fuster, 1989). It should be remembered that dopamine is abundant and plays an important role in other motor structures as well (motor cortex, basal ganglia). Not surprisingly, dopamine seems to mediate prefrontal neuronal transactions in motor memory and the temporal organization of motor behavior.

Brain imaging in the human has provided further evidence of the involvement of prefrontal cortex in the representation of movement. During the ideation of serial skeletal movement or during speech, which is a special form of serial movement, increases of cerebral blood flow have been detected in prefrontal and motor areas but not in primary motor cortex (Ingvar and Philipson, 1977; Larsen et al., 1978; Lassen and Larsen, 1980; Roland et al., 1980a,b; Frith et al., 1991). Prefrontal activation is especially marked when the subject is mentally planning motor sequences (Ingvar and Philipson, 1977; Roland, 1985; Roland and Friberg, 1985).

Can the memory of the future make the future happen? I already have referred to indications that motor networks of prefrontal cortex are not only representational but also operational, that they not only contain the engram of the movement but set the motor system to enact it. (This issue will be discussed further in chapters 8 and 9.) However, whereas the directional specificity of some prefrontal cells indicates their involvement in representation and execution of movement, so far there is no evidence of somatotopic or kinematic organization in prefrontal cortex, with the exception of the frontal eye field (area 8). Stimulation experiments have provided hints of the organization of ocular kinematics within this prefrontal area (Bruce et al., 1985). Movement representation in more anterior prefrontal cortex is most probably idiosyncratic to the individual, context-dependent, and poorly defined topographically. In general, motor representation appears better organized in premotor cortex.

Premotor Cortex

The nonprimary motor cortex, or premotor cortex, which is topographically and, to some extent, connectively interposed between the prefrontal and the primary motor (MI) cortex of the precentral gyrus (area
4), largely coincides with area 6 (FB) and includes what has been termed
MII (see chapter 4). It is conventionally divided into two portions with
somewhat different anatomical and physiological characteristics (figure
7.9): a lateral area (6b) or premotor cortex proper (PM) and a medial
area (6a of Vogt) (Wiesendanger, 1981; Tanji and Kurata, 1989). The
latter also is known as the *supplementary motor area* (SMA). Unit and
stimulation studies show that both are, to some degree, somatotopically
organized and contain separate kinetic maps (Alexander and Crutcher,
1990a,b; Crutcher and Alexander, 1990; Fried et al., 1991; Kurata, 1992).
Because of the presence within them of cells that show anticipatory
discharge before movement, both premotor areas are assumed to be
involved in the preparation for movement or motor set (Tanji et al.,
1980; Godschalk et al., 1981; Wise and Mauritz, 1985; Di Pellegrino and
Wise, 1991). It is important to note, however, that the anticipatory
discharge of premotor neurons generally begins after that of prefrontal
neurons and before that of motor (MI) neurons. This order of initiation
of anticipatory discharge before movement, which coincides with the
order of development of slow local surface potentials, strongly suggests
that the processing of motor set begins first in prefrontal cortex, then
involves premotor cortex, and finally moves to motor cortex (Fuster,
1989; also see chapter 9). At each cortical stage, motor set undoubtedly
engages the connective loop of that cortical stage with subcortical structures (basal ganglia and lateral thalamus). The order of recruitment of
frontal areas before movement, however, in no way implies that the
processing of movement or the control of its execution takes place

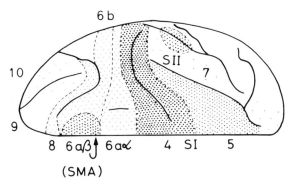

Figure 7.9 Macaque's cortex, viewed from above, with several cytoarchitectonic areas
designated (the stippling refers to density of corticopontine projection). (From Wiesendanger, 1981, with permission.)

serially from area to area in cascade fashion. There is enough temporal overlap in the discharge of the three regions to cast serious doubt on this inference and to favor, instead, parallel and "heterarchical" processing (Kalaska and Crammond, 1992; Alexander et al., 1992). Here, again, the latter view is not incompatible with a hierarchical order of motor representations and of their activation in the setting up of the motor apparatus for action.

Lesions of premotor cortex lead to a variety of deficits in learning or execution of motor sequences (Wiesendanger, 1981). In the monkey, lesions of SMA have been noted to induce deficits in self-initiation of limb movements (Passingham et al., 1989), whereas those of PM cortex disrupt movements triggered by sensory cues (Halsband and Passingham, 1985). Petrides (1986) has shown that lesions of the premotor arcuate region induce deficits in performance of conditional association learning—that is, learning of motor responses contingent on associated stimuli of two sensory modalities. A review of human lesion studies led Goldberg (1985) to postulate a role of the SMA in the organization of motor sequences based on internal programs. Imaging studies have also indicated the participation of premotor cortex, the SMA in particular, in the initiation and organization of such sequences (Ingvar and Philipson, 1977; Roland et al., 1980a; Colebatch et al., 1991; Deiber et al., 1991; Grafton et al., 1992a,b). Neither lesion nor imaging studies, however, shed light on the nature of the mnemonic representations of movement that are based in premotor cortex and from there exert control on behavior. More revealing in this respect have been electrophysiological data.

The so-called *Bereitschaftspotential* (BP) or readiness potential (Kornhuber and Deecke, 1965), which is a negative DC potential preceding motor action by 1 to 2 seconds, appears to originate in the SMA. It is temporally continuous with the contingent negative variation (CNV), the slow negative potential of prefrontal origin that precedes deliberate action by an even longer time than the BP (Walter et al., 1964; Brunia et al., 1985; Birbaumer et al., 1990). Both potentials are probably manifestations of the underlying activation of massive populations of frontal neurons. It is on the basis of electrical phenomena such as the BP, as well as the neuropsychological and neuroimaging evidence of SMA participation in the initiation of voluntary movement, that the SMA has been attributed a critical role in volition (Eccles, 1982; Mushiake et al., 1991). By contrast, the PM cortex, on the basis of lesion studies and some of the unit studies discussed later, has been thought to be essential for the control of externally referenced and automatic movements (Evarts and Wise, 1984; Passingham, 1985; Rizzolatti et al., 1983).

Single-unit studies show that, in general, motor representation in the premotor cortex is not defined in terms of particular effectors, muscles, or muscle groups, but in terms of global movement, trajectory, or target.

It has been said that premotor neurons encode motor acts rather than individual movements (Rizzolatti et al., 1988). What defines the motor act that the premotor neuron encodes is not the mere physical parameters of the movement with regard to the body but the coordinates of external space, the motor sequence, and the goal. Indeed, units have been described in PM and SMA that anticipate motor acts defined by their goal, their temporal gestalt, or their trajectory. Let us review them by order of motor abstraction, from the highest to the lowest.

At the top of the premotor hierarchy of representation are those units that are activated before and during the reaching to a target of biological significance (Mann et al., 1988; Rizzolatti et al., 1988; Alexander and Crutcher, 1990a,b). These are units that could be called *teleokinetic*, to use a word coined in another context by Hess (1943) that seems especially appropriate here. They are activated in anticipation of a purposive movement to attain a certain goal, not in relation to the same movement out of the task or for another purpose; for example, one such unit will be excited in relation to finger flexion to grasp an object but not in relation to the same flexion to push an object away (Rizzolatti et al., 1988). Some units will be activated in relation to the grasping of an object with the mouth, with one hand, or with the other. Remarkably, some units will be activated by simply the *sight* of the grasping performed by a person (Di Pellegrino et al., 1992) (figure 7.10). Of course, units of this kind, capable of such degree of abstraction as is required to *class* within one category such diverse movements to a goal, can hardly be supposed to encode specific movements. It seems more reasonable that the units in question are the premotor components of widely distributed associative networks that span both posterior and anterior cortex. The units would belong to networks encoding (i.e., classing) a wide array of sensory inputs as one perceptual category and extending to frontal cortex, there to encode (i.e., to class) a wide range of movements into a corresponding motor category.

At a lower level in the premotor representational hierarchy would be those neurons that fire in relation to specific *sequences of movement* (Mushiake et al., 1990). Here, the motor category is strictly defined in the time and space domains. Figure 7.11 shows an example of one such unit. The unit fires at a high rate just before and during the execution of a certain series of movements but not during any of the component movements. It seems to abstract the sequence. That sequences are represented in premotor cortex is underscored by the evidence that premotor lesions impair the human subject's ability to reproduce motoric rhythms from memory (Halsband et al., 1993).

Somewhat lower and more concrete in their relation to movement are the premotor cells that are activated preferentially in relation to the kinematic properties of impending movement—that is, to body-centered spatial coordinates (Weinrich and Wise, 1982; Tanji and Kurata,

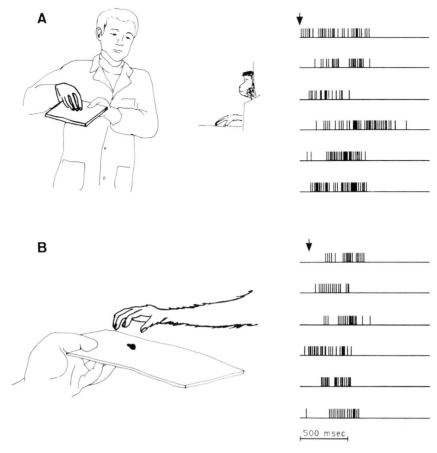

Figure 7.10 Activation of a premotor cell (A) by the monkey's observation of a grasping movement by the experimenter and (B) by the animal's grasping of a piece of food. Arrows indicate initiation of grasping. (From Di Pellegrino et al., 1992, with permission.)

1985; Riehle and Requin, 1989; Crutcher and Alexander, 1990). Units of this kind, characterized by directional tuning, constitute the majority of premotor units. They are hierarchically one step above the units of the next area, the primary motor cortex (MI), most of which are characterized by activations immediately preceding and accompanying the movement and selectively attuned to its dynamic properties (muscles involved, load, etc.) (Tanji and Kurata, 1982; Lamarre et al., 1983; Kalaska et al., 1989; Crutcher and Alexander, 1990).

Unit studies have not yet yielded any clear-cut functional map of premotor cortex or any systematic topography of the types of neurons described. Whereas the relationship of premotor cells to motor representation are better established than those of prefrontal cells, we are not here any closer to a topography of motor memory than we were in prefrontal cortex. Attempts to establish differences between SMA and PM cells have been largely unsuccessful (Okano and Tanji, 1987; Romo

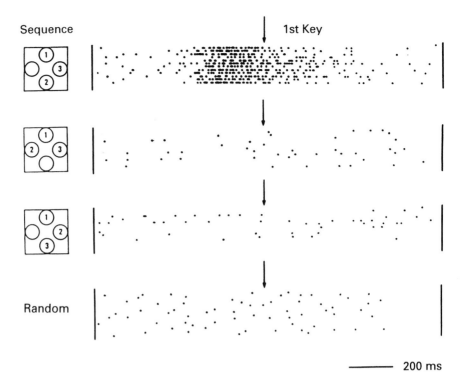

Sequence   1st Key

Random

——— 200 ms

Figure 7.11 Discharge of an SMA unit during a sequence of key-pressing movements. The cell is activated by the particular sequence on the top left panel but not by others. (From Mushiake et al., 1990, with permission.)

and Schultz, 1987; Thaler et al., 1988). One exception is the study by Mushiake and colleagues (1991) which showed that, during an instructed delay before movement, the majority of task-related SMA units were especially activated if the movement was self-initiated instead of initiated by a visual stimulus, whereas the reverse was true for PM units. Premotor neurons seem more accessible to visual input than other frontal neurons (Okano, 1992). By contrast, MI unit activations are closely linked in time to movement execution and are invariant regardless of trigger or other conditions. These findings coincide well with the lesion data mentioned earlier (Halsband and Passingham, 1985; Passingham et al., 1989). In conclusion, it appears that the signals activating PM representation and motor set come mostly from external receptors, possibly through posterior association cortex, whereas the signals activating SMA representation and set come mostly from internal sources, possibly from the prefrontal cortex just above.

A recent study of Tanji's group (Aizawa et al., 1991) has provided evidence of premotor neuronal plasticity and for the principle of motor memory migration, deduced (in the previous section) from behavioral recovery after prefrontal lesion. SMA units, the study shows, are normally activated before movement during learning of a visuomotor task. With extensive overtraining, however, SMA activation disappears. If MI then is ablated, task performance deteriorates markedly and, during relearning of the task, SMA-activated cells reappear. Evidently, SMA cells, no longer needed after overtraining, presumably because there has been a displacement of the task engram to a hierarchically lower level (perhaps PM cortex or basal ganglia), are recommissioned with the need to relearn the task. This neuronal evidence of premotor plasticity agrees with neuropsychological and imaging studies of premotor involvement in human motor learning (Halsband and Freund, 1990; Grafton et al., 1992a).

In sum, the premotor cortex contains neurons that seem to belong to representational networks of different hierarchical position. It is not possible to subdivide this cortex hierarchically because cells of different categories seem intermixed within it. Not even the SMA-PM separation is clear-cut, because cell types are mixed in both subareas. However, judging from the prevalence of different cell types within them, it appears that the SMA is hierarchically somewhat higher than PM cortex. Units in the SMA seem to represent more general, voluntary, complex, and goal-oriented actions than PM-area units, although probably less than prefrontal units. Moreover, SMA units show a degree of plasticity in their commitment to a task.

Motor Cortex (MI)

By having earlier ascribed the primary motor cortex to phyletic motor memory and by extrapolating to this cortex the gradients of increasing motor concreteness that we have followed down from the prefrontal regions, we have been led to the classic picture of MI as a functionally rigid, somatotopically highly organized cortex with small parcels (modules) controlling specific muscles. This picture, we now know, is not accurate. The recent regional mapping of MI by stimulation, unit study, and metabolic methods has led instead to a picture of extensive functional overlap and distribution, where somatotopy is defined mainly by neuronal innervation of synergic muscles (Alexander and De Long, 1985; Cheney and Fetz, 1985; Buys et al., 1986; Gould et al., 1986; Sato and Tanji, 1989). Muscle synergy would be defined by desired effect. MI thus can represent a wide selection of patterns of movement that are only loosely organized in topographical fashion.

By virtue of interaction and overlap of movement representations, any given pyramidal cell may participate in several kinds of movement, and any given movement results from the global output of a widespread population of cells, by ensemble coding. Thus, in a reaching movement, the discharge of certain clusters of neurons in MI is tuned broadly to the direction of that movement, suggesting that the movement results from the joint action (vector) of all the cells in the cluster, and thus from a population code (Georgopoulos et al., 1982, 1986, 1993; Schwartz et al., 1988). Depending on the range of the movement and the musculature involved, it is again possible to discern within MI a hierarchy of movement representations much as the one we have found in premotor cortex, but now in more concrete dynamic terms.

Another misconception deriving from the classic picture of MI is that it is structurally and functionally fixed by genetic rule. However, we now know that its neuronal substrate preserves considerable plasticity after birth (see chapter 3). New patterns of connectivity can be formed in MI as a result of training and experience. Rearrangements in that connectivity may result from synchronous synaptic convergence of inputs from higher up in the motor hierarchy (e.g., from premotor cortex) and inputs of somatosensory and proprioceptive origin (Asanuma, 1981; Iriki et al., 1989; Sanes et al., 1992; Pavlides et al., 1993). Again, imaging studies of motor learning show that MI is a plastic structure (Seitz et al., 1990; Deiber et al., 1991; Grafton et al., 1992a).

Having attended to these necessary modifications of the conventional notions of MI, however, this cortex still is viewed, overall, as a representational stage under premotor cortex. MI is a hierarchically lower level in that in it, motor representation is more organized somatotopically, more related to dynamic and kinematic aspects of movement, and less determined by postnatal experience than motor representation in prefrontal or premotor cortex.

Concluding Outline

Now let us recapitulate the organizational principles of cortical motor memory in light of the evidence just reviewed and within the framework of motor representation in the nervous system outlined at the beginning of this chapter. In this summary, I must emphasize two closely related points: First, the various frontal areas, from the prefrontal cortex down to the motor cortex, constitute a representational continuum without abrupt transitions. Second, any frontal representation of novel and complex behavior constitutes a blend of representations at various levels of the motor hierarchy.

None of the experimental or clinical evidence so far available and reviewed in this section suggests that frontal areas specialize in the exclusive representation of distinct movements. Only for heuristic reasons have we divided the discussion into presumed hierarchical levels of motor memory. Rather than indicating discrete levels or stages of representation, the neuropsychological and functional data indicate a continuous gradient of representation within frontal cortex along the dimensions mentioned previously: acquired-genetic, general-concrete, and voluntary-automatic. In all three dimensions, the transitions between the major frontal regions appear to be gradual. The replication of somatotopy at various hierarchical levels is not incompatible with that gradualism but is a manifestation of it. There are, however, hints that various general categories of action (e.g., skeletal movement, oculomotor movement, speech) are principally represented in certain frontal domains (area 8, Broca's area, etc.).

It all likelihood, the most novel representations of voluntary action, the most novel programs and plans, are formed and stored by the organism in the prefrontal cortex. The clinical evidence of this, though indirect, is very persuasive. There is no comparable animal evidence, but the delay-task deficits of the monkey with prefrontal lesion certainly support the idea that the prefrontal cortex is needed for new motor representations with a substantial temporal dimension. Whereas a delay task itself, after being learned, is an old procedural memory that prefrontal lesion does *not* eradicate, the representations of the cue and response for every trial are new and profoundly affected by that lesion. They are new, that is, for every trial. A delay task is devised in such a manner that every trial must be treated by the animal as unique and independent from other trials: That is, the game is old but the play is new.

Thus, the delay task illustrates the mixture of old (automatic) and new (voluntary) memories in behavior, and the prefrontal deficit in the task suggests that those memories are represented at various levels of the motor hierarchy. To repeat, a delay task is a complex behavior that requires at least two categories of memory: the procedural memory or basic rules of the task and the trial-specific memories of the cue (retrospective) and of the motor response (prospective). At first, on learning the task, both kinds of memory are new and the animal needs the prefrontal cortex for both. After the task has been well learned, however, the animal no longer needs this cortex for the procedural memory of the task, which has become automatic and relegated to lower structures, probably the basal ganglia and premotor cortex. Nonetheless, the animal still needs the dorsolateral prefrontal cortex for the trial-specific memory of the cue and the response, which are new for every trial. If that part of prefrontal cortex then is removed, the monkey can perform the task but not correctly; with delays beyond a certain duration, the animal fails to retain the perceptual memory of the cue and, what is most interesting, it fails to evoke the prospective memory of the motor response and to prepare for it (short-term set).

Delay-task performance also illustrates the operational blend of motor memories and motor structures in motor processing and control. There must be, in that performance, a continuous interaction of different hierarchical levels through the reentry loops of the system. The lower levels, where the procedure is represented (though a scheme of the trial may well remain represented in prefrontal cortex), must interact with the prefrontal cortex, whose networks are activated to retain the trial-unique memories of cue and response. The plan of action for the individual trial, which is new in the sense just noted, is nested within the old and automatized program of the task; the latter is mostly, if not completely, represented in lower levels, the former in dorsolateral prefrontal cortex. Plenty of parallel processing and reentry must take place between levels during performance of the task.

In premotor cortex, we are theoretically one step down the cortical motor hierarchy. The SMA may lie there somewhat higher than the postarcuate PM area, yet by descending from prefrontal cortex to SMA and from there to PM cortex, it is very doubtful that we are successively stepping down from one sharply defined category of motor representation to another. Rather, the descent is probably smooth and gradual—to wit, the temporal overlap of voluntary actions apparently represented in prefrontal and SMA cortex, the overlap of goal-oriented and direction-tuned cells (and their networks) in SMA and PM, and the overlap of motor anticipatory cell discharge in prefrontal, SMA, and PM cortex.

There is no question, however, that the transition down into primary motor (MI) cortex is somewhat more abrupt. Learning and conditioning have here a lesser role. Lesion causes paralysis. Unit activity is closely related to specific movements and dynamics, and unit discharge rarely precedes movement by more than half a second. We are at the cortical stage for microrepresentation of the action. Even here, however, representation is distributed and, to some degree, amenable to plastic change with learning and experience.

Thus, as we make our way down from prefrontal cortex to MI, neuronal networks generally appear to represent motor actions that are progressively less voluntary and more automatic (i.e., stimulus-bound), less abstract and more concrete in both space and time, less new and more firmly established in the experience of the organism or the species. We should keep in mind, however, that the representations of normal behavior of any degree of complexity contain elements of representation at several levels and, therefore, are widely distributed throughout the hierarchy.

SPEECH REPRESENTATION

This chapter would not be complete without discussion of the representational role of the cortex of the frontal lobe in the highest and most characteristic of human actions, the spoken language. Again, our aim is limited to extracting from available knowledge whatever principles of organization appear well-founded and amenable to further research. Nothing close to a frontal map of speech representation is possible. Anyway, the quest for such a map is probably pointless, because speech is the epitome of integrative action and seemingly involves vast areas of the cerebral cortex, which is to say it is represented in widely distributed and interactive networks of anterior and posterior cortex.

The first and most elementary principle of speech organization is the preponderant, if not exclusive, localization of linguistic representations and mechanisms in the left or dominant hemisphere. The second principle is the division of speech functions between posterior (postrolandic) and anterior (prerolandic) cortex (Geschwind, 1970).

As noted in chapter 6, a large region of posterior association cortex (PTO), which contains several hubs of polymodal confluent connections, is involved in semantic memory, which includes the perceptual memory of the meaning of words and sentences (Luria, 1966; Barbizet, 1970; Walsh, 1978; Mayes, 1988). Within that region, Wernicke's area is a critical focus for semantic language representation, in the posterior extremity of the superior temporal gyrus. This would be the focus of representation of the sensory, or receptive, aspects of language. The cortex of the frontal lobe, on the other hand, is involved in the motor, or effector, aspects of language. Nevertheless, this division of the cortical substrate of language into a sensory and a motor component is somewhat artificious and has only very general validity. It is barely tenable in functional terms, because normal speech requires the continuous and intimate cooperation between the two cortical sectors of language representation. Let us now briefly concentrate on the frontal sector, which is the one closer to speech action.

The spoken language is hierarchically organized like any other goal-directed motor action, with which it develops ontogenetically in parallel (Kimura, 1979). Basic sounds or phonemes are combined to form words, words to form sentences, and sentences to make discourse (Hockett, 1960; Chomsky, 1965). In normal discourse, words and sentences are organized in treelike hierarchical fashion by the underlying grammatical structure. Indeed, that hierarchical organization, with its supraordinate and subordinate or nested elements, is a powerful argument against sequential, chainlike language processing.

One can easily visualize, in the structure of language, a pyramid of categories of meaning, from the most elementary and concrete at the bottom to the most general and abstract at the top. If we substitute *meaning* for *goal*, we have an analogous hierarchy to that of motor action. Much as in motor action, we have in speech a stacking of syntheses of progressively higher class. In the production of spoken language, as in the execution of motor behavior, the higher assemblies govern and sequence the lower ones, which are nested under them like motor subroutines. The need for higher guidance in the sequencing of speech and action was first recognized by Lashley (1951) in a masterful article in which he refuted the argument that serial behavior consists simply of the chaining of successive acts. (This may hold true, however, for automatic and routine speech or behavior.)

Is there a hierarchy of frontal areas to match and support that hierarchy of speech assemblies and their corresponding representations? The answer is yes, in rough terms. Here, to describe it, we revert to the bottom-to-top order.

At the lowest level of the neural hierarchy for speech is the motor cortex (MI) that controls the oropharyngeal musculature, in the inferior portion of the precentral gyrus (see figure 6.14). This constitutes the most peripheral component of the cortical apparatus for the articulation of speech. It is the cortical substrate of phyletic memory for speech and represents the most elementary phonemes. Whether that contains all the genetic apparatus of speech is debatable, however. Chomsky (1980), based in part on the universality of grammar rules that emerges from cross-cultural and developmental studies, argues for the hereditability of those rules. This nativistic point of view would seem to imply a degree of neural complexity and associative power more conceivable in higher cortex than in MI. Greenfield (1991) postulates that the innate fund of ability for speech and for manual behavior lies in Broca's area and the areas of premotor and prefrontal cortex that phylogenetically and ontogenetically derive from it.

Broca's area is the next step above MI. It is the cortex of Brodmann's areas 44 and 45, in the inferior frontal gyrus of the left hemisphere. Injuries of this area typically result in the form of aphasia that carries Broca's name, for he was the first to describe it (Broca, 1861). It is the best known of all disorders of the effector mechanisms of language (Geschwind, 1970; Luria, 1970; Passingham, 1981). The patient's speech is ordinarily slow, effortful, and poorly articulated. It is a form of language that has been called *agrammatism* because of the common lack in it of articles and liaison words, as in telegraphic style.

From the nature of the disorder that results from its injury, Broca's area can be inferred to support the most elementary representations of propositional speech. However, we encounter here a common methodological problem of lesion studies. The effects of a lesion in a given cortical area do not tell us much about the function of the area in normal conditions. In terms of our current interest, they do not tell us anything about the program or representation that the area supports for the spoken language. In any case, it seems reasonable to infer, from the effects of its lesion, that Broca's area mediates the most elementary forms of syntax and, therefore, represents the most elementary syntheses of speech. In support of these inferences is the evidence from imaging studies that Broca's area is invariably activated not only during overt speech (Ingvar and Schwartz, 1974; Larsen et al., 1978; Ingvar, 1983; Roland, 1985; Hinke et al., 1993) but also during internal speech (Larsen et al., 1978; Lassen and Larsen, 1980; Roland, 1985; Hinke et al., 1993) or during the listening to simple onomatopoeic words (Nishizawa et al., 1982).

Broca's aphasia, although a most dramatic speech disorder, is far from being the only aphasia that can result from frontal injury. Understandably, however, from a hierarchical point of view, lesions in frontal areas of higher rank and later development result in more subtle disorders, for they affect higher speech syntheses of less common use.

The premotor cortex is developmentally and hierarchically about on a par with Broca's area (Fuster, 1991b). In the hierarchy for skeletal movement, we have seen it interposed between MI and the prefrontal cortex. It, too, however, seems to play a role in the spoken language, although it remains unclear precisely what this role may be. The electrical stimulation of the SMA has been reported to elicit rhythmical sequences of syllables (Penfield and Roberts, 1966). Damage to premotor cortex, especially the SMA, causes an aphasia in some ways similar to Broca's, but of lesser magnitude (Luria, 1970; Masdeu, 1980; G. Goldberg et al., 1981); here the patient's speech is reported to be less spontaneous and fluent than normal. Furthermore, premotor cortex, including SMA, is activated during both overt and covert speech (Roland, 1985; Roland and Friberg, 1985). However, neither the clinical lesion nor the tomographic image of premotor cortex can be easily assumed to be strictly circumscribed to this cortex, for it may encroach on Broca's area, which lies immediately under it, or on the prefrontal cortex in front. Thus, it is possible that some of the speech disorders or activations ascribed to premotor cortex are attributable to lesion or activation of those other portions of frontal cortex that are more within the domain of the speech hierarchy. Conversely, however, prefrontal lesions and images not encroaching on either Broca's area or premotor cortex can be more readily identified, as can the speech representations associated with them.

Although Broca's area can be considered part of the prefrontal cortex by reason of its connectivity with the nucleus medialis dorsalis of the thalamus (the conventional criterion to define prefrontal cortex), language disorders from prefrontal lesion outside of Broca's area are markedly more subtle and difficult to define than Broca's aphasia. Prefrontal speech disorders vary substantially, depending perhaps on such imponderables as the precise localization of the lesion, but typically have certain common features that can be summarized as follows. The first characteristic is their laterality: Prefrontal speech disorders from damage in the left or dominant hemisphere generally are more severe than those resulting from damage in the right or nondominant hemisphere (Barbizet et al., 1975; Ramier and Hécaen, 1977; Kaczmarek, 1984; Miller, 1984).

Among the most typical abnormalities of prefrontal damage are the aspontaneity and poverty of speech. In this respect, the speech disorder is somewhat similar to the disorders of skeletal motility commonly observed in prefrontal syndromes. The prefrontal aphasia, which Goldstein (1948) called "central motor aphasia" and Luria (1970) "frontal dynamic aphasia," is characterized by a severe diminution of spontaneous speech and speech fluency. The quantity and range of narrative production are markedly curtailed. The patient seems to suffer a loss of what Jackson (1915, 1958) called the "capacity to propositionise." In the patient's generally constricted speech production, sentences are short and simple and dependent clauses scarce (Lhermitte et al., 1972; Albert et al., 1981). There seems to be a lack of utilization of language recursiveness (Chomsky, 1975). Whatever speech the patient generates is riddled with stereotypical, ready-made expressions and is commonplace. There is an obvious dearth of creative and synthetic language. For these reasons, it is appropriate to attribute prefrontal speech disorders to a breakdown of the so-called syntagmatic properties of language (Pei and Gaynor, 1954). In this sense, these disorders are not qualitatively different from Broca's aphasia. They share with the latter the difficulty in establishing syntheses of speech, except that in prefrontal cortex the failed syntheses seem to be of a higher order, of a more abstract category, than in Broca's area.

The apparent inability of the prefrontal patient to form syntheses of speech was deemed, by Luria and Homskaya (1964), to be at the root of prefrontal disorders in planning and in the temporal organization of behavior. According to those authors, one of the critical functions of the prefrontal cortex is to form syntheses of internal speech that represent the plan of behavior and that guide it to its goal. The concept is debatable on several grounds (Drewe, 1975), mainly because of the difficulty in objectifying it. There seems to be little doubt, however, that substantial prefrontal damage is an impediment to the formation of high-order syntheses of speech, as it is to the formation of high-order syntheses of motor action. Are both speech and action synthesized and represented by the same prefrontal networks? There is no way of knowing, but this remains a reasonable possibility. Certainly the patient with prefrontal damage has difficulty not only verbally formulating the plan of the action but also implementing it according to its goal. The patient probably is missing the prefrontal network or networks that represent the synthesis of the plan, the goal, and the action.

Additional evidence of the role of prefrontal cortex in speech representation is provided by imaging studies (Nishizawa et al., 1982; Ingvar, 1983; Roland, 1985; Petersen et al., 1990; Posner et al., 1988; Frith et al., 1991). Prefrontal foci of activation have been observed in silent reading, in active listening to speech, and in generating lists of words.

In conclusion, then, neuropsychological and functional data suggest that there is, in the human frontal cortex, a representational hierarchy of spoken language paralleling that of motor action. The two hierarchies extend from primary motor cortex to prefrontal cortex and represent progressively higher syntheses (classes) of speech and motor action. It is unclear to what extent the two coincide or interact in behavior. It seems clear, nonetheless, that strictly sequential processing down the frontal cortical hierarchies is out of the question. Rather, different levels in either representational hierarchy continuously interact in the course of speech as in motor behavior, though the mechanisms of interaction are still a mystery. In either case, the interactions may involve subcortical loops—through basal ganglia, lateral thalamus, and cerebellum. By these interactions between layers, high-level programs can control subordinate and nested routines and thus support the continual interplay of voluntary and automatic action that makes up normal sequential behavior, both in the motor and in the speech domain.

8 Dynamics of Cortical Memory: Retrieval and Attention

Although largely based on functional data, the previous two chapters were meant to define the structural organization of memory. In them, I attempted to outline the cortical topography of established perceptual and motor memories. To sketch the structural base for the self-organized associative networks postulated in chapter 5, I used, in addition to the data on connectivity presented in chapter 4, the findings from a variety of neuropsychological, electrophysiological, and imaging studies. None of these sources of evidence, however, can provide more than indirect and partial support to any notion of the structure and topography of memory and, because of this, any resulting conceptual scheme of where memory is could not possibly be complete at this time.

Nevertheless, the scheme that has thus far emerged provides a suitable platform for empirical attempts to establish the general principles of how memory works in behavior and in our daily life. These attempts are the subject of this chapter and the next. Now that we have some reasonable ideas of how the organism has formed certain memories and where they are located, we can begin to deal with the questions of how they are retrieved, attended to, and held temporarily active and, more generally, how they control behavior.

The neural mechanisms of retrieval and attention seldom are discussed in the context of the neurobiology of memory, yet they are extremely relevant to it. By queries and stimuli of all sorts, we routinely force our experimental subjects to retrieve memories in order to assess how they are acquired, where they are stored, and for low long. However, rarely do we focus on the process of memory retrieval per se though, obviously, after a memory has been formed in the cerebral cortex, the most critical question for us here is how it will be mobilized to reenter behavior and the stream of consciousness. Retrieval is the first question concerning the dynamics of established cortical memory and thus the first topic of this chapter. Forgetting, or the failure of retrieval, will follow.

Somewhat less obvious than that of retrieval is the importance of attention in memory dynamics, which is the subject of the second part of this chapter. Again, as in dealing with relations between perception and memory, or action and memory, our problem is the natural but misleading tendency to compartmentalize cognitive and cortical functions. All too often we see attention as another box in a box diagram or on a cortical map. True, the connecting arrows with a memory compartment may be there too, but it is difficult to avoid the impression that attention and memory are meant to occupy different and separate functional or structural domains. This is highly implausible. Attention is intimately related to memory, structurally and functionally. Even from a superficial perspective, who will deny that the behavioral and phenomenal fate of retrieved memory depends on the strength and selectivity of the focus of attention? Efficient behavior requires a mechanism that selects and allocates active memory to perceptual and motor systems, for both have limited processing capacity. At the phenomenal level, no two engrams can be simultaneously maintained in consciousness at any given time, and no single engram can be kept there for any length of time without an attention mechanism and a persistent focus of representation. As we shall see, attention can be plausibly considered a property of any active memory network. There is no need for a cortical area exclusively devoted to attentive function.

Here for the discussion of retrieval and attention in memory dynamics, we must draw material from a variety of methodologies. I hope that the text's frequent shifts from human to animal and vice versa, and from method to method, will not blur my line of reasoning. One line of empirical approach, however, that will be found consistent through this chapter and the next is as follows: To substantiate the dynamics of cortical memory, I shall often make use of neural data obtained during behavioral tests of sensory discrimination. This use of data from discrimination paradigms to clarify how memory works—after it has been formed—may surprise some readers, for in neurobiology we employ such paradigms primarily to study sensory functions, or learning and its deficits, but not the dynamics of established memory. However, the use of discrimination for studying retrieval and activation of memory should surprise no one who has followed my argument for perception and behavioral action as the classing (which implies discrimination) of stimuli and responses based on memory (see chapter 5). In fact, sensory stimuli in well-rehearsed discrimination tests are the best means to expose those top-down and endogenous factors from prior memory that play a critical role in memory retrieval, selective attention, and active short-term memory.

MEMORY RETRIEVAL

Retrieval is the act of getting at stored information. The concept comes from cognitive psychology and subsumes, generically, all that is understood by recall, recognition, and remembering. There are valid operational distinctions between these three retrieval functions which, in the human, can be independently tested to some extent (Klatzky, 1975). They may be differentially affected in disorders of memory. On phenomenal and experimental grounds, however, all three share the associative character that is the essence of cortical memory and its retrieval. Memories are retrieved by associative access through their component representations, by reconstruction from fragments. The act of retrieval depends on eliciting those representations by stimuli, external or internal, that have somehow been previously associated with them, however tenuously and however remotely in the past. The memory-eliciting stimuli need not be identical to those originally incorporated into the memory; they may simply be similar in some way or perceptually equivalent to them (see chapter 5). Those retrieving stimuli can be enormously diverse, like the memories they evoke. An effective stimulus might be, for example, a word or command, a visual image, an odor, an instinctual urge, or even an internal representation or thought, abstract or concrete. That stimulus, in a broad sense, is like the hand in the basket that picks out one cherry and makes others follow.

The association of an evocative stimulus with the memory it evokes may have been formed at any previous time. Whether that time is remote or recent marks the only distinction between the retrieval of long-term memory and that of short-term memory. Whether the context of retrieval is structured by a psychometrist or not is immaterial to the nature of the process. The retrieval is basically an associative process, whether the subject is asked or prompted by circumstances to elicit the memory of an event from a date or from any other clue, or the name of a person from a photograph or from a social encounter, or urged by hunger to recall the name of a restaurant.

Short-term memory, of course, can be tested in a more structured situation than long-term memory, but there too retrieval is by association, whether rehearsal is allowed or not, whether distractors are interjected or not into the retention period. Even in so-called free recall, the subject is asked to elicit, in any order, items of a previously presented list that are associated by co-occurrence with one another and with stimuli in the testing environment. Retrieval in that case is no less associative than in a test of paired associates. The phenomenon of priming (see chapter 2) also is based on associative retrieval, even though there the association between the retrieving stimulus and the priming cue may be covert, unconscious, and part of long-term memory.

The retrieval of motor memory is basically no different from that of perceptual memory. Motor memories are elicited by stimuli associated with the motor actions they represent. This is the case whether the stimulation is external or internal and whether it has been recently or

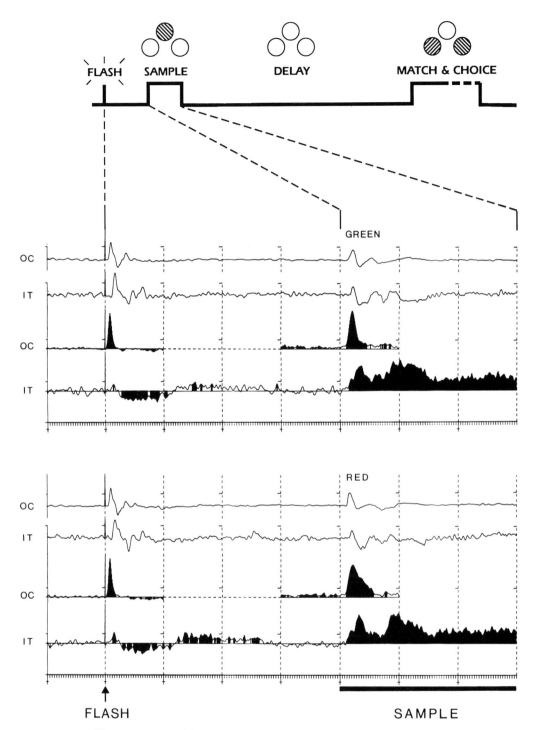

Figure 8.1 (*Top*) Schematic diagram of a delayed matching-to-sample task with two colors, each trial preceded by an alerting flash. (*Middle, bottom*) Average evoked potential and multiple-cell records from visual (striate) cortex (OC) and from inferotemporal cortex

remotely associated with the memory which, when retrieved, may or may not lead to the action itself. Of course, when the test material is verbal, the action is often the spoken word. Furthermore, all tests of retrieval of perceptual memory require actions based on some aspect of motor memory.

To summarize, despite vast differences in the circumstances and difficulty of memory retrieval, all processes of recognition, recall, and remembering in the human appear to have one common feature: *the access to a memory through a stimulus or set of stimuli that at one time or another has become, by co-occurrence, an associated element of the memory and presumably, therefore, of the neural network that constitutes it* (see chapter 5). Now let us explore which stimuli are involved, how they gain access to the network, and how the network reacts when that happens.

Retrieval Mechanisms

Recognition is the form of memory retrieval that lends itself best to neurobiological study. Behavioral recognition tests of many kinds have been used for this purpose in the human as in animals, but most are variations of a simple test that can be described as follows. The subject is first trained or instructed to perform certain discriminant actions in response to certain discriminant stimuli in a given context. Thus, a set of memories is formed by association of the stimuli with the context (i.e., with other stimuli) and with their corresponding motor (may be verbal) responses. Thereafter, every time one of the stimuli is presented, it will be recognized and acted on accordingly. The speed and accuracy of the response will provide evidence of the efficacy of retrieval.

The first methodology to reveal the recruitment of neuronal networks in the act of retrieval was the study of event-related or evoked potentials in discriminations—that is, the field potentials recorded from the brain immediately after sensory stimuli that elicit discriminatory motor responses. John (1967), in the cat, was probably the first to discover that in some regions of the brain, such potentials become synchronous and coherent (i.e., attain similar morphology and time course) as the animal learns a discrimination and those brain regions become engaged in the process of behaviorally discriminating. Comparable findings were made by Freeman (reviewed by Freeman and Skarda, 1985).

In monkeys trained to perform delayed matching to sample with colors, Ashford and Fuster (1985) observed the synchronicity and coherence of neuronal activity elicited by visual stimuli in different cortical

(IT) in the period before and during the presentation of a green (*upper graph*) or red (*lower graph*) sample stimulus. (Evoked potentials are in the upper two records of each graph, multiple-unit histograms of spikes in the lower two; vertical dash lines are 0.5 seconds apart.) (From Ashford and Fuster, 1985, with permission.)

areas (figure 8.1). In the context of the task, the stimuli could be assumed to serve two related purposes: to retrieve the perceptual memory of the stimuli, well established in long-term storage by prior learning, and to guide the monkey to the appropriate motor response on each particular trial. Here we focus on the first. Both the alerting flash that begins a trial and the subsequent color stimulus that is to be memorized for a few seconds activate almost simultaneously two widely separated areas of visual cortex, one primary and the other associative: the striate (occipital) cortex and the inferotemporal cortex. Activation of the latter lags by only a few tens of milliseconds behind that of the former, after which both cortices remain activated together for some time—approximately 250 msec after the appearance of the memorandum (sample); for a while, their respective multiunit discharge and evoked-potential records show similar configuration and time course. This finding can be understood only by assuming coherence of activation and mutual influences via reciprocal connections between the two cortices, which are conventionally considered separate stages of the visual processing hierarchy (see chapter 4). Recently, in monkeys performing visual discriminations, Bressler and coworkers (1993) have demonstrated the coherence of potentials in widely distributed and separated locations of posterior and frontal cortex.

Gevins and his colleagues (Gevins, 1989; Gevins et al., 1989a, b) developed and applied to the human a powerful computational method for studying covariance and correlation of event-related potentials. Their data give further credence to connectivist concepts of memory dynamics such as ours. Let us briefly review the data. Gevins's experimental paradigm basically conforms to the one outlined at the beginning of this section but with a somewhat more elaborate discrimination procedure (figure 8.2): instead of one stimulus per trial, the subject must act in accord with three successive stimuli. A brief visual cue (the letter V) appears first in the center of a screen; it has a rightward or leftward tilt to cue the subject as to which hand to use to respond. A second stimulus, a number, indicates the amount of pressure the subject must apply on a surface with the index finger of that hand (*1* to *9*, for 0.1 to 0.9 kg). The response of the subject follows and, after that, the subject is provided with numerical feedback (a third stimulus on the screen) on the accuracy of the response. By high-resolution electrical recording from the surface of the skull, the experimenters measure event-related covariances (ERCs)—namely, the covariations of evoked-potential course and magnitude in all the recording locations (26 electroencephalographic channels) during and between the four events: cue, stimulus, response, and feedback.

The three visual stimuli—the cue (slanted V), the pressure-indicator stimulus, and the feedback—induce within fewer than 100 msec a focus of activity in the occipital region that rapidly becomes covariant with

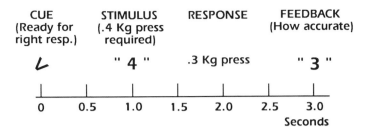

CUE (Ready for right resp.)	STIMULUS (.4 Kg press required)	RESPONSE	FEEDBACK (How accurate)
∠	" 4 "	.3 Kg press	" 3 "

0   0.5   1.0   1.5   2.0   2.5   3.0

Seconds

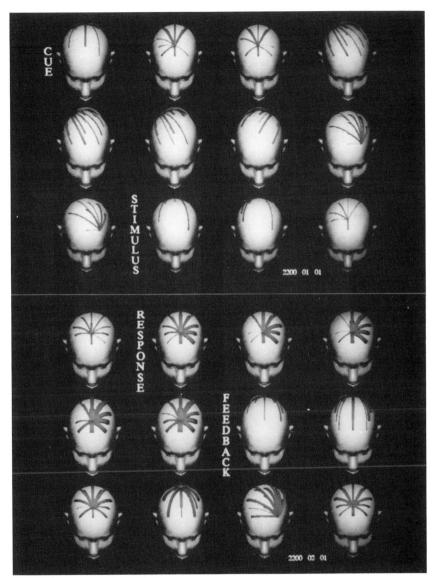

Figure 8.2 (*Top*) The task used by Gevins and colleagues, as described in the text. (*Bottom*) Head diagrams showing event-related covariance between electrodes at various times during the task. The thickness of each connecting band is related to the degree of covariance between the two interconnected locations. (From Gevins, 1989, with permission.)

     Dynamics of Cortical Memory: Retrieval and Attention

activity in parietal regions (see figure 8.2). There, new foci are established. Then the latter become covariant with locations in the prefrontal region, where the activity becomes transiently concentrated. Thus, each within a period of 500 msec, all three stimuli successively induce a pattern of covariance in temporoparietal and prefrontal regions. To some extent, especially in its later components, that pattern is related to the laterality of the response. The patterns observed suggest *waves of covariance* (i.e., joint excitation) that migrate from visual areas into parietal cortex and eventually into prefrontal cortex. These findings are consistent with the notion that all three stimuli elicit successive retrievals of their respective perceptual memories in postrolandic cortex, followed by their respective motor memories and motor set in prefrontal cortex. It may be inferred that three large and somewhat overlapping components of a preformed network of perceptual and motor memory are successively activated as the test requires. Furthermore, the temporary covariance of excitability in areas successively recruited is consistent with two important concepts: first, that large cortical regions are almost simultaneously recruited, possibly by correlated inputs, as suggested by Von der Malsburg (1985) and discussed in chapter 5 and, second, that cortical regions jointly activated *remain* jointly activated for some time (possibly by reentrant inputs between them).

The findings by Gevins and coworkers (Gevins, 1989; Gevins et al., 1989a, b), like ours in the monkey (Ashford and Fuster, 1985), cast serious doubts on the notion of strictly serial processing between cortical areas, whether or not they belong to the same sensory processing hierarchy. However, some serialization of processing does apparently take place in memory retrieval, inasmuch as (1) differences in onset latency can be observed between areas after any given memory-retrieving stimulus, (2) the activity of some areas (e.g., inferotemporal) outlasts that of others (e.g., occipital), and (3) covariances are subsequently seen to move over the surface of the cortex.

Also by single-unit analysis, retrieval of memory can be shown to entail the rapid and almost simultaneous activation of many cells in cortical areas involved in distributed representation. Chapters 6 and 7 provide some evidence of this while arguing for the participation of associative areas in perceptual and motor memory. Unit records, however, make the rapid and simultaneous activation of memory networks more evident on the perceptual than on the motor side. This is the case, of course, because the neurons of perceptual networks are more likely to be recruited in synchrony after a discrete sensory stimulus than are the neurons of motor networks before the motor response to it, unless that motor response is temporally separated from the stimulus and can be easily timed and anticipated by the animal. Thus far, as previously noted, the recruitment of cells in memory networks has been most clearly observed by recording from parasensory association areas for the modality of the retrieving stimulus (e.g., inferotemporal areas for vision).

An important question remains unanswered: How dependent is the activation of associative neurons from *endogenous factors* (i.e., from their belonging to a given memory network) and how dependent is it from *exogenous factors* (such as the physical attributes of the retrieving stimulus)? Technical difficulties in holding neurons through a training period prevent us from answering that question with certainty, but we do know that neuronal responses in the associative areas we have explored (e.g., inferotemporal cortex) are modulated to some degree by both exogenous and endogenous influences. The cells in our experiments can be inferred to respond to physical attributes because they differentiate them, and this is true also for cells of the same areas in acute experiments on untrained animals (e.g., Gross et al., 1972). At the same time, the responses of some cells to a memory-retrieving stimulus depend on their participation in the network it activates. There is evidence that those responses are greater if the stimulus is familiar to the monkey than if it is novel (Miyashita, 1988) and also, greater if the monkey attends to the stimulus than if he does not (Fuster, 1990; see below). Furthermore, those responses to the stimulus are attuned in magnitude and time course to the need of the animal to retain it in short-term memory (Fuster and Jervey, 1982). Inasmuch as a cell is more strongly activated and for a longer time by a memory-retrieving stimulus than by others, we can assume fairly that the participation of that cell is greater in the memory network of that stimulus than in those of others.

Sakai and Miyashita (1991) trained monkeys to respond behaviorally to visual stimuli presented temporally and spatially in pairs (paired associates) (figure 8.3). Subsequently, exploring the inferotemporal cortex, the authors found cells that responded specifically not only to a given stimulus but also to the associated stimulus, even though the two might be physically very different from each other. This finding is entirely consistent with the principle of memory formation by synchronous convergence and with the concept that retrieval consists in the activation of a memory network by any of the stimuli that, by mutual association, have contributed to its making.

Hints of evidence are beginning to emerge, also in unit records from task-performing monkeys, that a given memory network can be accessed by stimuli from several modalities if such stimuli have contributed to the making of the network. This has been observed, for example, in monkeys performing a tactile memory task (see chapter 6) in which the presence of the tactile stimulus is signaled at the beginning of every trial by an acoustic stimulus (click). In this situation, cells of somatosensory and posterior parietal cortex are seen to respond with very short latency to that acoustic signal and, in addition, to subsequent events related to manipulation of the test object (Koch and Fuster, 1989).

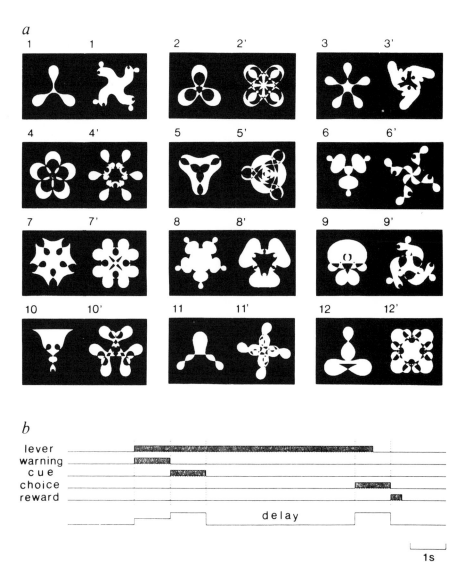

Figure 8.3 (*a*) Twenty-four visual stimuli (Fourier descriptors) experimentally paired by training and later treated by inferotemporal cells as paired associates. (*b*) Training paradigm: One stimulus is presented as the cue in a trial; after a delay, the same stimulus is presented with its associate, and the monkey must choose the first. (From Sakai and Miyashita, 1991, with permission.)

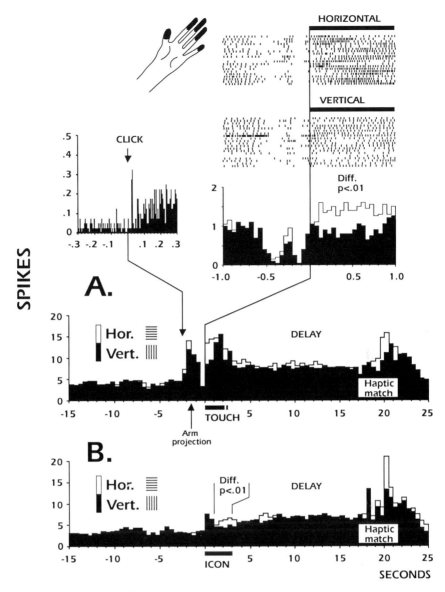

Figure 8.4 Discharge of a parietal cell during performance of a haptic-to-haptic (*A*) and a visual-to-haptic (*B*) delayed matching task. The cell's receptive field is shown above (in black) on the monkey's hand. (*A*) A click initiates the trial, signaling that a cylinder with horizontal or vertical edges (the sample) is accessible for palpation in an invisible compartment in front of the animal. The animal palpates the object (*TOUCH*) and a delay follows, at the end of which two cylinders are made available for palpation (one vertically and the other horizontally ridged), and the animal must choose the one matching the sample. Note that the cell is activated by the click (expanded record above), by arm projection, and by touch (differentially, more by horizontal than by vertical edges); sustained elevated discharge is recorded through the 18-second delay. (*B*) The monkey is now presented with a picture (ICON) with horizontal or vertical stripes, which he must memorize through the delay for a matching choice of cylinder. Note that the cell continues to favor the horizontal (now visual) pattern, however slightly, over the vertical and to exhibit sustained activation during the delay.

The unit in figure 8.4 shows prompt activation by the click, subsequent activation as the animal moves the hand toward the test object, and differential activation (higher for horizontal than for vertical edges) during the touching of the object (Zhou and Fuster, 1992). Furthermore, the cell is activated, differentially and with equivalent direction selectivity, by a visual image (icon) showing the direction of the edges of an object that the monkey must choose, by palpation, some 18 seconds later (see figure 8.4B). (The cell also shows activation during the delay, which will be discussed in the next chapter when we discuss active memory.)

Data of this kind suggest that four categories of stimuli (auditory, kinesthetic, cutaneous, and visual) can activate a cell in a network that all four have previously shaped by association during the learning process. More precisely, in dynamic terms, the cell may be part of several networks that are activated at different times as behavior dictates. All these networks, with common nodes of interaction, would be components of a larger network of polymodal perceptual memory (see chapter 6) engaged in the perception-action cycle (see chapter 9) and at the service of the temporal integration of behavior. The reader undoubtedly will recall the principles of network composition and interaction postulated in chapter 5. In any case, it is by such interactions that, as in the preceding example, auditory and visual stimuli may gain access to the network territory of another modality (somesthesia) and activate its neurons. A cross-modal phenomenon comparable to those described has been observed in inferotemporal cortex (Iwai et al., 1987); visually responsive cells in that cortex were noted to respond to an auditory signal associated with, and preceding, a visual discrimination.

Attempts have been made to visualize cortical memory retrieval by neuroimaging. In an experiment by Roland and Friberg (1985), human subjects were required to perform mental operations while their regional cerebral blood flow was measured and compared with resting baseline levels. Three forms of silent thinking were performed: (1) 50-3 thinking—that is, successively subtracting 3 from 50 and from each resulting number (47, 44, etc.); (2) jingle thinking—that is, mentally omitting every second word in a well-known circular jingle; and (3) route-finding thinking, in which the subjects had to imagine themselves at their front door and walking alternatively to the left and then to the right every time they reached a corner. During all three forms of thinking, all subjects showed activations of various degrees in multiple cortical areas. Despite considerable variability between subjects, some significant findings emerged (figure 8.5): All areas activated were in the cortex of association, not in the primary sensory or motor cortex (the striate cortex could not be imaged by the method). Different forms of thinking activated different and discrete cortical patches. Most all activated areas were within two general regions, one in posterior and the other in

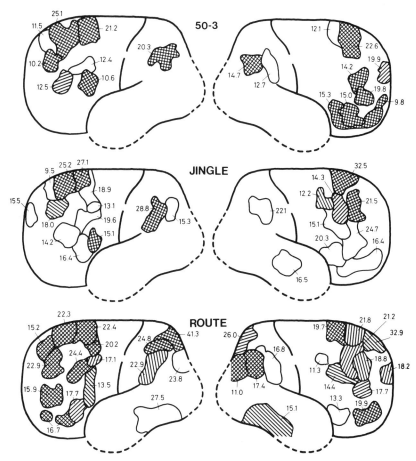

Figure 8.5 Average increase (percent) in regional cerebral blood flow during three types of thinking (see text). (*Left*) Left hemisphere, six subjects. (*Right*) Right hemisphere, five subjects. Crosshatching indicates statistical significance at $p < .005$ level; hatching, statistical significance at $p < .01$ level; white (outlined), statistical significance at $p < .05$ level. (From Roland and Friberg, 1985, with permission.)

anterior cortex: These were the supramarginal-angular-posteroparietal region and the dorsolateral prefrontal region. The third mental task (route finding), which required organized recall of visuospatial information, produced extensive activations in those two regions and, in addition, in the right inferotemporal area. In the recognition of visual patterns, another imaging study (Roland et al., 1990) showed activations (increased blood flow) of parietooccipital areas and, among other subcortical regions, the posterior hippocampus.

Petersen and colleagues (1990) investigated with positron emission tomography the cortical areas activated by visual stimuli with various degrees of *semantic load:* (1) real English words, (2) pseudowords that obeyed English rules, (3) nonsense strings of letters, and (4) letterlike forms. Real words and pseudowords activated left medial and lateral extrastriate areas in addition to the visual cortex. Nonsense words and letterlike forms failed to activate extrastriate areas. Real words, unlike the other stimuli, activated also prefrontal loci. These findings reveal that the recognition of words entails the recruitment of areas that neuropsychology has implicated in semantic processing. However, it should be noted that, outside the visual cortex, the areas activated by recognition were, in this study, rather small and their activations relatively low. This is surprising in view of the extensive associations of words. It certainly defies connectionist views of language and the wide cortical distribution of semantic memory that we envisioned in chapters 5 and 6. The reasons for the apparent discrepancy may lie in methodological problems of neuroimaging. The most serious problem is the mismatch between the relatively large time window of the brain image and the short duration of cognitive acts and their neural correlates. The problem is compounded in this study, as in many others, by the necessity to average observations. Asynchronies within and between subjects in the recognition of any given word during imaging time may weaken the cortical image of retrieval and tend to restrict the areas activated. Thus, stimuli with semantic load may appear to have less activating impact than they actually have. The results are nonetheless the more remarkable for what they show with a seemingly conservative method of assessment.

Imaging methods, no less than macropotential methods or even the neuronal recording method as currently employed, undoubtedly miss the subtleties of neural processing in memory retrieval. These methods tell us little about such matters as the mechanisms of parallel and serial access to memory and the conscious awareness of it once it has been retrieved. Here, these issues can be touched on only lightly and primarily as potential research subjects.

In everyday life, both serial and parallel processing of sensory information must be constantly ongoing in the brain on a massive scale. Many sensory channels undoubtedly have access to any given memory network and, conversely, many memory networks may be activated by a given stimulus which, in one form or another, happens to be represented in all. Which stimulus or stimuli will prevail and which memory or memories will be activated at any given time must depend on innumerable imponderables of the situation. It is possible, in any case, that several stimuli reach the same memory in parallel and, also, that several memories are activated in parallel. Furthermore, neither a stimulus nor the memory it evokes need be conscious. When dealing with these matters, we should always keep in mind that the experimental situation in which memory ordinarily is tested in the human, as in the animal, is necessarily contrived and biased toward serialization of processing, attentive selectivity, and awareness. None of them need be a constraint to the retrieval of memory.

Although we cannot yet even fathom the neurophysiology of it, *unconscious retrieval* warrants some mention here. In the course of our daily life, the processing of myriad stimuli takes place outside our awareness, while we concentrate seriatim and attentively on a narrower set of stimuli to pursue our goals. Through their preestablished channels, those stimuli of which we are not aware (some perhaps from the internal milieu) are conceivably capable of eliciting memories at the unconscious or preconscious level—to use psychoanalytical concepts and lingo—and mobilize their networks to influence our behavior in more or less subtle ways. Covert recognition (Cowey, 1991; Goodale et al., 1991) can certainly determine our decisions, create changes of mind and mood, and possibly even engender symptoms and illness.

Consider for a moment *state-dependent learning*, which epitomizes learning and memory by co-occurrence or near-co-occurrence of external and internal stimuli. The phenomenon has been extensively studied in animals but no doubt takes place also in humans. The coyote (Gustavson et al., 1974) is exposed to lithium-poisoned lamb's meat, which makes it sick. Thereafter, the sight, taste, or smell of lamb, whether dead or alive, will make the animal sick. No one knows for sure what may have happened in the coyote's nervous system for that to occur, but it is a reasonable guess that both limbic and cortical structures, as with any kind of memory, have played a role in that learning process. Here, however, associations have been formed between visceral and sensory inputs at a high cognitive level, involving a cortical network that can eventually be accessed through any of the originally participant senses (Garcia and Holder, 1985). In a similar manner, some people become sick at the mere sight or mention of a boat. It is important to note that in state-dependent conditioning, as in aversion learning, the relationship between the retrieving stimulus and the memory itself may be highly symbolic and need not be conscious.

Priming is another phenomenon in which the latter is true. Almost certainly, priming involves retrieval under unconscious influences. That is to say, the primed recognition is probably influenced or mediated by a hidden—unconscious and symbolic—association of the retrieving stimulus.

Forgetting

Forgetting is the inability to retrieve memory despite conscious effort to do so. This is certainly a topic of great interest to the neurologist, the psychiatrist, the jurist, and the common folk. It is, however, another of those neuroscientific topics in which ignorance and misconceptions prevail over facts.

For no obvious reason, we forget dates and facts, names and events, persons and places, what we see, hear, read, and so on. We forget items of perceptual memory and motor memory as well; not only may we forget to sign the document, lock the door, or write the number, but we forget whether or not we did it. Forgetting is a source of frustration, mishap, altercation, and humor. Fortunately, in our daily lives, we do not normally forget other than trivial things and then only under certain circumstances. Age and pathological processes, however, can make forgetting serious and common. Let us briefly examine these issues, if for no other reason than to set another agenda for neuroscience.

The retrieval of short-term memory, whether it is that of a recent item that is still in the process of consolidation or the active short-term retention of a previously consolidated item, may fail for essentially two reasons: decay and interference. Among the essential features of short-term memory is the passive decay of recently acquired information (Peterson and Peterson, 1959; Klatzky, 1975). This is true for working memory and, as we shall see later, has an apparent correlate in the behavior of cortical cells. Thus, we forget what, by consolidation, rehearsal, or both, has not survived that normal decay.

Another characteristic of short-term memory is its vulnerability to interference, proactive or retroactive. A previous item of perception, memory, or action can impede retention of the current memory; alternately, a current item, a distractor, can retroactively interfere with memory that was recently acquired. All forms of interference are potentially deleterious for the same reason: the limited capacity of short-term memory. There is a limit to what can be retained at any given time in short-term memory and, for that reason, whatever is in that state is potentially subject to displacement or obliteration by interference.

The forgetting of long-term memory is more complex, more erratic, and less well understood. Initially poor fixation of the memory, because of inattention or lack of rehearsal, is a common cause of poor retrieval. Obviously, affective state and motivation at the time of acquisition are significant factors. The disinterest that accompanies even mild depression or the scattered attention of euphoria may adversely determine how effectively we later remember facts, events, faces, names, and so on. The psychoanalytic tenet that no memory is ever lost, although it can be temporarily repressed and irretrievable (Freud, 1930/1961, p. 69), is unprovable, but there is no question that emotional conditions can block or prevent the retrieval of certain memories, especially if they are associated with strong emotions.

None of the factors mentioned above can account easily for the mystifying phenomenon of *infantile amnesia*. No one of us is capable of remembering distinctly the experiences of early infancy, especially if they took place before age 30 months. It appears that one of the reasons for infantile amnesia is that, before that age, the mechanisms of active memory have not developed. There is no evidence of recall capacity before 8 months. Indeed, before 12 months, the short-term memory of infants is ineffective or nonexistent (Mandler, 1990). It is in the course of their second year of life that children acquire the capacity to recall simple events and sequences of actions (Bauer and Mandler, 1989; Bauer and Hertsgaard, 1993). The rate of memory processing increases progressively with age, though in early stages both acquisition and recall remain spotty, and it is difficult to characterize a memory system or store that develops faster than others (Rovee-Collier, 1990). Motor memory (including habits) seems to develop faster than perceptual memory. Both undoubtedly develop pari passu with the development of the connective apparatus of, respectively, frontal and posterior cortex of association. Perhaps perceptual memory lags behind motor memory because the former, more than the latter, relies on the associative power of words, which is undeveloped in the prelingual child.

If memory and its retrieval are based on association, it follows that the enrichment of the associative network of a memory eventually should permit easier retrieval. All *mnemonic rules and strategies* are based on this assumption and amply validate it. The best strategy for retrieval of a recalcitrant memory is to use alternative associations as lines of access to its network. The more lines available, the better. We remember the name of an occasional acquaintance much better when we re-encounter him or her in the same context in which we made the acquaintance than in any other setting. Faced with the embarrassing mental blocking of a name in a different environment, it helps—sometimes—to recreate in our mind the context in which we first met the person. The *free-association method* (Freud, 1943) is essentially a strategy to reach repressed memories by successive approximations, and unwittingly, through various lines of association.

The potential access to memory through multiple associative lines is congruent with our notions of the self-organized memory network (see chapters 3 and 5). The various lines of access are nothing other than associations that the network acquired, concomitantly or at different times, as it developed. When one fails, others may be tried for retrieval. They may be of one or more sensory modalities, as many as contributed to the making of the network.

The pathology of memory is, in operational terms, the pathology of retrieval, but retrieval may fail for many reasons. Normal aging commonly is associated with some degree of memory loss, but it is not clear whether the forgetfulness of the elderly is mainly due to poor memory fixation, loss of stored information, or loss of the capacity to recall. All three may play a role. It is a common assumption that, with age, there is a general decrement in the connectivity of the cortex, in the numbers of neurons and synapses available, and in the capacity to form new connections. However, the evidence for these generalities is soft, and much of the literature on the neurobiology of aging memory is hard to evaluate. Let us review some of it briefly.

Age-related memory dysfunctions have been well documented in the rat, especially with regard to various forms of spatial memory (Barnes, 1979; Toledo-Morrell et al., 1984; Barnes and McNaughton, 1985; Gallagher and Pelleymounter, 1988), and in the monkey (Moss et al., 1988; Rapp, 1990; Bachevalier et al., 1991). Practically every study, however, emphasizes individual variability. Some animals lose memory with age and others do not; among those that do, some lose it at an earlier age than others. The situation obviously is analogous to that of the human. On close analysis, it becomes clear that variability is also the rule in the neurobiology of aging memory. There are, however, some consistencies of age-related deterioration of neural stucture and function that may be at the foundation of the cognitive deficits of the aged. Insofar as impaired memory is the most prominent of these deficits, those consistencies deserve attention here.

The hippocampus has been noted to undergo involutional changes. In rodents, there is an age-related loss of synapses by entorhinal axons on dendritic spines of hippocampal cells (Geinisman and Bondareff, 1976). This synaptic loss of terminal contacts of the perforant path appears to correlate with the magnitude of the age-related loss in spatial memory. A related finding is that of diminished persistence of long-term potentiation, induced by perforant path stimulation (Barnes, 1979; Barnes and McNaughton, 1985). Granular cells of the dentate, the recipients of neocortical inputs through the perforant path, seem to be the most directly affected elements of the hippocampus (Geinisman and Bondareff, 1976). However, some of the dentate cells exhibit increased reactivity to those inputs, possibly through gap junctions (Barnes and McNaughton, 1980; Barnes et al., 1987) and to compensate for the loss of other synaptic contacts. Neurochemically, the most affected synapses in the hippocampus are those from cholinergic neurons of the septal region (Fischer et al., 1989, 1991; Koh et al., 1989). Septal cholinergic cells are reportedly smaller in old monkeys with memory deficits (Stroessner-Johnson et al., 1992). This evidence is in accord with the reported deterioration of cholinergic systems in the human as a function of age (Lacalle et al., 1991) and in Alzheimer's disease (Whitehouse et al., 1982).

Clearly, functional disorders of the hippocampus could be the basis of the age-related troubles of the human in memory acquisition as well as memory recall. Normal aging would bring about a gradual deterioration of hippocampal structure and mechanisms resembling the one that can be observed, more dramatically, in pathological aging (Hyman et al., 1984; Perani et al., 1993). However, that process of decay would take place with marked individual variability, as in lower animals. Moreover, considerable variability might also determine whether the impairment of hippocampal connectivity affects memory acquisition or memory retrieval, both evidently impaired in most of the aged to one degree or another.

However, much of the impaired capacity to recall that affects some of the aged may be attributed to the loss of stored information—in other words, to the deterioration of cortical memory networks. Here again, though, we must deal with uncertainty and inconsistency. The structure of the human neocortex does not seem to age uniformly. There are reports of age-related and generalized cortical cell loss (e.g., Brody, 1955), but these have been disputed mainly for reasons of methodology (Cragg, 1975; Haug et al., 1981, 1983). Nonetheless, it seems indisputable that cell shrinkage and death do normally occur in the cortex   and that they accelerate with involution in certain regions of the neocortex. Especially affected appear to be associative areas of the frontal and temporal lobes (Huttenlocher, 1979; Haug et al., 1981, 1983; Terry et al., 1987). Similar changes have been observed in monkeys (Brizzee et al., 1980; Cupp and Uemura, 1980). Size, volume, and density of neurons in those regions generally decrease, possibly because of defective protein metabolism (Uemura and Hartman, 1978). The involution seems to affect most severely the dendrites and the synaptic contacts on them (Scheibel et al., 1975; Uemura, 1980). Notably impaired in the human, especially after age 50, are the basilar dendrites of pyramidal cells in supragranular layers of Wernicke's area, in the superior temporal gyrus (Jacobs and Scheibel, 1993). Given the importance of this area for semantic memory (see chapter 6) and of corticocortical connections with supragranular termination for the activation of cortical networks (see chapter 4), it is reasonable to infer that the dendritic degeneration observed is at the root of the often-observed age-related impairment in recall of names.

Normal aging also is accompanied by a general decrease in numbers and functional viability of cortical neurotransmitters. The evidence is especially strong for monoamine transmitters, which have been shown to decline in the rat (Finch, 1978), the monkey (Goldman-Rakic and Brown, 1981), and the human (Carlsson, 1981). In the monkey, the decline is particularly severe for dopamine in prefrontal cortex and may be related to the age-dependent deficit in learning and performance of delay tasks, for it can be reversed by clonidine, a norepinephrine agonist (Arnsten and Goldman-Rakic, 1985). In all likelihood, the cortical neurotransmitter decline of normal aging, and the cognitive deficits that accompany it, reflect the gradual involution of the subcortical nuclei that provide the neocortex with chemical transmitters. This is probably true particularly for the cholinergic system and the nucleus basalis of Meynert (Lacalle et al., 1991), which is most affected in Alzheimer's dementia. This point was emphasized in chapter 3 in the context of memory consolidation.

This section concludes by referring more generally to the importance of all neurotransmitter systems for the converse process: memory retrieval. These chemical modulators are essential not only for the making of the network but for its activation in memory recall. Logically, any weakening of the connective infrastructure of the network, as from losses of transmitters and synaptic contacts, is going to render the network less available for reactivation and recall.

Another index of the lesser availability of memory networks to retrieval as a function of aging is the general diminution of neocortical metabolism (Kuhl et al., 1982; Smith, 1984). The cause of this metabolic decline is obscure, but it may be related to the general decrease in cortical vascularization that also accompanies normal aging (Gustafson et al., 1978; Shaw et al., 1984). The evidence of involutional decrease of cortical blood flow, however, has been contested in subjects with total absence of vascular disease and risk factors (Mamo et al., 1983; Duara et al., 1984).

Memory failure in focal cortical pathological processes has been discussed in previous chapters in the context of localization and structure of memory. To emphasize the probable importance of the hippocampus and parahippocampal cortex for memory recall, the reader is reminded here of the interesting case presented by Schnider and colleagues (1992) and discussed in chapter 6. Whatever role the hippocampus plays in the retrieval of memory must be compatible with its better-established role in memory formation (see chapter 3). Carpenter and Grossberg (1993) have developed a network model, based on what they term *adaptive resonance theory* (ART), which accommodates both recognition and memory formation and resolves what they call the "stability-plasticity dilemma." Their hippocampal model incorporates novelty-detecting and memory-search mechanisms of interaction between hippocampus and self-organizing feature maps (Grossberg, 1972) of the neocortex.

A well-known general observation (Klatzky, 1975; Tulving, 1983) is that, regardless of pathology, semantic memory is more resistant to cortical damage, and thus more available to retrieval, than is declarative memory. The reason seems obvious and was discussed in chapters 5 and 6. The memory of facts, word meanings, and ideas is determined by varied and multiple associations; it is much more solidly anchored in cortical networks than the memory of events and concrete associations. Semantic networks probably have many more lines of associative access (including verbal associations) than episodic or declarative networks, which is probably what makes the former less vulnerable than the latter.

MECHANISMS OF ATTENTION

Attention, like memory, is a property of systems. It makes no more sense to speak of a special neural system for attention than it does to speak of one for memory. Both sensory and motor systems are endowed with the means for selecting information among alternatives. That is the hallmark of what we call *selective attention* (somewhat redundantly, because attention is selective by definition). Memory and attention are intimately interrelated. What we remember and for how long we remember it depends closely on that selective function of attention, as do the dynamics of active memory, which we will discuss in the next chapter.

The term *attention* has a phenomenological origin. William James (1890, pp. 403–404) defined it as

the taking possession by the mind, in clear and vivid form, of one out of what seem several simultaneously possible objects or trains of thought . . . It implies withdrawal from some things in order to deal effectively with others . . .

Obviously, James was referring to more than sensory stimuli as the potential object of attention, by this reflecting introspective—and popular—knowledge. His notions, however, largely because they were resistant to behavioral testing, generally were dismissed by the behavioristic psychology prevailing in the first half of this century. In fact, the entire subject of attention was considered, during that time, to be an almost illegitimate subject of study. In recent years, thanks to information theorists and cognitive psychologists, the study of attention has regained remarkable impetus and produced a large body of literature, although the neurobiology of attention has advanced only piecemeal. Little is known about attention's neural mechanisms, yet functionalist and even neurological theories of attention have proliferated at an increasing pace.

Here we will deal with the role and mechanisms of attention in perceptual and motor memory, particularly as they involve the cerebral cortex. I will make no attempt to substantiate or refute with neural data every plausible concept of attention in the literature but will consider cortical data obtained by use of suitable paradigms in the light of commonly held concepts, especially if the data bear on the relationship between attention and memory. The question of motor attention or "set" was discussed somewhat in chapter 7 and will be further discussed later.

"[R]ecognition and attentional selection consists in making perceptual categorizations" (Bundesen, 1990). This basic assumption, in a recent theoretical article on visual attention, points to the essence of attentive function in the sensory retrieval of perceptual memory. It needs only two important qualifiers to distinguish it from perception itself, for which we have accepted Hayek's (1952) definition as an act of classifying the world: Those qualifiers are time and selectivity. *Attention* is the perceptual categorization that, at a given time, the organism actively selects to fulfill its adaptive needs. This definition of attention, *mutatis mutandis*, could be applied to motor categorizations just as well. The *set for action* (motor attention) is the mirror image, on the output side, of the categorization of the sensory world that is required on the input side to make efficient use of limited system capacity. With these ideas in mind, we can resume the discussion where we left it off in the section on memory retrieval.

Once a stimulus has been recognized and a fragment of memory retrieved by it, whether consciously or unconsciously, two things can happen to the stimulus. One is that it is dismissed by the organism as inconsequential or disruptive and, along with a multitude of other stimuli, prevented from influencing behavior or entering subjective experience. Whether this involves some kind of neural filtering or inhibition will be discussed later. The other thing that can happen is that the stimulus, having been recognized as part of a memory which it helped retrieve and which calls for further action and analysis, enters selective processing within what is commonly understood as the focus of attention. The focusing of attention, however, need not be the separate function or mechanism that some postulate but rather an intrinsic property of the network that holds the memory and is mobilized to process information selectively and in an orderly manner. Indeed, if selective attention is merely perceptual (or motor) categorization, all we need for it is a memory network that does the job of associatively processing and channeling information within itself. This would take care of the selectivity of attention and of perception. For good reason, the terms *selective attention* and *selective perception* can be used interchangeably (Horn, 1965), although both are somewhat redundant. Later, we will deal with cortical manifestations of that selectivity.

There is, however, another aspect of attention, in addition to selectivity, that must be considered first in neural terms. It is the intensive aspect of attention that we commonly call *alertness*. The reasons for addressing it before the issue of selectivity are twofold: First, a certain minimum level of alertness is a precondition of attention and can be, at the same time, an enhancer of all inputs regardless of their source (Posner and Boies, 1971). Second, the substrate of alertness seems to lie in primordial subcortical structures of the brain stem, from where it can modulate the entirety of the cerebral cortex.

Alertness

The reticular core of the upper brain stem has long been considered the essential neural substrate of alertness or vigilance (Moruzzi and Magoun, 1949; French et al., 1952; Magoun, 1958). The electrical stimulation of what came to be called the *reticular activating system* awakens animals from sleep, inducing cortical electroencephalographic activation (fast frequency, low voltage) and behavioral arousal. Conversely, reticular lesions induce coma and lethargy. Several neurotransmitter systems (monoaminergic and cholinergic) with widespread cortical modulating influences are now known to have nuclei of origin or pathways within the reticular formations of the upper brain stem (Felten and Sladek, 1983; Hedreen et al., 1984).

The stimulation of those systems by electrical or chemical means activates widespread cortical regions. This activation not only can awaken the organism from sleep but, in the awake animal, can increase alertness, thereby enhancing attention. Here it is appropriate to refer to early data from my laboratory (Fuster, 1958; Fuster and Uyeda, 1962). In monkeys, the electrical stimulation of the mesencephalic reticular formation with a mild current facilitated the performance of a tachistoscopic test, a visuomotor task that required a high degree of attention (figure 8.6). The animal under stimulation was better able to discriminate visual stimuli presented with short exposure time, and its reaction time was shorter, than without stimulation. Higher currents had the opposite effects. The reticular facilitation of visual discrimination or other behaviors was demonstrated subsequently by other investigators (Mahut, 1964; Sterman and Fairchild, 1966; Frizzi, 1979).

In a theoretical paper, Deutsch and Deutsch (1963) recognized the necessity for a diffuse nonspecific system, such as the reticular activating system, as the basis for the mechanism of selective attention. However, instead of accepting that the role of the reticular system in attention might be secondary to its role in general alertness, they attempted to explain the selectivity of attention as an internal reticular mechanism. They postulated interactions between different levels of global activation of the system and variations in strength of different inputs from specific discrimination mechanisms, the net result of which would be the selective potentiation of certain discriminations above a "shifting reference standard" marked by the system. It is difficult to understand, however, how a system with such overlap of different plexuses (Scheibel and Scheibel, 1958) and such diffuse distribution of efferents could adjust its output to fit the selective and shifting necessities of attention.

In the 1960s and 1970s, many studies were conducted to clarify in humans the relationships between selective attention to sensory stimuli and the cortical macropotentials evoked by them. Clever paradigms

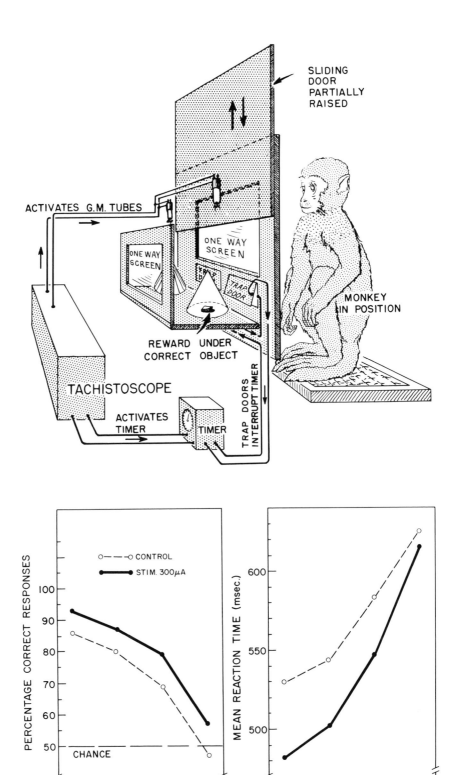

were designed to bring out correlations between attention and the magnitude of stimulus-evoked potentials that were presumed to reflect cortical involvement in sensory processing. Direct relationships were demonstrated between attention and evoked-potential size (Spong et al., 1965; Donchin and Cohen, 1967; Eason et al., 1969; Hillyard et al., 1973). Attention was shown to augment, in particular, potentials that had late-onset latency after the stimulus (e.g., the P300). The findings of these studies are consistent with the notion, expressed by Näätänen (1975) in an excellent critical review, that the observed evoked-potential enhancements were, for the most part, due to general nonspecific alertness, which is a precondition for selective attention, but not due to selective attention per se. In accord with this view are our earlier findings that, in lower organisms, cortical visual potentials were enhanced by electrical or chemical activation of the mesencephalic reticular formation and were depressed by an anesthetic or by reticular lesions (Reinoso-Suárez and Fuster, 1961; Fuster and Docter, 1962). Late potentials were particularly susceptible to changes in reticular activity.

Whereas increased alertness or vigilance, probably through brainstem modulating systems, enhances attention and its cortical mechanisms, it is clear that waning alertness or vigilance results in deterioration of attentive performance (Mackworth, 1970), and this too has its electrocortical manifestations. In the human, as vigilance diminishes during performance of a difficult visual detection task, the cortical potentials evoked by the detected stimuli diminish in amplitude, and performance deteriorates (Haider et al., 1964). Especially liable to waning vigilance, from fatigue or other factors, are the long latency potentials, such as the *P300* (Mane et al., 1983). Also liable is the contingency negative variation (CNV) or expectancy wave, a slow surface-negative cortical potential that occurs, mainly in frontal areas, after a stimulus, preparing the subject for a second stimulus and a motor response (Walter et al., 1964). Fatigue from sleep deprivation makes the CNV disappear (Naitoh et al., 1971). In accord with this, frontal lesions are known to diminish the capacity for sustained attention (Wilkins et al., 1987).

Gevins and coworkers (1990) have further substantiated some of the neural phenomena of decreased alertness by investigating event-related covariances during performance of a difficult memory task demanding fine motor-coordinated responses. As fatigue sets in, not only do

Figure 8.6 (*Top*) A monkey performing tachistoscopic discriminations. Two similar objects (a cone and a 12-sided pyramid) are presented in brief exposures, their relative position changed at random, and the animal must choose the correct object (the cone) immediately after each exposure. *Below:* Graphs of average performance under normal conditions (CONTROL) and under mild electrical stimulation (STIM) of the mesencephalic reticular formation. (From Fuster, 1958, with permission.)

evoked potentials and the CNV diminish but the topographical cortical patterns of covariance change in distribution and generally diminish in strength (figure 8.7). The latter phenomenon suggests that the memory network activated by the stimulus becomes less effective in its spatially and temporally selective operations. This attrition of the orderly recruitment of network components in space and time, on which selective attention is based, probably reflects the diminution of modulatory influences from the brain stem on the cortex.

Inputs from limbic structures can affect cortical activity in attention, although less massively and more selectively than brainstem inputs. The hippocampus and the amygdala which, as noted in chapter 3, play a critical role in the formation of cortical memory networks, may play a no less critical role in these networks' activation after they have been formed. In the previous section, I alluded already to the possible involvement of the hippocampus in memory retrieval. I shall conclude this section with a note on the involvement of both limbic formations in attention.

A simple alerting stimulus, before a monkey has to make a visual discrimination, can activate hippocampal cells with a short latency (fewer than 40 msec; Coburn et al., 1990); conceivably, those cells could, in turn, contribute to the preactivation of inferotemporal cortex before the discriminant stimulus arrives, after it has been processed in V1 and other extrastriate areas. The hippocampal input may prime the inferotemporal network for the latter to be selectively activated by subsequent visual input.

Furthermore, the reactions of some hippocampal cells to a given stimulus feature (color) are enhanced and prolonged by attention if the animal must retain that feature in memory for a short term (Fuster, 1991a). Thus, the hippocampus, which presumably helped establish the inferotemporal network that represents the visual stimulus, is apparently again involved in activation of that network as the animal attends to it and needs to retain it in active memory.

The amygdala, on the other hand, most likely plays a role in recognizing the motivational significance of any external stimulus. It too may be involved in cortical network activation. Amygdala units in the monkey have been noted to differentiate appetitive and aversive visual signals (Fuster and Uyeda, 1971), which indicates that those units are attuned to drive or motivation. Now, because of the preestablished associations of a cortical network with internal inputs related to those variables, the amygdala can activate that network (i.e., sensory association areas) retrogradely on arrival of the memory-retrieving stimulus, thus facilitating its analysis and categorization (LeDoux, 1989; 1993). Anatomical studies indicate that connections between amygdala and association cortex are numerous, reciprocal, and widespread (Turner et al., 1980; Van Hoesen, 1981; Barbas and De Olmos, 1990).

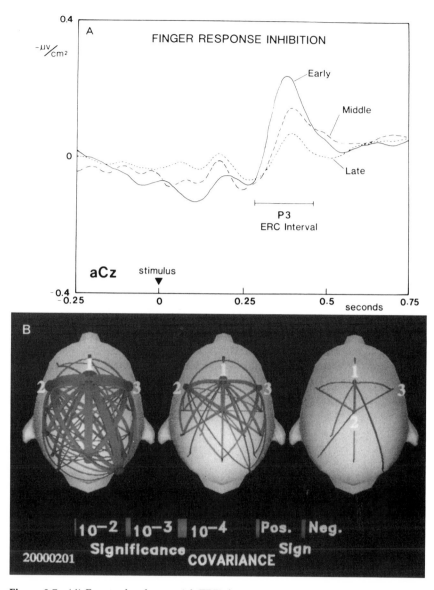

Figure 8.7 (*A*) Event-related potential (ERP) from a vertex electrode site (aCz) in a task in which the subject continuously has to attend to stimuli requiring the inhibition of a finger response. The amplitude of the P_3 component (long latency) of the evoked potential diminishes from an early to a late stage of performance. ERC, event-related covariance. (*B*) Event-related covariance in three stages of performance (early, middle, and late). Covariance diminishes globally as a function of task stage and, presumably, fatigue. (From Gevins et al., 1990, with permission.)

Selective Attention

Having considered the contributions of brain-stem and limbic structures to the more general (alertness) and motivational aspects of cortical attention mechanisms, we come to the discussion of the selectivity of those mechanisms. Let us now discuss the selective activation or inhibition of cortical areas and networks beyond their more general modulation related to arousal, alertness, and biological drive.

Before proceeding further, one important distinction of attentive selectivity is necessary because, as we shall see, it has cortical manifestations, especially evident with regard to vision. An animal can heed two general aspects of a stimulus: (1) its location (selectivity by location) and (2) its qualities or attributes, such as color, shape, pitch, and texture (selectivity by property). It will be remembered that two separate cortical systems have been proposed, one for spatial vision and the other for object vision (see chapters 4 and 6). Location, however, can be legitimately viewed as just another attribute of a stimulus—present, expected, or remembered—and not by itself as a categorical entity without object. Thus, spatial attention can be subsumed under attention to property (Posner, 1988): One would be a special case of the other and nested within it. Yet, as mentioned earlier, spatial attention probably has its own cortical map, most likely including parts of parietal cortex (see chapter 6).

Now the basic assumption about attention, articulated earlier, can be modified and expanded to make it a neurally testable hypothesis: *Attentive selectivity* is the categorization of sensory stimuli and motor responses that the activated memory network implements in accord with a temporal and spatial order inherent in the network. Much of the selectivity of cortical areas and networks in perceptual and motor categorization was already discussed in the previous two chapters, where we gathered evidence for the cortical structure of representational networks. There, we inferred structure from function. Here, we deal with function itself, with those networks in operation, thus attempting to substantiate our postulate and better understand the dynamics of memory.

As we have seen in the discussion of memory retrieval, a memory network apparently is not activated all at once and to the same degree. Immediately following a retrieval stimulus, patterns of activation and covariance have been noted to migrate over the cortex in some experiments (e.g., Gevins et al., 1989a,b). Here, a few words on methodology are appropriate. Of course, if the memory retrieved simply leads to internal representations without motor consequences, the tracing of cortical activation is difficult, if not impossible. Neuroscience does not yet have the means to trace trains of internal representations outside of structured behavior. When, however, as in experiments previously mentioned, the retrieved memory is a temporally extended structure of behavior (a behavioral *gestalt*) with component sensory and motor representations, then we can trace, by electrical means, the activity of the network as it becomes operational and as behavior is implemented. Once the perception-action cycle (see chapter 9) has been set in motion, the internal dynamics of the network become traceable from one categorization to the next. The focus of attention (or of representation) can thus be followed from one part of the network to another. Experimentally interjected delays between stimuli and responses, as in memory tasks, help to separate in time, and thus better to distinguish, categorizations of perception from those of action.

At every step along the way, as processing goes from one part of the network to another and the focus of attention shifts with it, the network must reach back into previous stages for finer analysis. That turning of the network on itself (closing a kind of internal perception-action cycle) probably makes use of recurrent collaterals in a manner we cannot yet understand precisely. Through them, as was postulated (see chapter 5), feedback (up-down) excitation has the effect of enhancing discrimination at lower levels and sharpening the focus of attention.

Until now, we have assumed that categorization proceeds forward and backward through the activated network as an excitatory wave, recruiting in orderly fashion its neuronal aggregates, arranged in modules or otherwise, and selectively increasing their firing level. Orderly and selective cortical excitation would be the essence of the process, allowing for covariant and sustained activation of numerous network components simultaneously. Later, neural evidence for this view will be presented. There is, however, a reverse and complementary side to attentive focusing that probably is based on the opposite of excitation: *inhibition*.

When we attend to something in particular, everything else seems to be suppressed by our nervous system and removed from awareness. A good example is the proverbial selective listening at a noisy party. Ever since psychologists became interested in information theory, that suppressive component of attention gained preeminence, and experiments with focused, divided, or overloaded attention lent it support (Cherry, 1953; Mowbray, 1953; Webster and Thompson, 1954; Moray, 1959; Treisman, 1960). All this led to the *filter theory* of attention (Broadbent, 1958; Treisman, 1964). It was argued that because of the limited capacity of sensory processing systems, attention is, above all, a filtering process. Only what is attended gets through, and all else is filtered out. To be sure, there is also preattentive or early scrutiny of what comes in (Treisman and Gormican, 1988), a kind of fast, parallel, and unconscious processing that selectively can retrieve material from unattended messages if relevant cues are embedded in them (Moray, 1959; Treisman, 1960). There is also a short-term memory store or buffer to take care of possible overload of information (Broadbent, 1958). Nonetheless, the essence of the postulated attention system is the rejection of what is *not* attended, not the enhancement of what *is* attended.

Both selective enhancement and suppression, however, are compatible in neural terms, at least theoretically, if we combine the excitatory process of categorization with lateral inhibition or something akin to it. Be that as it may, the first neural data obtained on the focusing of attention reflected the inhibition of the unattended. When the cat is attending to a mouse in a jar, click-evoked potentials in the cochlear nucleus diminish in size (Hernández-Peón et al., 1956). Auditory habituation was reported to have the same effect (Galambos et al., 1955). Some investigators (Marsh et al., 1962; Worden and Marsh, 1963), using careful control procedures, were unable to reproduce the latter phenomenon and others argued that, if real, the neural effects inferred might take place at rather peripheral levels of sensory systems (reviewed by Horn, 1965). In any event, psychophysical experiments indicated that, in a visuomotor task, filtering takes place on the perceptual and not on the motor side of the processing chain (Treisman and Geffen, 1967).

Single-unit data obtained by Moran and Desimone (1985) provide some support for the concept of attentive filtering in the extrastriate cortex of the monkey. In their experiment, the animal is forced constantly to fixate vision on a central spot on a screen. A small stimulus, to which the animal must attend without moving its gaze from center, is presented within the receptive field of a single cell in area V4 or inferotemporal cortex, eliciting a strong excitatory response of the cell. When the animal is forced to attend a second stimulus some distance away but still in the receptive field, then the response to the first stimulus drops substantially in magnitude. It is as if the receptive field had shrunk to accommodate the second stimulus and thus almost excluded the first. An attenuation index (ratio of response to unattended over attended first stimulus) reflects the amount of the attention-related descent in unit response. The authors of this study conclude that their data are evidence of attentive gating within the receptive fields of extrastriate units. An important methodological problem is that the behavioral paradigm utilized in these experiments is somewhat unnatural; the monkey is forced to attend to stimuli out of the center of gaze, thus splitting attention between the fixation spot and peripheral stimuli in a task that is essentially a test of spatial attention. Nonetheless, the data constitute reasonable prima facie evidence of attention-related neuronal selectivity in paravisual cortex. These data are compatible with the concept of inhibitory filtering in selective spatial attention. A subsequent unit study (Chelazzi et al., 1993) supports this concept further.

Inhibitory filtering is also an important element of Crick's conceptualization of the neural basis of selective attention (Crick, 1984). According to his *searchlight* idea of attention, inhibitory influences from the reticular nucleus of the thalamus would modulate cortical synapses to sharpen the encoding of certain stimuli and stimulus configurations.

More congruent with the view that attention basically consists in perceptual categorization (with lateral inhibition possibly playing a supportive or ancillary role) is the evidence of attentional enhancement of unit responses in association cortex. Using behavioral paradigms similar to the eye-fixation paradigm mentioned previously, cellular responses to visual stimuli have been seen to be facilitated by selective attention in posterior parietal cortex (Bushnell et al., 1981; Mountcastle et al., 1981; Goldberg and Bruce, 1985), inferotemporal cortex (Richmond and Sato, 1987; Sato, 1988; Spitzer and Richmond, 1991), and prefrontal cortex (Goldberg and Bushnell, 1981). Conversely, expected tactile stimuli have been noted to produce smaller unit responses than unexpected tactile stimuli in the polymodal cortex of the depth of the superior temporal sulcus (Mistlin and Perrett, 1990). In this observation, however, it is difficult to exclude the possible influence of alertness and emotional factors that have a nonselective role in attention.

Using a delayed-matching paradigm, I attempted to clarify the functional involvement of neurons of the inferotemporal cortex in selective nonspatial visual attention (Fuster, 1990). My objective was to find out whether inferotemporal neurons, which are known to detect certain visual features in the environment, would respond selectively to one such feature when the animal must selectively attend to it (i.e., must extract it from a complex stimulus for behavioral use). The stimulus at the start of each trial, always presented in the same central position, was a large colored disk (8 degrees of visual angle) with a gray symbol in the middle (figure 8.8). Depending on the symbol, the monkey was required to memorize the symbol itself or else the background color, and then appropriately respond after a 10 to 20-second delay. Thus, in some trials the color was relevant, and in others it was irrelevant. An important objective of the study was to compare the reactions of inferotemporal units to a given color when the animal attended to it and their reactions to the same color (identical size, brightness, position) when the animal did not attend to it. What role does attention play in inferotemporal cell response to a stimulus dimension (color) even if its value as a behavioral cue is not spatially defined? A purpose in using nonspatially defined cues was to circumvent problems of ocular motility by taking advantage of the large receptive fields of inferotemporal units (Desimone et al., 1984).

Many cells responded indiscriminately and with short latency to all stimuli, regardless of their features. Others responded preferentially to one given feature, a symbol or a color. Among those that selected color (red or green), there were some on which attention had no effect: They differentiated the colors equally well whether color was relevant or not. Others, however, showed greater responses to their preferred color

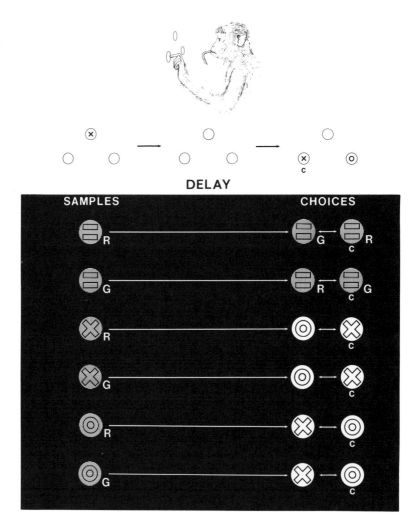

Figure 8.8 Schematic diagram of a task demanding selective attention to visual features (color or shape). Each trial begins with brief presentation, on the top button, of one of the six sample stimuli, each a combination of color and symbol. After a delay, two stimuli appear in the lower buttons for matching to the sample and for choice. The pressing of the correct button (c)—that is, the button with the distinctive feature of the sample (color or symbol)—leads to juice reward. That feature's position changes at random between the left and the right button. The = symbol on red (R) or green (G) sample is followed by the same symbol on the two colors at the choice; the animal must choose the color of the sample. The X or O symbol at the sample is followed by the two symbols on white background; the animal must choose the symbol in the sample. In the trained animal, = forces attention to color, whereas X or O forces attention to symbol. (From Fuster, 1990, with permission.)

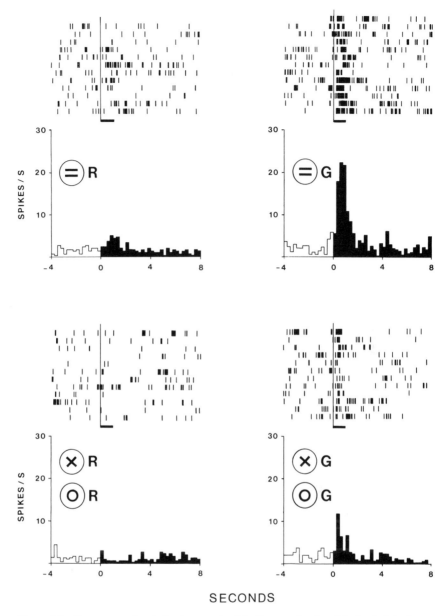

Figure 8.9 Responses of an inferotemporal cell to the sample stimuli in the task in figure 8.8. The cell responds more to color, especially green, when color is relevant (top graphs) than when it is not (bottom graphs). (From Fuster, 1990, with permission.)

Dynamics of Cortical Memory: Retrieval and Attention

when color was relevant than when it was not (figure 8.9). These cells had the longest response latency (most had an onset latency longer than 200 msec). An attention index (the reciprocal of the attenuation index of Moran and Desimone, 1985) was calculated for all color-selective cells and applied to their responses to the preferred color. That index was found to be directly related to the latency of the response to color. In other words, the greater the attention-related enhancement of a cell's response to color, the longer was the onset latency of that response (figure 8.10).

These findings indicate that the reactions of inferotemporal neurons to a nonspatial stimulus quality such as color are enhanced when that quality, without changing physical properties, becomes relevant and the animal must attend to it. The results further indicate that the enhancing effect of attention is most pronounced in cells that have long latency of response. This suggests that these cells, which categorize color as a behaviorally relevant feature and seem therefore involved in selective attention (categorization) for color, lie in deeper stages of sensory information processing. Not only are these findings in accord with the basic assumption that sensory attention consists in perceptual categorization guided from the top down by endogenous factors, but they support the notion of serial processing in attention (Koch and Ullman, 1985). After the rapid screening and parallel processing of early or preattentive stages, processing of a stimulus would enter a serial processing phase, during which contextual cues (e.g., the symbol in my experiment) would be analyzed before the neural substrate for the behaviorally relevant category is reached. All this would take place under the guidance of endogenous factors that at this time cannot be specified but must be assumed to derive from long-term memory. From where could they stem but the history of the stimuli and their context?

Neuroimaging has also contributed to the neurobiological knowledge of selective attention. For example, a study by Roland (1981) revealed that while human subjects attended to an expected light touch on the tip of their index finger, regional cerebral blood flow, which is an indirect measure of local metabolic rate, increased (by some 25 percent) in the contralateral somatosensory cortex (figure 8.11). A lesser increase was observed in dorsolateral prefrontal cortex.

Positron emission tomography has been used as well to image cortical metabolic activity in selective attention. Corbetta and coworkers (1990) had human subjects discriminate different attributes of visual stimuli (shape, color, and velocity). While the subject paid attention to a given stimulus dimension, activity increased in a restricted region of extrastriate cortex in both medial and lateral aspects of the cerebral hemispheres. Attention to stereognostic features of tactually perceived objects activates somatosensory cortex (Roland and Larsen, 1976). When attention is focused on spatial rather than qualitative aspects of the

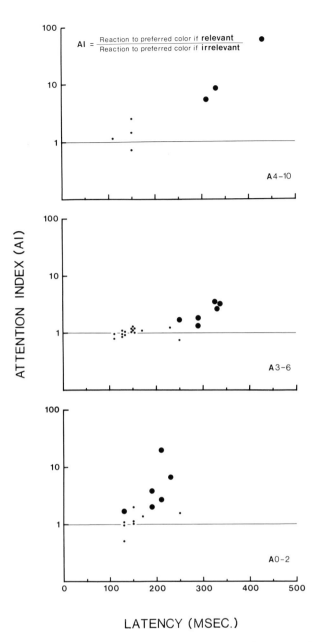

Figure 8.10 Relationship between attention index (see text) and inferotemporal cell–response latency in three animals. Cells from each animal, and a different inferotemporal position, are plotted in each separate graph. Cells that prefer one color, especially when it is relevant (so-called color-attentive cells), are represented by large dots. (From Fuster, 1990, with permission.)

Dynamics of Cortical Memory: Retrieval and Attention

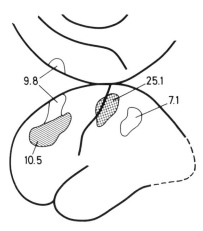

Figure 8.11 Increased percentage of blood flow in somatosensory cortex ($p < .001$) during expected touch of the index finger. (From Roland, 1981, with permission.)

visual environment, superior parietal and superior frontal cortex are activated (Corbetta et al., 1993), in keeping with the surmised importance of these two regions for spatial attention (see chapter 6).

In conclusion, the available evidence gathered thus far points to the notion that perceptual attention is based on the selective activation of certain areas of cortex involved in representation and categorization of behaviorally relevant sensory features. Furthermore, the evidence is consistent with the possibility that the activation of neuronal groups in those areas is accompanied by inhibition of neuronal groups that represent nonrelevant features. This filtering function would sharpen, in cortical representation, the contrast between an attribute that is relevant and those that are not. Lateral or recurrent inhibition may play a role in this filtering function.

Can we speak of *motor attention* as motor categorization in the same way as we speak of perceptual attention as perceptual categorization? I believe we can, but by disregarding the common phenomenological view of attention exclusively as a sensory selective function.

There are classes or *categories of action* much as there are classes or categories of perception. In chapters 4 and 7 we have seen that frontal areas (i.e., areas in front of the central [rolandic] fissure) constitute the cortical levels of the neural hierarchy for representation and processing of motor action. All classes of action are represented in that hierarchy, from the most general to the most concrete. At the lowest cortical level, in motor cortex, the finest and most specific movements are represented. Conversely, the most complex, global, and temporally extended structures of behavior are represented in prefrontal cortex, which constitutes the highest level of the motor hierarchy. The processing of those behavioral structures commences when the networks that represent them cease to be merely representational and become operational—in other words, when they channel information to lower levels for motor enactment. That processing generally continues downward, engaging successive subcortical loops, toward motor cortex and the pyramidal tract. Lower stages of the processing hierarchy feed back to prefrontal cortex, where that behavior is not only represented in schematic fashion but is organized in the temporal domain (Fuster, 1989).

There is, therefore, a symmetrical cortical organization for representation and processing of sensation, on the one hand, and for representation and processing of action, on the other. Perceptual categories are represented and processed up their hierarchy, from the lowest and most concrete to the most general. Action categories are represented and—within the limits noted in chapter 7—processed down their hierarchy, from the most general to the most concrete. In both hierarchies, as we proceed from the center of the system to the periphery, large classes include smaller classes, the smaller nested within the larger, in perception as well as in action.

The word *set* comes closest to characterizing motor attention. It connotes the qualities of adaptation and preparation for movement. Of course, there is set, as there is planning, for large action as well as for small action. All classes of action have corresponding neural structures and mechanisms for motor set, although neither have been identified with precision. Frontal areas, however, are stacked from the top down (prefrontal, premotor, and motor) for progessively more concrete and immediate set and action (see chapter 7). The structural (connective) symmetry with perceptual processing areas is preserved in functional terms, as we noted, even with regard to the temporal order of processing. Perceptual attention succeeds the alerting or memory-retrieving sensory stimulus, whereas, motor set precedes the consequent motor action. There is an intimate functional relationship between perceptual attention and motor set. For one thing, orienting movements of the eyes and head are clearly at the service of perceptual attention and are guided by it. For another, motor set is strictly dependent on sensory cues and proprioceptive inputs (consider haptics). There is a constant interplay of the two at all levels in the perception-action cycle (see chapter 9).

Precisely because of that sensorimotor interdependence, the neurobiology of motor set is difficult to study. For experimental purposes, it is easier simply to time-lock perceptual attention to a discrete sensory stimulus (as I did in the inferotemporal experiment cited earlier [Fuster, 1990]) than it is to time-lock motor set to equally discrete and well-controlled movements. Nonetheless, as pointed out in the previous chapter, the set-related activity of neurons before movement has been substantiated in motor cortex (Evarts and Tanji, 1976; Lecas et al., 1986), premotor cortex (Godschalk et al., 1981; Wise and Mauritz, 1985; Di Pellegrino and Wise, 1991; Riehle and Requin, 1993), and prefrontal cortex (Kubota and Funahashi, 1982; Watanabe, 1986a, b; Quintana and Fuster, 1992; Di Pellegrino and Wise, 1993).

The most convincing evidence we have thus far of prefrontal neuron involvement in motor attention (set) comes from the use of a delay task with thorough separation of cue and response, not only in time but in space (Quintana and Fuster, 1992). This feature is methodologically essential, because it allows us to clarify whether the activity of a given cell is correlated with the sensory or the motor aspects of the task; sensory and motor correlations are mutually confounded in most unit studies that make use of spatial delay tasks, whether manual or oculomotor. Our task (figure 8.12) fulfills the requirements of spatial and temporal dissociation and, in addition, imposes different strengths of behavioral contingency between stimuli (colors) and the directionality (right or left) of manual response. In this manner, the two neuron types described earlier (see chapter 7) have been better exposed than with other tasks: sensory-coupled cells whose activation decreases in the

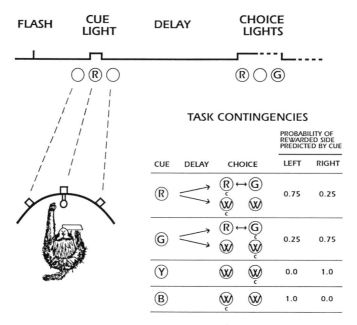

Figure 8.12 Schematic view of task with temporal and spatial separation of cue and response (choice). The monkey faces a panel with three small stimulus buttons. Following a diffuse warning flash, the cue, one of four colors, appears in the central button. After a delay, the two lateral buttons turn either red (R) and green (G) or both white (W). If the buttons are colored, the monkey must choose the one matching the cue; if white, the animal must choose left for red cue, right for green cue, right for yellow (Y) cue, and left for blue (B) cue. Consequently, yellow and blue cue predict the response side (right and left, respectively) with 100 percent probability, whereas red and green cue predict the response side with 75 percent probability (left if red, right if green). Colors and position of choice are changed at random. (From Quintana and Fuster, 1992, with permission.)

course of the delay, and motor-coupled cells that concomitantly accelerate their discharge as the motor response approaches. Furthermore, we have observed that the acceleration of discharge is proportional to the strength of contingency between stimulus and response. The stronger the contingency, and thus the better the animal can predict the direction of the motor response, the steeper is the accelerating slope of the discharge that precedes it (figure 8.13). The cells seem to reflect the probability of the motor act to which they are attuned and for which the animal is preparing.

Summing up, in the dorsolateral prefrontal cortex, which is the highest stage for sensorimotor integration in the time domain, we have suggestive evidence of a neural basis for the transfer of the focus of attention from perception to movement. This transfer is revealed by a shift of excitation from cells encoding the memory of the stimulus to cells encoding the memory of the response. Moreover, the relation between the firing of the response-coupled cells and the probability of

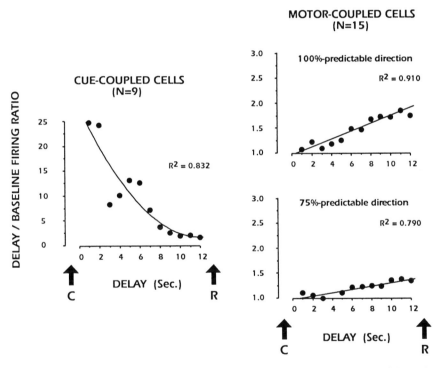

Figure 8.13 Average discharge of cells in prefrontal cortex during the delay of the task in figure 8.12. C, cue; R, response. (*Left*) Descending discharge of cue-coupled cells (perceptual memory activation). (*Right*) Accelerating discharge in anticipation of the response (motor memory activation). Note that the slope of acceleration of firing is related to the predictability of response direction. (From Quintana and Fuster, 1992, with permission.)

the response they encode is, in itself, an argument for the participation of the prefrontal network they constitute in the making of that response. While the response is still in preparation, that network is most likely engaged in motor set. We can only speculate about the underlying mechanism, which probably includes the excitatory priming of lower cortical and subcortical stages of the motor hierarchy for the impending movement. This will be explored further in the next chapter.

9 Dynamics of Cortical Memory: Active Memory

An evoked memory or the memory of a recent event can continue in our awareness well after we have retrieved the memory or experienced the event. The memory stays within an internal focus of attention that I have earlier named the *focus of representation*. Such a memory, to which we persistently attend, is what is here called an *active memory*. This is an anthropocentric concept of memory, not defined by content or duration but by phenomenal state—that is, by the fact that a given memory can remain attended to, in consciousness—and, in that state, capable of controlling behavior, speech, and the trend of thought. (Of course, unconscious or marginally conscious memories, which are out of the focus of representation, can also do that to some extent.) Clearly this state of memory is akin to what James (1890) called *primary memory* (see chapter 2).

The trouble for neuroscience and for experimental psychology is that a concept such as that of active memory, as I have introduced it, is not amenable to objective study without easily falling into tautological reasoning or trivial measurement. Yet the concept cannot be dismissed as an intractable issue of subjective psychology. Above all, it is useful because it leads to a useful hypothesis in studies of primate memory with human relevance—namely, the hypothesis that *an* active memory is an active cortical network, its neurons active above certain baseline or spontaneous level of firing. At the very least, the idea of active memory as a dynamic state of cortical representation comes closer to explaining a wide range of neural phenomena of mnemonic storage (reviewed later) than does the construct of yet another memory system. Indeed, as we have seen in previous chapters, there is no evidence of separate cortical systems for long- and short-term memory, for memory in permanent storage and memory in transient storage. There is, however, ample evidence that the two stores are one and the same but in different dynamic states.

In previous chapters, I have attempted to objectify the substrate of established memory—that is, the cortical layout of what we could call passive or latent memory. Here the goal is to objectify active memory and to examine that layout in the active state. I will attempt to substantiate the hypothesis, stated in chapter 5, that under certain conditions a memory network becomes and stays active above a certain level or threshold and, in that state, remains useful for current behavior as a temporary store of information. To a degree, my colleagues and I have already done this by employing functional methods to trace experimentally the topography of established memory contents on the surface of the neocortex (see chapters 6 and 7). We are going to do it again to explore further the dynamics of cortical memory in behavior.

So-called working memory (Baddeley, 1983) is an operational concept of active memory and, as such, useful for its neural analysis. It can be defined as the ad hoc memorization of a discrete item of information for a motor or cognitive act to be performed in the short term; thus, working memory has been construed as one kind of short-term memory. (Another kind, as discussed in chapter 2, would be the short-term process of consolidating permanent memory.) However, active memory, which need not have a behavioral purpose, subsumes and transcends working memory. It does not have a specific cortical locus or system, although the frontal cortex, as we shall see, is exceedingly important for it.

Delay tasks are the best and most widely used tests of working memory, and their value for investigating the neural aspects of active memory is, as we shall see, unequaled. Before proceeding with this discussion, however, it seems necessary to reemphasize that neither the concept of working memory nor the means to test it (delay tasks) can provide more than a limited view of active memory, however useful to the experimenter. At the same time, we must not underestimate those tasks or misinterpret them as irrelevant or unnatural. To appreciate fully their importance and the generality of the memory process they require, one need consider only how indispensable that process is for the making of any new and temporally extended structure of behavior, speech, or thought. All sequential behaviors that are nonroutine necessitate a mechanism of temporal information storage to attain their goal. No creative speech is possible without that mechanism. Without it, logical thinking cannot reach its conclusions. Active memory is part and parcel of any behavioral or cognitive gestalt that we may wish or need to construct in the course of time. The individual trial of a delay task is the simplified epitomy of such a gestalt.

TOPOGRAPHY OF ACTIVE MEMORY

The delay task is also a practical means to activate working memory for a well-controlled period of time (i.e., the delay period of each trial). Thus, the method opens up active memory to rigorous neurophysiological study. Obviously, one of its first objectives is to define the cortical distribution of activated memories, which we can assume to vary widely depending on their content. A direct, though not necessarily precise, approach to this issue is to test the effects of selectively inactivating cortical areas of association, by lesion or otherwise, on the animal's performance of memory tasks. For this purpose, a procedure of reversible inactivation clearly is preferable to the traditional method of surgical ablation, because the first, unlike the second, allows the use of the animal repeatedly as its own control. Furthermore, reversible lesions avoid the imponderable effects of ablation (e.g., secondary degeneration) on neural structures at a distance from the area ablated.

Regional cooling is a convenient method to inactivate or depress the cortex reversibly and thus to test the involvement of any given cortical area in active memory. All our studies with this method have been conducted by use of implanted cortical cooling probes (figure 9.1) in monkeys trained to perform one or more delay tasks.

When a large portion of their inferotemporal (IT) cortex is bilaterally cooled to 20°C, monkeys exhibit a reversible impairment of a visual delayed matching task for color (figure 9.2). The procedure affects only minimally, if at all, the performance of a spatial delayed-response task. These findings implicate IT cortex in the active retention of colors while suggesting that active memory of spatial information is retained elsewhere, possibly in parietal or frontal cortex.

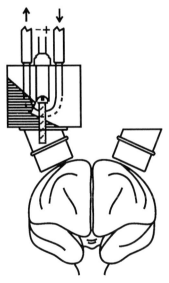

Figure 9.1 Diagram of two cooling probes over a frontal view of the monkey's brain. A thermoelectric (Peltier) cooler is attached to one of them. The probes are permanently implanted in the animal, lying over the dura mater above the cortical area to be cooled. Also implanted are subdural thermistors to monitor and control the local cortical temperature by electrically regulating the cooling power of the coolers. The latter are attached to the probes only for the experiment.

Dynamics of Cortical Memory: Active Memory

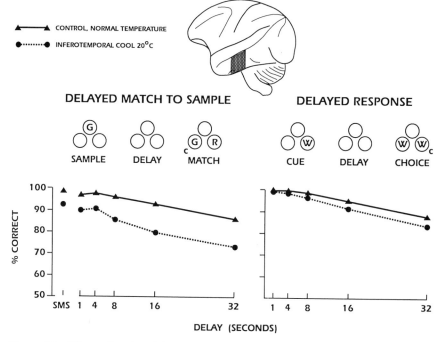

Figure 9.2 Effects of cooling bilaterally a portion of inferotemporal cortex (shaded area in the brain diagram) on performance of the two delay tasks. Control testing is done with coolers in place but inoperative. c, correct response; SMS, simultaneous matching to sample; G, green; R, red; W, white.

Note, however, that in addition to impairing delayed matching, IT cooling induces a statistically significant deficit in simultaneous matching to sample (SMS); see the two isolated points at the left of the graph in figure 9.2. This observation, which was considered only cursorily when my colleagues and I first published the data (Fuster et al., 1981) and which was replicated in another cooling study with zero delay (Horel and Pytko, 1982), indicates that the cooling impairs not only visual short-term memory but also discrimination. This may mean that IT inactivation causes some kind of perceptual defect in addition to the defect in active memory (delays of 1 second or longer). A sensory defect is unlikely, however, because cooling fails to impair visually guided behavior outside of the testing situation and the visual delayed-response task with short delays. The most likely explanation for the SMS deficit is that it reflects the monkey's difficulty in eliciting the long-term engrams of the discrimination of colors in the context of the task; in other words, the animal has trouble retrieving associative long-term memory stored in IT networks.

This interpretation is consistent with the assumption that the same IT cortex that ablation studies have shown to be important for acquisition and long-term storage of visual memory (see chapter 6) is important for its short-term activation. It also is consistent with my general hypothesis, further supported by neuron-discharge data (see chapter 6 and text following), that long-term memory and active short-term memory share the same cortical substrate. It would be wrong to conclude, however, that IT cooling either wipes out the memory trace or completely blocks its activation, because the cooling effects noted earlier, although highly significant, are relatively mild. It is more reasonable to infer from the results that the cooling merely depresses IT function so as to weaken both the retrieval and the short-term activation of visual memory.

In conclusion, the cryogenic depression of a modality-specific associative area of posterior cortex seems to hinder the activation of a modality-specific memory (for color). Now the question is whether and to what extent, in the context of the behavioral task, the prefrontal cortex takes part in the active representation of that memory and its behavioral consequences. If our thinking is correct (see chapters 5 through 8), perceptual memory networks associated with behavioral action extend to, and link with, motor memory networks in frontal cortex. Thus, the cryogenic depression of this cortex ought to depress the latter networks and interfere with the tasks they mediate. Moreover, given the convergence of pathways from posterior cortex on dorsolateral prefrontal cortex (see chapter 4), and given the neuropsychological evidence of the supramodal (i.e., modality-nonspecific) role of the dorsolateral prefrontal cortex in the temporal organization of behavior (see chapter 7 and text following), we reasonably can predict that the cooling of this cortex will adversely affect all delay tasks, regardless of the sensory modality of the memorandum.

Thus far, we have observed cooling-induced prefrontal deficits in tasks with visual (Fuster and Alexander, 1970; Fuster and Bauer, 1974; Bauer and Fuster, 1976), tactile (Fuster et al., 1990), and auditory (Sierra-Paredes and Fuster, 1993) memoranda. A prefrontal deficit occurs whether or not what the monkey has to remember is spatially defined (Bauer and Fuster, 1976; Quintana and Fuster, 1993). This is particularly interesting in view of the commonly held notion, derived from ablation studies, that the dorsolateral prefrontal cortex is specialized mainly in the processing of spatial information; this seems to be a misconception, although a spatial role may still obtain (in addition to the temporal role) for a portion of dorsolateral prefrontal cortex, such as the cortex of the sulcus principalis (Goldman-Rakic, 1987; Fuster, 1989).

Let us look at a few graphic examples of reversible prefrontal deficit. Figure 9.3 illustrates such a deficit with the same visual tasks used earlier to test IT cooling (see figure 9.2). Mark that prefrontal cooling impairs almost equally the nonspatial (delayed color-match) and the spatial (delayed-response) task.

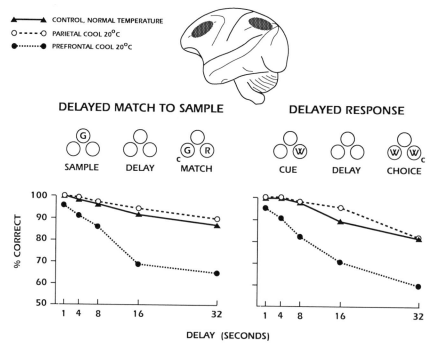

Figure 9.3 Effects of cooling bilaterally portions of dorsolateral prefrontal cortex or posterior parietal cortex (*shaded area* above) on performance of two delay tasks. C, correct response; G, green; R, red; W, white.

Figure 9.4 shows three delay tasks that involve the haptic sense. The top two require a cross-temporal transfer of information between touch and vision (Di Mattia et al., 1990). The lower task is performed by exclusive reliance on haptics. Prefrontal cooling reversibly impaired the performance of monkeys on all three tasks (figure 9.5), whereas posterior parietal cooling failed to do so (Fuster et al., 1990; Shindy et al., in press). It should be noted that reaction time was not affected by either prefrontal or parietal cooling, thus practically ruling out the possibility that the performance deficit might be caused by a cooling-induced lowering of motivation. The failure of parietal cooling, in our experiment, to affect haptic behavior is somewhat surprising but understandable because that cooling did not directly affect the areas that are seemingly most critical for haptics, SI and SII (see chapter 6).

Thus, the inference has been supported, and so far not contradicted, that perceptual networks of posterior cortex blend with associated motor networks of frontal cortex. A delay task relies on the activation of a posterior network for the modality of the memorandum and, in addition, on the activation of an associated prefrontal network essential for organizing the motor response called for by the memorandum. A delay task depends on both and can be impaired by depressing either. Having

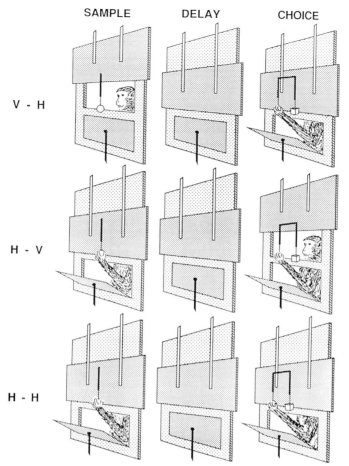

SAMPLE   DELAY   CHOICE

V - H

H - V

H - H

Figure 9.4 Three delayed matching tasks with visual and tactile stimuli. V–H, visual to haptic; H–V, haptic to visual; H–H, haptic to haptic. (From Di Mattia et al., 1990, with permission.)

considered these generalities on the topography of active memory, let us now consider its neural dynamics.

CORTICAL DYNAMICS AND MEMORY CELLS

While a monkey waits to perform a motor act in accord with a recent sensory stimulus, as in a delay task, innumerable neurons in widespread areas of its neocortex undergo sustained elevations of firing. The degree of such neuronal activation and the distribution of activated neurons, which are mainly, I suppose, pyramidal cells (the largest and easiest to detect with a microelectrode), depend on the nature of both the stimulus and the required motor response.

Such are the cells that have been dubbed *memory cells*. I call them this not only because they are active while the animal is memorizing infor-

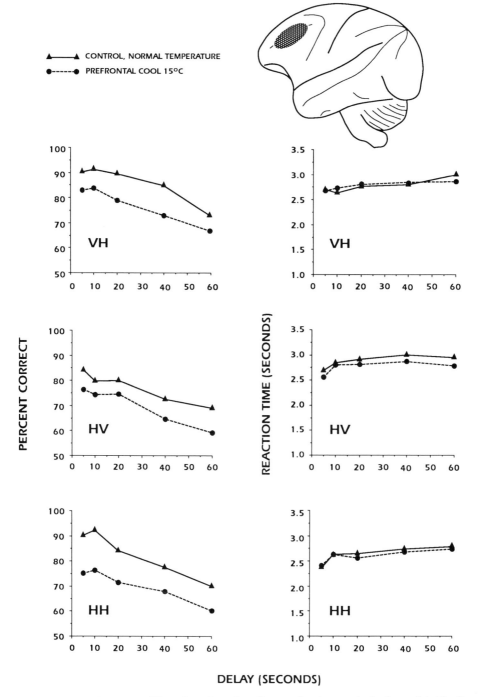

Figure 9.5 Bilateral prefrontal cooling on the three tasks in figure 9.4. Shading marks prefrontal area cooled. VH, visual to haptic; HV, haptic to visual; HH, haptic to haptic. (From Shindy et al., in press, with permission.)

mation but because their activation is contingent on a number of variables related to that information and the ability of the animal to retain it for the short term. These features strongly indicate that the cells in question are constituents of the activated network representing that information.

The concept of memory cells is useful for characterizing the properties of certain units in certain behavioral settings, as well as for drawing inferences from those properties, as I do here. However, the name may be misleading and requires a note of caution. Memory cells may be involved not only in temporary memory but in other cortical functions as well. Conversely, memory cells are but one category of units, among others, in any given cortical area. Hence, the concept does not contradict our basic position, that all cortical areas are involved in several aspects of information processing, memory being just one of them.

The first memory cells were discovered in the prefrontal cortex of monkeys performing the classic delayed-response task (Fuster and Alexander, 1971; Fuster, 1973). Figure 9.6 shows the spiking record of one of the earliest examples and illustrates some of the main properties of these cells. In summary, they are as follows:

1. Firing is elevated above intertrial spontaneous baseline during most or all of the retention period or delay (in our tests, usually 5–20 seconds)—that is, during the period between the cue stimulus to be remembered and the consequent motor response. Some cells are inhibited during that period and thus, in operational terms, are not considered memory cells; they may belong, though, to a memory network uninvolved in memorization of that particular cue, a network activated by a stimulus different from those of the present task. Some cells are delay-activated after one task cue and delay-inhibited after another.

2. The delay activation can be shortened or lengthened by changing, in either direction, the duration of the delay. In other words, the motor

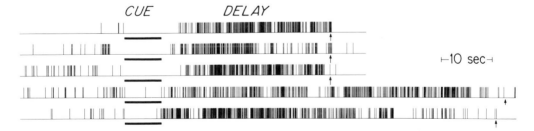

Figure 9.6 Discharge of a cell in prefrontal cortex of a monkey during five trials in the classical delayed response task. Arrow marks monkey's response at the end of the memorization period (delay). Note that the cell is inhibited during presentation of the cue but persistently activated throughout memorization (30 seconds in upper three trials, 60 seconds in lower two). (From Fuster, 1973, with permission.)

choice and the end of the need to remember the cue determine the end of discharge above intertrial baseline.

3. Delay activation commonly follows an excitatory reaction at the time of the cue and is followed by a comparable reaction at the time of the choice-stimulus that prompts the motor response. In some cells, however, the delay activation is preceded and succeeded by inhibition at the cue and at the choice-stimulus.

4. The occurrence of delay activation is related strictly to the presence of a cross-temporal contingency between the cue and the response, and thus the need to remember. Mock trials or trials with incomplete cues fail to elicit delay activations.

5. The magnitude of the activation in the delay period is related to the accuracy of the animal's performance. Both delay activation and performance accuracy can be diminished by distracting stimuli during that period.

In addition to these general properties, memory cells may show specific relationships to the stimulus to be remembered or the response to be performed in a particular delay task. These properties depend, of course, on the nature of the task and the cortical area from which the units are recorded. I will refer to these properties as I proceed with the neuronal correlates of active memory.

Because memory cells were first seen and most extensively investigated in the prefrontal cortex, the mistaken notion (originating in lesion studies) was reinforced that this cortex is a center or depository of short-term memory. It has become increasingly evident, however, that memory cells are present also in other areas of association cortex, although in these areas they generally are less common and tend to be more particular about the sensory properties of the memorandum (cue). It has also become evident that the reason they are so numerous in dorsolateral prefrontal cortex (where they may reach 40 percent or more) is because of the supramodal (polysensory) nature of this cortex and its involvement in motor memory and motor processes that all delay tasks share in common.

Having found memory cells in several and separate neocortical areas during any given delay task, I now believe that such cells are component elements of widespread memory networks that extend into both anterior and posterior cortex of association; whereas the posterior components of those networks support the perceptual representations, their anterior components support the motor representations that the animal must use in the task. In no case, however, can this split of representation and labor be considered clear-cut. The associative character of the networks and the memories they support determines that both anterior and posterior memory cells are, to some degree, involved in both perceptual and motor memory and thus in the memory aspects of the perception-action cycle (see later discussion).

ACTIVATION OF PERCEPTUAL MEMORY

In chapter 8 we discussed how, by association, sensory stimuli retrieve perceptual memories that are part of the fund of long-term memory. We also discussed how retrieved memories, and the stimuli that elicit them, can become the object of categorization and discrimination under the focus of attention. We used single-unit data, particularly records of memory cells, to make the point that these cells belong to established cortical memory networks. Now I will argue that such cells and their networks continue to be activated after retrieval if behavior requires the active memory of percepts under the focus of representation.

Perceptual Networks in Active Storage

If a monkey is to retain a visual cue through a delay, then, as expected from results of reversible lesions (Fuster et al., 1981), memory cells can be found in IT cortex that are evidently involved in the active retention of that cue (Fuster and Jervey, 1981, 1982; Miyashita and Chang, 1988; Fuster, 1990). They can easily be detected there during a visual task, such as delayed matching to sample (DMS), in which the cue is non-spatially defined (e.g., a color) and the memory not confounded by directionality of impending motor response. In chapter 6, to illustrate the discriminating properties of IT neurons, I showed one such neuron (figure 6.6) that exhibited memory features after a discriminant activation at the cue (sample). However, the mnemonic activation of a cell during the delay need not be preceded by its activation while the cue is present. Activation may be absent at the cue even though the firing during memorization is elevated above baseline and clearly selective for one of the memoranda (figure 9.7). Even more remarkably, some units exhibit an inhibition at the cue before their discriminant discharge during memory (figure 9.8). It is as if that inhibition reflected the operation of a gate that would open only for the loading of the information into short-term memory or, more precisely, for the activation of its representational network. Miller and colleagues (1993), in a variant of DMS, observed a similar suppressor effect on IT units and interpreted it as the expression of what they called an "active reset mechanism." Such a reset or gate mechanism is an important feature of our computational models of active short-term memory (see Zipser et al., 1993, and text following).

Note also that the cell in figure 9.8, which seems to engage in retention of the red color, shows a gradual decay of firing during the delay of red-sample trials. This decay is reminiscent of the well-known decay

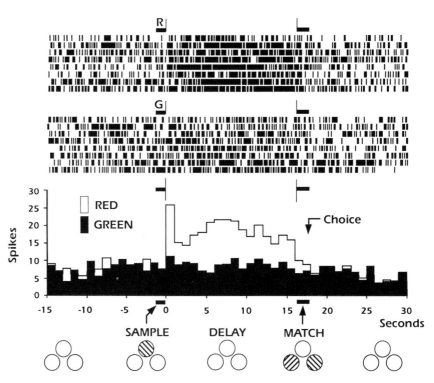

Figure 9.7 Rasters and frequency histograms of a cell in inferotemporal cortex before, during, and after trials in a delayed matching-to-sample task with colors (task paradigm below). Note activation during memorization of red (R) sample and return to baseline firing after match and choice. G, green.

of human short-term memory (Peterson and Peterson, 1959). However, such a smooth descent in firing is relatively rare, and the sustained delay activation of IT memory cells may adopt a considerable variety of temporal patterns (Fuster and Jervey, 1982). In any event, the average discharge of all cells during the delay has a tendency to decline. A perhaps related decline has been observed in the reactivity of IT neurons to visual stimuli of decreasing novelty (Fahy et al., 1993; Li et al., 1993). Decreasing novelty, however, cannot be equated to memory decay. In accord with this statement is the recent observation that, in the human, the reactions of temporal cells to a visual cue diminish gradually as the cue is used repeatedly to retrieve—successfully—an item of verbal memory (Haglund et al., 1994).

Another feature of memory cells in IT cortex, already mentioned in chapter 6, warrants reemphasis here: Regardless of the course and magnitude of the memory cells' activation during the delay, this activation disappears shortly after the monkey has made its choice at the end of the trial. It should be noted that, even though at the time of that choice the animal must look again at the sample color (to wit, eye movement records), the firing of a memory cell reverts to intertrial

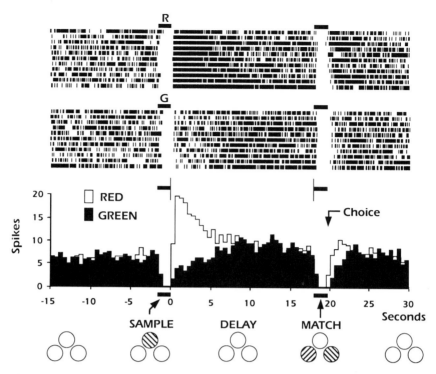

Figure 9.8 Discharge of an inferotemporal neuron during a visual memory task. The cell (like the prefrontal neuron in figure 9.6) is inhibited during "loading" of input to memory and markedly activated during memorization of red (R). G, green.

baseline shortly thereafter (see figures 9.7, 9.8). Thus, when the animal is no longer in need of memorizing the color, the neuron fails to be reactivated in a sustained manner by its preferred color. This is one more reason to attribute the delay activation of that neuron—and the network of which it is a part—to its memory function and not simply to the sensory features of the stimulus.

In conclusion, a sizable proportion (5–30 percent) of neurons in the cortex of the inferior aspects of the temporal lobe, which lesion studies have shown to be important for visual discrimination and memory, have memory properties. These neurons are most probably part of memory networks that are excited during active retention of visual information. The microelectrode evidence of a few memory cells in V1 (Fuster, 1990) and the tomographic evidence of V1 activation during active visual memory (Bihan et al., 1993) suggest that those networks extend from IT cortex to as far back as primary visual cortex. The mechanism is not yet clear by which the networks' neurons are activated to retain visual information or deactivated when its retention is no longer needed by the animal. This issue will be discussed after further description of neuronal correlates.

Dynamics of Cortical Memory: Active Memory

If the information the monkey has to retain is of the *tactile modality*, then the neurons to explore with microelectrodes are logically those of the parietal cortex, especially in areas that lesion studies have implicated in tactile discrimination and memory (see chapters 4 and 6). Here too we have found memory cells, for stimuli of the tactile modality (Koch and Fuster, 1989; Zhou and Fuster, 1992). Our search has been facilitated by use of haptic DMS tasks. In these tasks, the trial is begun by alerting the animal acoustically to the presence and accessibility of a stereometric object in an invisible compartment, straight in front of the animal and ready for sampling by touch. After the monkey has touched the object, the delay ensues, during which time the animal must retain in memory the surface features of the object for the upcoming match. The latter is prompted by a second sound, after which the animal reaches into the compartment and chooses, from two objects, the one that matches the sample. Under these conditions, some parietal cells, their number varying with area and object, show memory properties. Their discharge is elevated through most or all of the delay period, in some cases selectively with regard to certain tactile features (figure 9.9).

Tactile memory cells have two remarkable characteristics. One is their location: They are found not only in cortex of association (area 5) but also in primary somatosensory (SI) cortex (areas 3, 1, and 2). To be sure, visual memory cells have also been found in V1 (Fuster, 1990), but rarely. In SI, however, tactile memory cells are common. The reason for this is not clear but probably has to do with the fact that the tactile sense—much more than vision—depends heavily on successive sampling (palpating), on serial processing and, of course, on short-term memory. It is as if tactile short-term memory were an integral part of the phyletic memory of primary sensory cortex.

The other remarkable characteristic of tactile memory cells is that they commonly are excited not only by the touch and memory of an object but by the movements of reaching to and palpating the object. Like their responses to the alerting click, already noted in chapter 6, the movement-related activation of some parietal memory cells illustrates their cross-modal associative character. It also suggests that these cells are thoroughly embedded in the neural circuits of the perception-action cycle (elaborated on later)—that is, the continuous flow of neural impulses from the sensory to the motor sector and back, which is the essence of haptics (sensing by active touch).

Nevertheless, parietal cells, just like IT cells, may be inhibited at the sample or during the delay of delayed matching tasks. Again, this is suggestive evidence of gating into short-term memory and of the reciprocal inhibition of some cells because they are part of networks representing alternate cues and memories. In addition, like IT neurons, some parietal neurons show similar reactions to the sample as a memorandum

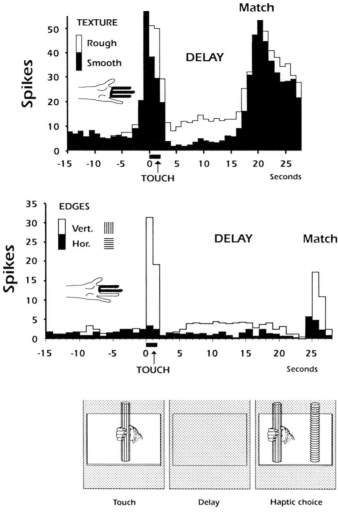

Figure 9.9 Frequency histograms from two units in parietal (S1) cortex during performance of haptic delayed matching (paradigm at bottom, see text). The units' receptive fields are indicated in diagrams of the monkey's hand. The *upper* cell is preferentially activated by touch and memorization of the rough-surface cylinder; the lower cell is activated by a vertically ridged cylinder.

and as a stimulus for choice, whether those reactions are excitatory or inhibitory.

Not surprisingly, in light of these observations, the internalized attention of a human subject to the expected touch of a fingertip produces a sustained increase of blood flow in the subject's contralateral somatosensory cortex, which can be detected by radiographic imaging (see figure 8.11) (Roland, 1981). That internal representation surely is not much different, qualitatively, than that of active tactile memory in a haptic memory task. The neuroimage, however, lacks the spatial or temporal resolution of the microelectrode.

The cellular manifestations of active memory of other modalities have not been explored electrophysiologically. It is to be expected, for example, that similar phenomena as those described in visual and somesthetic cortex will be found in the association cortex of the superior temporal gyrus during auditory memorization.

Our deliberate emphasis on the role of the neocortex in active memory should not lead anyone to ignore the role of other cortical or subcortical structures in it. We have seen already in the previous chapter how important limbic structures seem to be for memory retrieval and selective attention. There is now some evidence, from recent studies, that those structures may play a significant role in working memory as well. Although the participation of amygdala neurons in this memory process appears to be relatively minor (Nakamura et al., 1992a), that of neurons of the hippocampus and related diencephalic structures seems substantial. By autoradiography, Friedman and collaborators (Friedman and Goldman-Rakic, 1988; Friedman et al., 1990) observed a metabolic activation of the hippocampus, the dentate, the mamillary bodies, and some portions of anterior and dorsomedial thalamus during delayed-response performance. Fuster and Alexander (1973), also using a spatial delayed-response task, previously had observed the delay activation of neurons in the nucleus medialis dorsalis, which is closely linked to prefrontal cortex. More recently, I (Fuster, 1991a) have found memory cells in the hippocampus.

This evidence, taken as a whole, suggests that active memory is maintained by circulation of nerve impulses through circuits that are not restricted to the neocortex but include subcortical and limbic formations. As we have seen in chapter 3 and again in chapter 8, these circuits seem to play a decisive role in the formation and retrieval of memory as well as in selective attention. In any case, that role seems heavily determined by the phylogenetically anchored functions of those ancient subcortical and limbic structures in drive and in the evaluation of the motivational significance of external stimuli. It is not surprising that extraneocortical structures to which the neocortex is well connected should help maintain the activation of neocortical networks in active memory. We suppose that those ancient structures contain extensions of neocortical networks and that neurons in those structures contribute associations with drive and motivation that are essential to activate those networks and to keep them active in working memory.

Thus, increasingly pressing becomes the question of how memory cells maintain their activity or, in broader terms, how active memory is maintained in the networks that we assume those cells constitute. I will address this question now, directly after discussing the neuronal correlates of perceptual memory and before discussing those of motor memory, because it is within the framework of perceptual memory that the issue is most amenable to theoretical and empirical treatment.

Our search for specific answers on mechanisms can now depart from two basic hypothetical principles that I have attempted to establish in previous chapters: The first is that the cortical network that keeps a memory active is largely the same network that supports and defines that memory in its permanent and, at other times, passive state. The two may, in fact, be identical, as in the case of an internally evoked long-term memory or in the case of our monkey retaining a well-learned stimulus through an enforced delay. The activated network may indeed be new, if new is the event just experienced and still in active memory. However, even if that event is unprecedented, chances are high that it will take place in a known context or, at the very least, that by associations of similarity it will evoke and activate old memories or fragments of them (see chapter 3). The memory of a new stimulus in a delay task is inseparable from its context, which is thoroughly established in long-term memory. Just as there is no such thing as an entirely new perception, there is not an entirely new memory (see chapter 5). Thus, the new material in active memory may be considered an appendix of a large and preexistent cortical net, even though that recent appendix, at this time, commands the focus of representation. In more specific terms, all this means that the activated network has been largely preformed in the past by hebbian rules, especially that of synchronous convergence, and is now reactivated to meet present circumstances. If there is a new stimulus or event associated with that memory, it quickly becomes part of it, and if no motor response is required, the activated network may be restricted to perceptual memory areas of the posterior association cortex.

The second hypothetical principle is that recurrent excitation through reentrant circuits plays a critical role in the sustained activation of a memory network. Active memory essentially may consist in reverberating activity through the circuits linking neurons within and between the component assemblies of a network that represent the various associated features of the memory. As we now know, the morphological evidence of recurrent and reciprocal connections within and between cortical areas is formidable. It will be recalled that reverberating activity through local cortical connections was an essential features of Hebb's (1949) short-term memory and learning model. Here we are postulating that this mechanism is at the basis of not only the short-term process that leads to long-term memory but also active memory in general, whether or not it has a definite term. In addition, we are extending the applicability of the mechanism to the linkage between distant components of the associative cortical memory network in the active state.

Although consistent with a large body of empirical evidence and theoretical reasoning, the two principles just enunciated remain, for the moment, no more than working hypotheses. These hypotheses will guide our ensuing discussion and our future research.

In very general terms, the postulated mechanisms can be supposed to operate at two levels: at the *microlevel* of the local cortical network, within and between the assemblies of cells representing discrete memory features, and at the *macrolevel,* across cortical areas pulled together in the network for the representation of idiosyncratic and complex categories of perception and behavior (see chapter 5). The two levels of mechanism may blend inseparably into each other but here, for our discourse and analysis, it is convenient to keep them apart.

Computational Models of Active Memory

Whereas the cortical column (see chapter 4) may well be the irreducible processing and representational unit in sensory areas, we have no empirical basis for estimating either the magnitude or the architecture of the minimal memory network in cortex of association. The trion model of Shaw and colleagues (1985) is a theoretical attempt to identify such a network by computer simulation. That model is based on Mountcastle's columnar concepts (1978) and on the assumption of mnemonic encoding by firing patterns. As discussed in chapter 5, a trion would be a small ensemble of units capable of yielding hundreds of thousands of periodic firing patterns depending on minute changes in interaction strengths (weights) and according to a hebbian algorithm. A given stable pattern of the trion, within a given time period, would underlie the temporary activation of a given memory. The plasticity of the model, its statistical behavior, and its speed of adaptation are three of its most attractive features. The assumption of a temporal pattern code, however, remains in question, although it cannot be ruled out.

In collaboration with Zipser and others (1993), we have been developing somewhat more empirically based computer simulation models of active memory. These models have been essentially suggested by the behavior of memory cells, particularly those of IT cortex (Fuster and Jervey, 1981, 1982; Fuster, 1990). The models are designed to reproduce, in an artificial neural network, the *sample-and-hold* operation of real neuronal networks in active short-term memory.

All our models thus far consist of a pretrained neural network with a simple recurrent architecture, in which every unit is connected to all others, as illustrated in figure 9.10. Our network is first trained by use of the backpropagation algorithm (Rumelhart et al., 1986) incorporated in Zipser's (1992) neural system identification procedure. In essence, this is an optimization (error-reducing) procedure designed to allow the

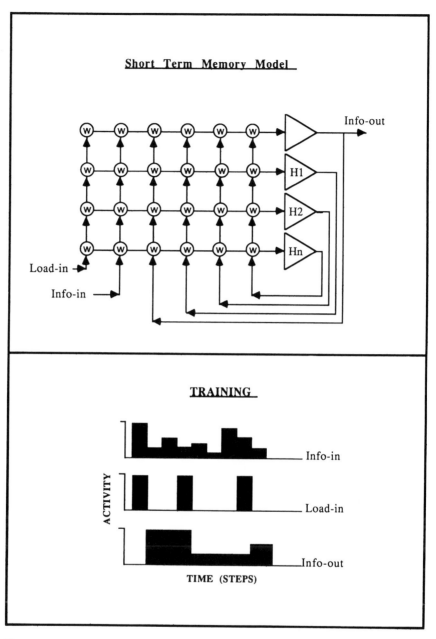

Figure 9.10 (*Top*) Structure of a model of short-term active memory. The soma of each idealized unit is represented by a triangle at right, and its input dendrite is shown at left with a row of synaptic contacts of a given strength or weight (w). The output unit is the blank triangle at upper right. The underlying triangles (H1, H2, Hn) represent hidden units—that is, units that mediate transactions within the network and determine its output at any given time in accord with the inputs it receives and its preestablished (i.e., pretrained) functional architecture. (*Bottom*) The training paradigm. (From Zipser et al., 1993, with permission.)

network, through successive iterations, to self-adjust synaptic weights to reproduce specified input-output relationships while input values change in time (see chapter 5). After training, those weights stay fixed, although they may differ widely for the various synapses of the network. Unlike conventional backpropagation models, our models incorporate the role of a periodic load signal or gating mechanism. When a postulated gate is open (load signal 0), the input of a given value is allowed into the network and held at that value. This loading mechanism mimics the operation of the hypothetical gate, explaining the inhibitory reactions of some memory cells at the cue and termination of delay trials. In the real brain, this load signal may come from limbic structures (e.g., amygdala) signaling what is important to be retained, or from the prefrontal cortex, which presumably determines what needs to be retained for subsequent action.

Our most realistic model to date is a spiking network model, in which input and output analog values correspond to spiking probabilities (Amit, 1990), whereby the stochastic character of real neuron firing is taken into account. The underlying assumption is that a neuron with constant input and output will fire randomly with a fixed probability. If the input frequency varies, the distribution of firing intervals should be the sum of exponential (Poisson-like) distributions, each corresponding to a different frequency (probability). By time-series analysis of neurons in the visual system, my colleagues and I (Fuster et al., 1965) were able to demonstrate both the randomness of firing and the sum of exponential distributions. The issue was further treated theoretically by Sejnowski (1976).

In the fully trained spiking model, single units are substituted by pools of n spiking neurons (also interlinked by reciprocal connections). The pools are networks within networks, as in our connectivist theoretical construct (see chapter 5). The set of inputs to a given pool at time t (time divided in steps or cycles) is defined by two vectors: $y(t)$, with components equal to the outputs of the network's other pools, and $z(t)$, with components determined by external inputs. Two additional vectors represent the weights of connection: w_i for inputs from other pools and v_i for external input. Thus, the output of pool i on time cycle $t+1$ is:

$y_i\,(t+1) = 1$ with probability $sf\,[w_i y(t) + v_i z(t) + b_i]$

where $f(x)$ is the logistical (sigmoid) function:

$f(x) = 1/(1 + e^{-x})$

and where b_i is a bias, s is a scaling factor ($0 < s < 1$) to keep the units away from saturation, as real neurons, and the values of w_i (weight) are adjusted for n (number of units in a pool) and s.

A delay-task trial can be simulated on the fully trained network by loading an analog input, which represents the memorandum, and holding it through the memory period by keeping at zero the load signal until the recall (choice), when the load signal is given a new value (gate closed again) without input signal. Under these conditions, the network's units behave much like real memory cells (especially if some internal noise, as real cells are subject to, has been introduced in the network). Of course, the behavior of output units is unremarkable because it is predetermined by definition of the model and the transfer function from input to output. What *is* remarkable is the behavior of the hidden units, which manifest a wide range of temporal patterns of discharge resembling those of real memory cells during acquisition and mnemonic retention of sensory information (figure 9.11). This suggests that those cells are components of similar cortical networks.

Our model shows another remarkable characteristic: Its units shift periodically, and as if spontaneously, between two or more frequencies or fixed point attractors. These shifts can be observed in the single-trial activity of a given unit, though not in averages of discharge from several trials. Having dealt in my work mainly with average discharge to assess the behavior of real neurons, I never suspected the presence of such frequency shifts (obscured by averaging). My colleagues and I were pleasantly surprised when, on the basis of what we observed in the model, we examined single-trial records of real neurons and found attractor frequencies there too, between which the units shifted at short intervals. A cell would be seen to relax to a certain frequency for a few seconds and then shift and relax to another, only to shift later to the first or to yet another. This might happen in baseline as well as delay (memory) periods (figure 9.12). A cell's attractor frequencies might be the same in both periods, but the cell might spend more time in a given high attractor frequency during the delay (i.e., during memorization) than during intertrial baseline.

This raises the interesting possibility that active memory simply enhances the tendency of cells to fire at their inherent attractor frequencies. The inherent frequency to which a cell is attuned would be built in by training and would be the marker of the cell's participation in a permanent memory-encoding network. The cell would be driven to that frequency more often than in baseline condition by the need to memorize the memory item that it, or rather its network, encodes. The empirical confirmation of this suspicion would support strongly our contention that short- and long-term memories largely share a common substrate.

In conclusion, the average discharge and spiking characteristics of memory cells in posterior association cortex are consistent with an active storage mechanism based on recurrent activity with fixed and preestab-

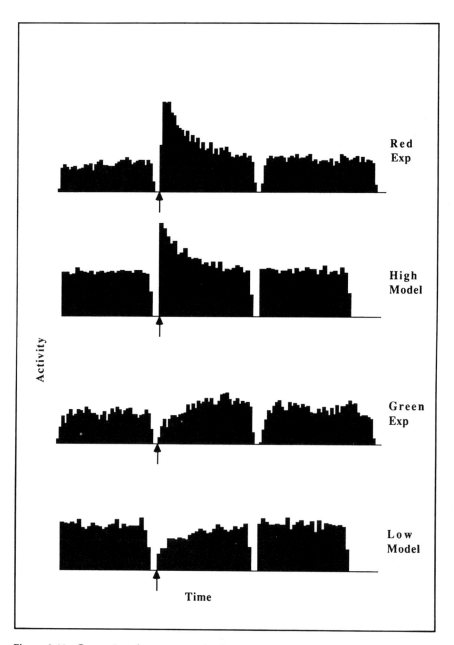

Figure 9.11 Comparison between a real inferotemporal cell (figure 9.8) and one of the hidden units of the spiking model in real or simulated memory (delayed matching) trials (see text). Red Exp, real cell during red-sample trials; Green Exp, real cell during green sample trials; High Model, model's unit (s = 0.3) gating in a high (0.99) initial stimulus; Low Model, model's unit (s = 0.3) gating in a low(0.01) initial stimulus. (From Zipser et al., 1993, with permission.)

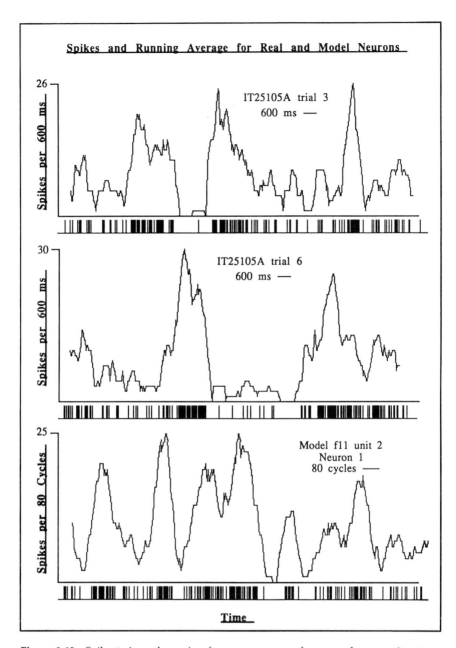

Figure 9.12 Spike train and running frequency average from a real neuron (top two graphs) and a model neuron (lower graph). Note in either case the sharp transitions between attractor frequencies. (From Zipser et al., 1993, with permission.)

lished synaptic weights—that is, fixed synaptic efficacy. Of course, in our model, the weights and the network have been previously established by a process of supervised (backpropagation) learning (see chapter 5). The learning is said to be supervised because it is determined by the training algorithm of the model builder (defining the input-output relationship). This kind of learning is entirely different from the unsupervised learning that is the hallmark of the associative self-organized memory network advocated in chapter 5. However, the difference in the process of formation of a network is immaterial to the issue of its behavior when active. Our model is not supposed to simulate learning or the acquisition of memory but rather the behavior of the already formed memory network when it is activated for temporary memory retention. Essentially, the model teaches us that once a gated input is loaded into a neural network, the network feeds on itself and the input is maintained until unloaded. The model also teaches us that, while maintaining the information, the units of the network adopt certain patterns of discharge that greatly resemble those of real neurons, including the tendency to shift between attractor frequencies.

Naturally, our model is provisional; all neural models are. It must be subjected to further tests in the real brain, with new analytical approaches and recording methods. Depending on the results of such tests, it may have to be modified or discarded. Empirical computational models of nervous function are like live creatures subject to darwinian evolution. Only the fittest survive in the empirical environment. No neural model is worth its salt that has not been tested and retested in the real environment of the functioning brain.

To better simulate the cortical microdynamics of active memory, we may have to adopt more realistic architectures, with better-defined constraints on connectivity, for example. It is possible, however, that our simple recurrent model, as is, has generic value that applies not only to the microdynamics but to the macrodynamics of cortical memory. Reentry, as a general principle, probably applies to the connectivity between widely separated components of the same cortical network. Most connections between associative areas are reciprocal (see chapter 4), although the reciprocity of connectivity is most certainly not directly between cells but between cell populations. Thus, a widely distributed cortical network may be almost instantly activated and kept activated by long-distance reentry between component neuronal populations that represent different aspects of the network's memory. One indication that IT memory cells are part of such broad networks is the higher–than–statistically expected incidence, in their firing, of complex spike sequences (Villa and Fuster, 1992). These are combinations of three or four spikes (triplets or quadruplets) separated by precisely the same two or three intervals (figure 9.13). Such recurrent patterns are consis-

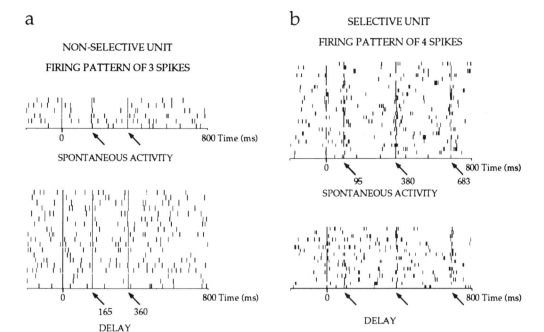

a

NON-SELECTIVE UNIT

FIRING PATTERN OF 3 SPIKES

0   800 Time (ms)

SPONTANEOUS ACTIVITY

0   800 Time (ms)

165   360

DELAY

b   SELECTIVE UNIT

FIRING PATTERN OF 4 SPIKES

0   800 Time (ms)

95   380   683

SPONTANEOUS ACTIVITY

0   800 Time (ms)

DELAY

Figure 9.13 Raster display of the activity of two inferotemporal cells between trials (spontaneous activity) and during the delay of a visual delayed matching task with colors (see figure 9.2). The measuring time was identical in both conditions. Both cells showed generally higher firing frequency in the delay than between trials. (*a*) Cell was nonselective with regard to the memorandum (color). Its spike trains showed higher-than-chance occurrence of triplets, especially during the delay. (*b*) Cell was color-selective. Especially between trials, it showed a high incidence of quadruplets. (From Villa and Fuster, 1992, with permission.)

tent with reentry. Because some of those cells show many of the patterns with long intervals (several hundred milliseconds long), it is reasonable to infer that the cells are part of wide networks, possibly extending far from IT cortex (e.g., into prefrontal cortex) and encoding several attributes (e.g., motor associations) of a visual memory. Supporting our suspicion is the recent evidence of complex spike sequences with similar patterns in the prefrontal cortex (Abeles et al., 1993). Abeles (1982) has shown that synchronous firing within a net of neurons tied by converging and diverging connections ("synfire chain") can generate those patterns in any given neuron for long periods of time. Those patterns are indicative of internal time locking in the net, but the time locking need not be determined only by convergence and divergence of synchronous input; it may be a product of recurrent connectivity, even though the synfire chain was designed essentially as a feedforward network.

ACTIVATION OF MOTOR MEMORY

Memory networks with motor components extend from posterior (perceptual) cortex, across the rolandic (central) fissure, into the cortex of the frontal lobe (see chapter 7). When one such network is activated by sensory input, the activation spreads into frontal cortex, recruiting there the motor component of the network (see chapter 8). The frontal network will stay activated for as long as sensory information needs to be retained for a consequent motor act and until that act has been performed. By reentrant corticocortical connections, frontal output will maintain activation of the perceptual network in posterior cortex, while neural processing within the frontal network will lead to the motor act. This is the essence of the reasoning that I will try to substantiate here using electrical and imaging data.

Frontal Networks in Active Storage

In a previous chapter (7), I have argued that motor memory resides in the cortex of the frontal lobe and in several other motor structures, including basal ganglia and cerebellum. I have also argued for the hierarchical organization of motor representations in the dorsolateral frontal cortex, which extends from the rolandic fissure (central sulcus in the monkey) to the pole of the frontal lobe. Different domains of action—skeletal, oculomotor, linguistical, and even perhaps the kind of internal action that constitutes logical thinking—appear to have separate areas of representation within that cortex, yet all of them seem organized hierarchically, with the most global schemes of action represented in prefrontal areas and the most specific in primary motor areas (intermediate schemes in premotor cortex.) Thus, the frontal hierarchy for motor memory looks like the mirror image of the posterior cortical hierarchy for perceptual memory. Now the issue is how, in the course of behavior, active memories of posterior cortex activate motor memories of frontal cortex, which in turn will lead to behavioral action. In our attempt to understand it, it is helpful to consider two important points: Posterior associative areas in the cortical perceptual hierarchy generally appear to connect to frontal areas of comparable level in the motor hierarchy, and the processing of action, in frontal cortex, appears to follow hierarchical gradients of representation, from the highest level (prefrontal) to the lowest (motor). With these two points in mind, let us resume our reasoning and review some supporting physiological facts.

When a perceptual memory is activated in posterior cortex and that memory has motor implications for the immediate or near future, motor memory is activated at almost the same time in frontal cortex. In connectionist terms, frontal neurons are recruited because they are part of the same network as those of posterior cortex that represent the sensory signals associated with and leading to the motor act. The frontal recruitment is almost certainly accomplished via long corticocortical connections from posterior to anterior cortex (see chapter 4). Motor memory thus is activated in the frontal sector of that wide memory network that extends forward from posterior cortex. Included in the frontal network is the representation of the scheme of the action in more or less precise terms. If the action is complex and has substantial dimensions in space and time, it is represented in the higher levels of the frontal hierarchy (i.e., in prefrontal cortex); if the action is a simple and direct reponse to a stimulus, then it is represented in premotor or motor cortex.

The neural process of transition from perception to action may be relatively simple if both the perception and the action are simple and the first leads directly to the second; then, supposedly, the transition engages only the lower stages of the frontal hierarchy—namely, the premotor and motor cortices. Even behavioral sequences, if they are simple and well rehearsed, may be processed at those stages in chainlike fashion—that is, with perceptions and actions immediately linked to one another in sequence and without temporal gaps between them.

However, if behavior contains contingencies between percepts and actions that are separate in time, then the processing must include mechanisms to mediate those contingencies. For that, the cortex must have the means to translate perception into action across time. It must represent not only a long and perhaps ill-defined sequence of behavior but also its individual components, and it must monitor the sequence while it is being executed. Essential to these operations is the ability to carry information from one time to another. Only through this ability can the cortex keep the sequence coherent and locked to its goal. That role of temporal transfer is shared, to some degree, by all three stages of the frontal motor hierarchy (motor, premotor, and prefrontal) but is best exemplified by prefrontal cortex (Fuster, 1985a, b).

As has been previously noted, to monitor a sequence of actions and to carry information across time, the dorsolateral prefrontal cortex appears to have at its disposal two complementary cognitive functions: short-term active memory and short-term motor set. These two functions help the animal to bridge temporal gaps between percepts and consequent actions—the first by keeping active the memory of recent events and the second by setting motor systems to act. Elsewhere (Fuster, 1989), I have reviewed the neuropsychological evidence from lesion studies for these two frontal functions in humans and animals. Briefly, prefrontal lesions interfere with the cross-temporal contingencies that are the essence of delay tasks (see the section, Topography of Active Memory) and that can be summarized in two simple logical statements: If now this, then later that action; if earlier that, then now this action. The animal with frontal lesion cannot reconcile these contingencies, apparently because it lacks clear representation of the recent past and of the impending action. The impairment of the two forms of representation can be recognized even better in the frontal patient, who cannot either remember recent events or plan for action. Let us now review the functional evidence for the involvement of frontal cortex in the first of these two kinds of active representation—namely, the perceptual memory of the recent past.

In accord with the anatomical evidence of projections from posterior to frontal cortex (see chapter 4), it is well-known that neurons in frontal cortex are physiologically accessible to sensory inputs of various modalities (Benevento et al. 1977; Bruce and Goldberg, 1985; Watanabe, 1992). The specificity of distribution of terminal fibers from posterior associative areas in the cortex of the sulcus principalis is consistent with the findings of corresponding functional specificity in target neurons of that prefrontal region, albeit with considerable overlap of modalities within it (Tanila et al., 1992). In the behaving animal, the reactivity of frontal neurons to sensory stimuli is known to be closely dependent on the significance of the stimuli for subsequent action. This is most obvious in tasks with temporal separation between the stimulus and the motor response to it, such as delay tasks (Fuster, 1973; Kubota and Komatsu, 1985; Yajeya et al., 1988; Funahashi et al., 1990). Thus, the cells of frontal cortex seem involved in sensory representation only or mainly insofar as this representation is part of motor memory and, as such, essential for motor control.

When, as in a delay task, the monkey must retain the memory of a stimulus through a period of time, many neurons of frontal cortex, especially in prefrontal areas, show sustained and elevated discharge (Fuster, 1973; Niki, 1974a, b; Fuster et al., 1982; Quintana et al., 1988; Funahashi et al., 1989). As in posterior cortex, that discharge may be specific for the kind of information that the animal must retain. In general, it tends to diminish in the course of the retention period (instructed delay). The presence of such cells is a clear indication of the participation of prefrontal networks in active perceptual memory for motor action. We should again note that the activation has been shown *not* to occur if the memorandum does not carry with it the need to act.

In recent years, neuroimaging also has provided evidence of prefrontal activation in active memory. Humans show metabolic activation in prefrontal areas during performance of delay tasks in which the memorandum is verbal (Paulesu et al., 1993; Petrides et al., 1993b) or spatially defined (Jonides et al., 1993). Petrides and colleagues (1993a) demonstrate activation of prefrontal cortex by short-term memorization of sequential information and of premotor cortex in conditional discrimination with delay.

By imaging the uptake of fluordeoxyglucose with positron emission tomography, my colleagues and I (Swartz et al., 1994) have explored metabolic activity in the brain of 18 human subjects in two conditions: a delayed matching task with abstract pictures and a control matching task, also with abstract pictures but without memory requirement (without delay) (figure 9.14). Despite considerable variability, we have been able to verify that prefrontal areas (9, 10, and 46) are significantly more activated during the memory task than during the nonmemory task (figure 9.15). Of particular interest with regard to motor set (see below) has been the finding of greater activation in premotor areas while the subjects perform delayed matching.

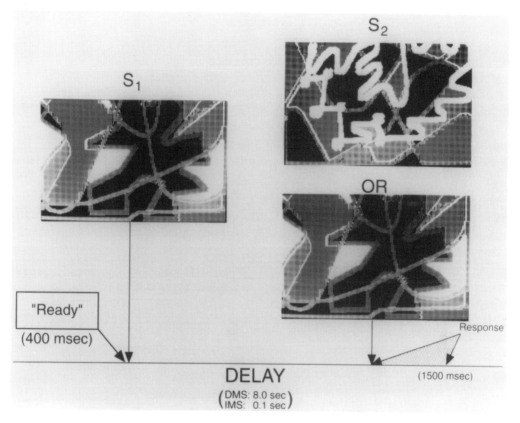

Figure 9.14 Diagram of the two tasks used for a brain-imaging study of active memory. The subject sits in a quiet, dim room and fixates gaze on a central spot of a color monitor. Each trial begins with a "ready" signal, followed by presentation of stimulus S_1, an abstract color picture on the monitor screen (diagonal subtending approximately 15 degrees of visual angle). An 8-second delay ensues in the memory task (delayed matching to sample), following which a second stimulus, S_2, appears. In the no-memory task (immediate matching to sample), the delay is practically nil. If S_2 matches S_1, the subject presses a button with the right hand; if it does not, the subject presses another button with the left hand. Brain activation (fluordeoxygluose uptake) is determined during performance of 80 trials of each task (approximately 30 minutes). (From Swartz et al., 1994, with permission.)

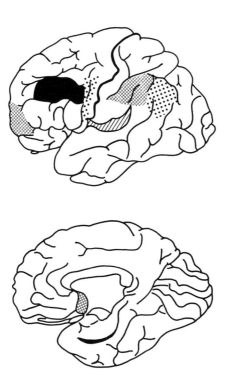

Figure 9.15 Areas in which activation during the memory task (delayed matching to sample) exceeded activation during the no-memory task (immediate matching to sample) (figure. 9.14). Black, F ratio > 11.0 (on discriminant statistical analysis); cross-hatching, F, 5.0–11.0; dotted, F, 4.0–5.0. (From Swartz et al., 1994, with permission.)

In conclusion, both single-unit research and neuroimaging show that prefrontal areas are activated during memorization of perceptual information for subsequent action. The supramodal nature of prefrontal activation, in contrast with the modality-specific activation of posterior cortex, is consistent with the notion that prefrontal neurons are common to many perceptual networks inasmuch as they have motor components. Conversely, the neurons in a modality-specific region of posterior cortex are part of a given network inasmuch as the stimulus in short-term memory is of the modality of the region.

COOPERATION OF POSTERIOR AND FRONTAL NETWORKS

Hence, we seem to have a vast cortical network with postcentral and precentral components engaged in the active memory of a sensory cue and a forthcoming motor response to it. What is the mechanism by which that network is maintained active during memorization? In the context of perceptual memory, I have attempted to provide an answer to this question at the microlevel—that is, at the level of the local cortical circuitry. Now, with a broader vision of the problem and of the network, let us try to find a complementary answer at the macrolevel. An attractive working hypothesis that I have been trying to develop is that the posterior and the frontal components of the network, while actively representing cue and response, feed each other excitation by reentrant connections. In chapter 4, we have provided evidence of a massive array of parallel and reciprocal connections between anterior and posterior cortex that could certainly serve the purpose. As we have repeatedly suggested, the initial wave of excitation elicited by the memory-retrieving stimulus would originate in posterior cortex and, via these corticocortical fibers, would recruit the frontal network. Thereafter, feedback and reentry would keep the totality of the network active. Corticocortical axons originating and terminating in prefrontal cortex would most likely be critical to that interplay of cortical regions (Goldman-Rakic, 1988). Mutual influences between prefrontal and postcentral regions would be especially important if the cue and the motor act are linked by a cross-temporal contingency (Fuster, 1985a, b), as in delay tasks.

My colleagues and I looked for evidence of those mutual influences in IT and dorsolateral prefrontal cortex during a visual delay task (Fuster et al., 1985). The objective was to reveal the functional relationships between two widely separated cortices that are part of a broad cortical network known to be engaged in visual delay tasks. On each trial, the monkey had to retain a color for a few seconds and then act on it with a choice of color. While the animal performed the task, we would, by means of implanted probes, cool one cortical area and record from the other (figure 9.16). As we had determined by prior experiments, cooling of either area, prefrontal (Bauer and Fuster, 1976) or IT (Fuster et al., 1981), induced a deficit in performance of the task. We reasoned that this was so because, by cooling, we depressed or inactivated either of two separate but essential parts of the network: the IT cortex, critical for discriminating and retaining visual information, and the dorsolateral prefrontal cortex, critical for delayed response. The question then was: What effect, if any, did the cooling of one area have on neuron discharge in the other? If the neurons of the two areas were indeed part of the same network, then the cooling of one should induce changes, possibly inhibitory, on the neuronal activity in the other. The cooling would, in effect, interrupt the reentry loops that we postulate are important for the active memory of visual information toward a delayed motor act.

The results of this work (Fuster et al., 1985) were confusing in some respects but revealing in others. Cooling of either area induced the expected behavioral deficit, but its effect on the cells of the other area could be not only inhibitory but excitatory. This was true for neuronal firing in reaction to the cue (sample) as during the retention period (delay). Figure 9.17 displays the average discharge of a unit in IT cortex under normal conditions and under cooling of dorsolateral prefrontal

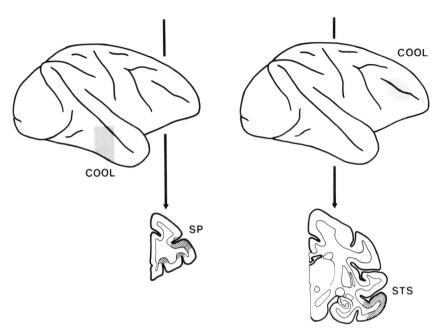

Figure 9.16 (*Left*) Inferotemporal cortex was cooled while recording single-unit activity from prefrontal cortex during performance of a visual delayed matching task. (*Right*) Prefrontal cortex was cooled and unit records obtained from inferotemporal cortex (same task). SP, sulcus principalis; STS, superior temporal sulcus. (From Fuster et al., 1985, with permission.)

cortex to 20°C. This unit, which shows inhibition (gating?) at both cue and choice, also shows, under prefrontal cooling, a depression of its activation during the delay. Other units, however, though clearly in the minority, show enhancement. Both IT and prefrontal cells exhibited a consistent and interesting effect of remote cortical cooling on them: a net diminution of color-dependent differences in the reactions and delay discharge (5–16 percent of the units, figure 9.18). In no cell did we observe an augmentation of color-differential reactivity or memory discharge. Thus, remote cooling had the effect, presumably, of damping the neuronal distinction of cues. In both cortices, the majority of cells affected by cooling of the remote area were found in supragranular layers (I–III). Because these are the preferred layers of origin and termination for corticocortical fibers (see chapter 4), that finding is an indication that interarea influences are normally transmitted through those fibers.

In summary, the results of our experiments are consistent with the idea that posterior and dorsolateral prefrontal cortices exert modulating influences on each other in active memory. This idea is in accord with neuroanatomical data and with our hypothesis that cells in both cortices can be part of one and the same network. In a visuomotor delay task,

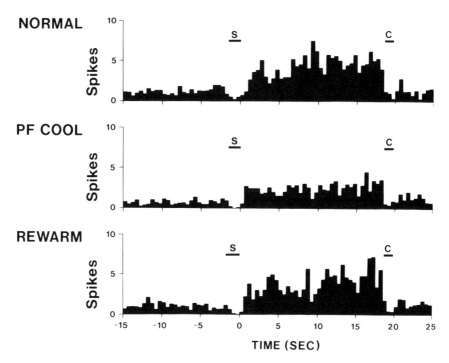

Figure 9.17 Discharge of a cell in inferotemporal cortex during delayed matching with colors. (*Top*) Normal temperature. (*Middle*) Bilateral prefrontal (PF) cooling to 20°C. (*Bottom*) Prefrontal cortex rewarmed to normal temperature. *S*, sample period; *C*, choice period. (From Fuster et al., 1985, with permission.)

such as DMS, the network represents the visual as well as the motor aspects of the task. The task requires the active memory not only of the cue but of the forthcoming motor response as well, however incomplete the latter memory may be, because in the delay of that particular task the animal knows only that it will have to move the arm in a general upward direction but does not know precisely whether it will be to the left or to the right. The network, we presume, keeps both memories active by reentry of impulses between the two cortices. That reciprocal reentry not only may keep the two representations active but also may allow the transfer of excitation from one to the other, from vision to action. Thus, in that task, the network would no longer be merely representational but would also become operational.

By way of reentrant connections, the activated frontal cortex presumably reciprocates posterior cortical input with excitatory output to the same portion of posterior cortex from which the perceptual input originates. Consequently, by feedforward and feedback, the entire perceptual-motor network, which spans portions of both cortices, is activated and maintained active, as is the memory it represents. At the same time, by a process we are far from understanding but that will be

Dynamics of Cortical Memory: Active Memory

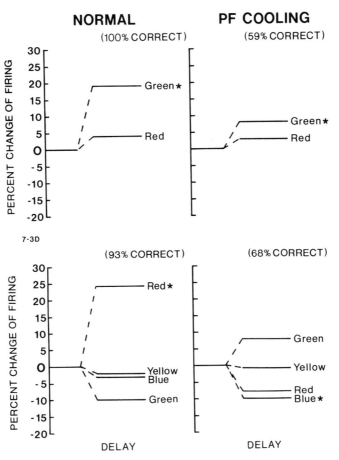

Figure 9.18 Average changes in discharge (percent of baseline, intertrial firing) induced by color samples in two inferotemporal cells during the delay of a delayed color-matching task. (*Upper graphs*) A cell in a task with two colors. (*Lower graphs*) A cell in a task with four colors. (*Left graphs*) Normal temperature. (*Right graphs*) Prefrontal (PF) cooling, 20°C. Behavioral performance level is indicated in parentheses. Asterisks mark firing significantly deviating from baseline. (From Fuster et al., 1985, with permission.)

discussed next, the focus of representation gradually shifts from the perceptual to the motor sector of the network and, as the frontal network representing the action reaches a certain level or threshold, it sets the subjacent levels of the motor hierarchy for execution of the action.

FROM MOTOR REPRESENTATION TO MOTOR SET

To better understand the mechanisms of translating perception into action, we must again consider different kinds of prefrontal cells. The analysis of the sustained activation of prefrontal units during memorization of the cue in a delay task reveals the presence of at least two distinct, though intermixed, cell populations (Niki and Watanabe, 1976;

Fuster, 1984; Quintana and Fuster, 1992; Funahashi et al., 1993). Cells of the first kind are usually activated to a maximum during or immediately after the cue. That activation, which is in some cases related in magnitude to a particular cue, tends to diminish as the delay progresses. Because their firing is temporally related to the cue, sometimes selectively, these cells seem to look backward in time and to engage in the perceptual memory of the cue. Conversely, cells of the second type tend to accelerate their discharge as the delay progresses and the monkey's motor response grows near. Furthermore, their firing often is related to a particular response movement. Thus, they seem to look forward in time and engage in representation of the motor response.

In line with previous discussion, the two groups of frontal neurons, which are most readily identifiable in prefrontal cortex, would constitute two different and complementary parts of the same cortical network, one representing the cue and the other the response. The first network component would represent perceptual memory and the second motor memory, both in the active state during the memorization period (delay). In operational terms, the gradual deactivation of the first as the second becomes activated suggests a transfer of excitation from the perceptual to the motor component of the network. Thus, as the cortical representation of the cue fades, that of the response would become progressively more vivid. In the previous chapter that transfer of excitation has been considered the basis of the shift of attention from perception to movement.

Therefore, the argument has become that the activation of the motor memory network in frontal cortex is essential not only for the representation but for the organization of the represented movement; accordingly, the neurons that represent the movement in frontal cortex seem to participate in the setting for and the execution of that movement. To summarize the evidence again, I shall begin by restating two important findings:

1. If a certain cue does not call for later motor response, then frontal cells fail to show the activation they normally show after cues that do call for that response (Fuster, 1973; Kubota et al., 1974; Sakai, 1974; Suzuki and Azuma, 1977; Joseph and Barone, 1987; Kubota and Komatsu, 1985; Yajeya et al., 1988; Yamatani et al., 1990).

2. Cells that, judging from their firing rate, are attuned to a particular response movement at the time of its execution are also attuned to it in the period that precedes it (Quintana and Fuster, 1992; Riehle and Requin, 1993); moreover, the degree to which a cell is activated in that period depends on the probability with which the animal can predict the particular characteristics (e.g., trajectory) of the coming movement (see figure 8.13).

Further analysis of motor-coupled cells reveals that, depending on their position in the motor hierarchy, frontal neurons intervene at different times before the delayed response to a cue (Di Pellegrino and Wise, 1991; Hocherman and Wise, 1991; Lurito et al., 1991; Riehle, 1991; Romo and Schultz, 1992; Smyrnis et al., 1992; Kurata, 1993). In addition, there seems to be an inverse relationship between the lead time of the anticipatory discharge of cells before movement and the specificity with which those cells encode it. Thus, in the highest levels of the hierarchy (prefrontal areas), cells show the longest lead times, their increased firing anticipating the response by many seconds, yet their firing is not precisely related to the movement or its trajectory. In a word, prefrontal neurons seem to encode global movements with long lead time (figure 9.19). Conversely, units in primary motor cortex (MI) are attuned closely to specific movements that they anticipate with lead times of less than a second, whereas premotor units show intermediate specificity and lead times.

At any level of the motor hierarchy, regardless of lead time, the representation of movement is maintained probably by reentry of impulses through local recurrent circuits. In fact, local recurrent activation may play no less a role in active motor memory than it does in active perceptual memory. Using the backpropagation algorithm, as we did for the perceptual memory model described in the previous section, Fetz and Shupe (1990) developed a recurrent model of motor representation. Their model's hidden units show sustained firing behavior that is remarkably similar to that of frontal neurons in memory tasks.

The progressively shorter lead times of motor-coupled cells between prefrontal and motor cortex suggest a gradual recruitment of neurons down the frontal motor hierarchy. That gradual recruitment of neurons from areas of broad representation to those of specific representation of movement, before the latter takes place, suggests, in turn, a progressive narrowing of the attentive motor set (see chapter 8), from preparation for global action to preparation for minute and specific action (e.g., from arm movement in a general trajectory to skillful finger movement). Thus, motor-set influences would flow down from the prefrontal cortex to premotor to motor cortex, successively priming them for increasingly more concrete action. The downflow of motor-set impulses would engage not only corticocortical connections but cortical-subcortical loops that involve the basal ganglia, the cerebellum, and the lateral thalamus. Consequently, when the action finally occurs, a network activation process is completed that begins with the sensory cue and its analysis in posterior cortex and proceeds through frontal cortex to the execution of movement.

Now let us briefly examine the gross electrocortical manifestations of the cellular phenomena of motor processing just described. As the human or the monkey prepares to act after a signal, a slow negative

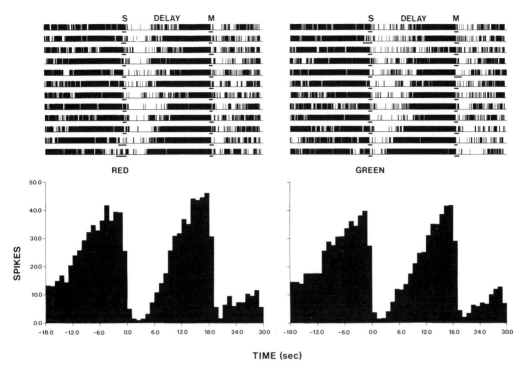

Figure 9.19 Firing rasters and histograms from a prefrontal cell during repeated trials of delayed matching to sample with colors. At the sample (S), the monkey is presented with a colored light on a stimulus-response button, which the animal must immediately press to extinguish, thus acknowledging the sight of the sample color. Through the ensuing delay, the animal must retain the color of the sample because, at the time of match (*M*), it is presented with two colors simultaneously on side-by-side buttons and must press the one matching the sample. Note the progressive acceleration of the cell's firing during the delay (18 seconds) in anticipation of the choice response, even though the animal can predict only the need for a hand movement but not its precise direction. (Because trials are presented at more or less regular intervals, the cell—like the monkey—apparently also is anticipating the motor response to the sample). (From Fuster et al., 1982, with permission.)

potential that can be recorded even extracranially—the contingent negative variation (CNV)—develops over the surface of the frontal lobe (Walter et al., 1964; Low et al., 1966; Loveless and Sanford, 1974; Kutas and Donchin, 1980; Libet et al., 1983b). This potential has been interpreted as a manifestation of expectancy or preparation for action (set) and seems to originate in prefrontal cortex (Jäervilehto and Fruhstorfer, 1970). Almost continuous with the CNV, and beginning approximately 500 to 1000 msec before the movement, is another negative potential with a somewhat more posterior origin, apparently in precentral cortex: It is the so-called readiness potential (*Bereitschaftspotential*), which has also been associated with the preparation for movement. At least one subcomponent of it, nearest in time to the motor act, has been attributed to the will or urge to move (Libet et al., 1982; Libet, 1985).

It is difficult to establish clear distinctions between those slow frontal potentials and to ascertain the functional significance of any of them. I have suggested that the distinctions may be unnecessary (Fuster, 1989). In my opinion, those potentials are components of one large wave of negativity that reflects underlying neuronal excitation and that, originating in prefrontal cortex, sweeps back toward the motor cortex following the anatomical gradients of frontal connectivity (see chapters 4, 7, and 8). That wave would reflect and accompany the previously discussed descending recruitment of frontal neurons, from the prefrontal cortex, through the premotor cortex, to the primary motor cortex (in the process engaging subcortical loops through basal ganglia). As the recruitment proceeds downward in the frontal motor hierarchy, progressively more concrete aspects of movement would be actively represented and anticipated, with preparation. This march from the abstract to the concrete, from the representation to the operation, from the macrogenesis to the microgenesis of the action, is well supported, as we have seen by single-unit data. It can be extended downward all the way to the muscle, for even there units (motor units, that is) show signs of preparatory set before final contraction (Mellah et al., 1990).

Of course, any perceptually induced movement causes some change in the environment, which in turn leads to further sensory input, thus completing a cycle of activation of cortical networks that is of critical importance for goal-directed, temporally extended behavior. As we see in the following section, the cortex of the frontal lobes, with its closely interrelated functions of memory and set, plays a crucial role in the operation of that cycle.

PERCEPTION-ACTION CYCLE

Any sequence of goal-directed behavior, from the instinctual and innate to the most unique and creative, is controlled by a circular flow of information processing for which I have proposed the term *perception-action cycle* (Fuster, 1989). The cycle's operation is a fundamental principle of biology that can be briefly described as follows: Sensory information is neurally processed, and the result of this processing is converted into movement, which induces changes in the environment (both external and internal). These changes, in turn, generate new sensory input, leading to new movement and that to more changes, and so on. This circular flow of information processing, with feedforward and feedback at every step, is what maintains the behavioral sequence smooth and on target. Without its proper functioning, behavior cannot proceed properly to its goal.

The principle certainly is not new. It may have been enunciated formally for the first time by Viktor von Weizsäcker (1950) who, not coincidentally, was a neurologist, as neurologists can best appreciate the innumerable possible malfunctions of the cycle—from disorders of proprioception to cortical disconnection syndromes, from ataxia to aphasia. He called it the *"Gestaltkreis"* (gestalt cycle). In more recent times, cognitive scientists have given it other names, such as the "perception cycle" (Neisser, 1976) and the "action-perception cycle" (Arbib, 1981).

The perception-action cycle has a neuroanatomy, which is stratified like the sensory and motor processing hierarchies of neural structures that it links together. Also like those hierarchies, it extends along the entire nerve axis, from the spinal cord all the way up to the neocortex. At all levels, the cycle links a sensory structure with a corresponding motor structure of roughly comparable hierarchical rank. Figure 9.20 depicts schematically the connectivity of the cycle's higher (i.e., cortical) levels. Simple as it is, the scheme represents, in abstract fashion, most major patterns of cortical connectivity discussed in chapter 4. Because the various hierarchical stages of sensory and motor function are linked

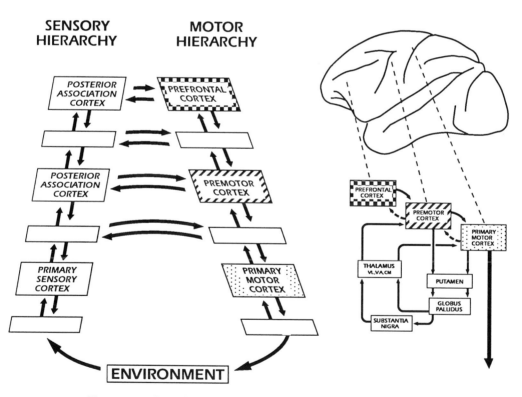

Figure 9.20 Cortical anatomy of the perception-action cycle (see text for description). (*Right*) The cortical motor hierarchy and its subcortical connective loops. (From Fuster, 1993, with permission.)

to each other, the perception-action cycle can be decomposed into a series of eccentric, partly overlapping and bidirectional circuits, closed at the bottom through the environment in one direction. This scheme of things has wide-ranging dynamic implications for the neurobiology of behavior.

Clearly, not all layers of the cycle need be involved in all behavioral sequences. In fact, only its lower layers may be active in most behaviors, which are made of routine and deeply ingrained sensorimotor integrations. Automatic, reflex, instinctual and thoroughly learned behaviors all can be formed by processing at lower levels. Whereas new patterns of behavior necessitate processing through neocortical structure, well-learned and rehearsed patterns do not; they can be executed by shunting at lower layers of the cycle. This is, of course, in line with the notions on the organization of motor memory discussed in chapter 7.

The prefrontal cortex, more specifically its dorsolateral aspect, is depicted in our scheme at the top of the cycle. It is there for two reasons: because it represents the newest and most complex schemes of behavior and because it supports the cognitive processes of active memory and motor set that allow the organism to bridge time between percepts and actions. Most of the evidence for the first point is clinical, whereas for the second it is neurophysiological (see chapters 7 and 8 and previous section).

At every neural layer of the perception-action cycle, there is forward flow from sensation to movement and feedback flow in the opposite direction (reciprocity of connections is the general rule). At lower layers, that output from a motor structure to a sensory structure has been called the "efferent copy" of movement (McCloskey, 1981). It is a form of *corollary discharge* that flows into the sensory sector and serves to adjust it for further sensory input in the presence of movement. I have already alluded to the importance of some of that feedback, which bypasses the environment, for haptic perception. That feedback crosses the central sulcus, from motor cortex to somatosensory cortex, and somehow aids the latter in the mechanisms of perception from active touch. This explains the activation of somatosensory neurons during hand exploration movement (Koch and Fuster, 1989; Zhou and Fuster, 1992).

At the highest levels of the neural perception-action cycle, the corollary discharge from dorsolateral prefrontal cortex to posterior association cortex presumably assists the anticipatory adaptation of perceptual processes during behavior. Teuber (1972) made of corollary discharge an important perceptual function of the prefrontal cortex but applied it to relatively low levels of sensorimotor integration (e.g., oculomotor influences on visual sensation). Instead, or in addition, the corollary discharge of prefrontal origin probably operates between higher categories of movement and perception, especially when time intervenes between them. Indeed, the reentrant input from prefrontal cortex on posterior cortex, which we have postulated to be important for preservation of active perceptual memory in anticipation of movement, can be construed as a form of corollary discharge. It would be high-level corollary discharge from a cortex organizing motor behavior in the temporal axis to a cortex that would thus be helped to maintain perceptual memory for upcoming actions.

This again brings into focus the essential role of the prefrontal cortex in the *temporal organization of behavior.* Clearly, this large expanse of cortex cannot be attributed any one function only: It is functionally heterogeneous. Nonetheless, two of its functions stand out: short-term active memory and motor set. To our knowledge, none of these functions has a clear-cut cortical topography. They seem to assist the processing in numerous domains of motor action (e.g., skeletal movement, eye movement). The prefrontal area for each of these domains is defined functionally by the nature of the information it handles and by its connectivity with other cortical and subcortical structures. A case in point is the prefrontal cortex of the frontal eye field where, within a small region (approximately coinciding with area 8), we can find cells that have short-term memory and motor-set properties in the context of a certain aspect of behavior (i.e., ocular motility).

In conclusion, a large territory of frontal association cortex appears to support two widely distributed functions, short-term memory and short-term motor set, at the service of temporal organization in a variety of behaviors. It is this supraordinate function of temporal organization that seems most characteristic of the prefrontal cortex and defines its place in behavioral neurobiology (Fuster, 1989). It is what makes prefrontal cortex a motor structure of sorts at the top of the neural motor hierarchy and of the perception-action cycle.

The structuring of motor behavior is manifest not only in skeletal and ocular movement but also in the highest expression of cognitive function, the *spoken language.* It is fitting and understandable that the prefrontal cortex reaches its maximum evolutionary development in the human brain, because this brain supports speech, which is supreme and uniquely human among all forms of temporally organized behavior.

Language is indeed unique to our species, and therefore unique must be its cortical organization. It is reasonable to suppose, however, that the functional dynamics of speech are not substantially different from that of any other form of sequential behavior. Speech's neural substrate is essentially analogous, if not identical, to that of other temporally structured behaviors. Language shares with these other behaviors a common cortical sensory base, beginning with primary sensory areas for the analysis of auditory, visual and, in the written language, tactile and kinesthetic information.

At higher levels of sensory processing, language has at its disposal large expanses of posterior association cortex (figure 9.21). They include areas that, by applying rough homological criteria, appear to correspond to polymodal association areas in the monkey. Notable among them is Wernicke's area in the posterior third of the superior temporal gyrus of the left or dominant hemisphere. All those posterior associative areas, including possibly some in the inferior occipitotemporal region, constitute the semantic substrate of language, the base for its perceptual and memory functions. Linguistic perception and memory are formed in these areas by experience and learning, much as other kinds of perception and memory (see chapter 6). In fact, it is likely, though not proved, that the representation of substantive names is enmeshed with the representation of the objects for which they stand and thus part of the same networks. This may also be the case for foreign words. Such a view is not incompatible with a certain concentration of semantic associations in and around Wernicke's area, which would account for the well-known sensory (semantic) aphasias from lesions of this area.

It is not hard to imagine a posterior cortical hierarchy supporting the perceptual categories of language. At the bottom would be the sensory cortex of three modalities. Above that would be a stack of progressively

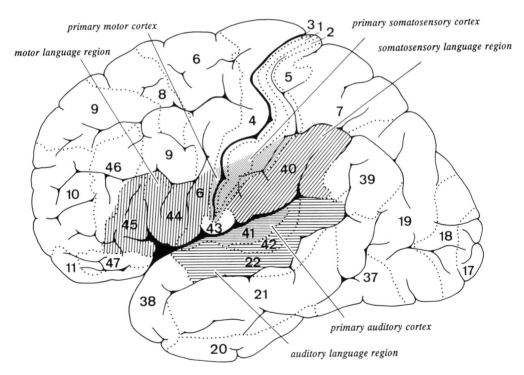

Figure 9.21 Language areas. This figure is almost identical to figure 6.14, but here area 40 has been added to Wernicke's area as among those of posterior cortex contributing to the perceptual aspects of language.

higher associative areas to support the representation of progressively higher categories of language, from the phoneme to the morpheme to the word to the sentence and the abstract concept. It is difficult to imagine, however, how such a linguistic hierarchy would relate to other perceptual categories. It seems plausible that, like these other perceptual categories, linguistic categories have been engraved in cell assemblies and networks by the principles of memory formation discussed in chapter 3. Once they have been formed, linguistic networks probably represent information according to basic connectionist principles (Pulvermüller and Preissl, 1991). As Braitenberg and Schüz (1992) have remarked, linguistic networks can best be conceived in statistical terms, constituted by weak, numerous, excitatory and plastic synapses tying together widely dispersed populations of cortical neurons supporting the associative framework of words and sentences.

To match that semantic hierarchy of posterior cortex, there is in frontal cortex, as we have seen in chapter 7, a symmetrical hierarchy of linguistical motor representations. The two are reciprocally connected by long fibers, which are part of the uncinate fasciculus. These connections between semantic networks and networks representing language expression are the horizontal links of the linguistical perception cycle, the various levels of which integrate spoken language of various levels of complexity, novelty, and abstractness (figure 9.22).

Like the cycle for skeletal action, the linguistical cycle is closed externally through the environment and internally through reciprocal connections feeding forward (perception to action) and feeding back (action to perception) at different hierarchical levels via horizontal links. Here, of course, the *environment* is the interlocutor or the written page. In a dialogue, our interlocutor's mind provides the feedback that shapes and modifies our speech (at least it should!). As I write, external feedback comes from what is already on this page, and it guides what I will write on the next. Both the interlocutor and the written page activate posterior cortical networks that partly determine, through frontal networks, subsequent language expression.

Internal feedback is more subtle and more hypothetical. It is well known that for its proper functioning, the speech apparatus requires feedback from hearing one's own voice. Presumably, there is corollary discharge at several neural levels of speech organization that is essential for modulation and control of language expression. How those feedback horizontal links operate is unknown, but their failure certainly is at the root of some of the aphasias that result from disconnection between Broca's and Wernicke's areas. Obviously, the root of much confusion concerning cortical aphasias is the difficulty in determining with certainty where the linguistical perception-action cycle is disrupted. In the testing of an aphasia, the diagnostician acts as the interlocutor, as the environmental link. It is difficult, in most cases, for anyone in that

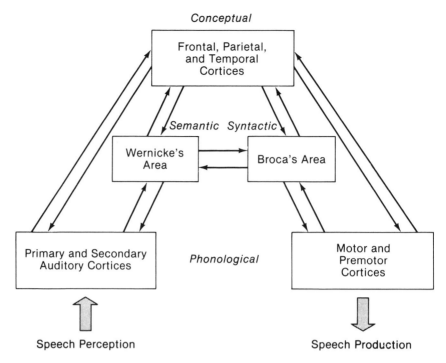

Conceptual

Frontal, Parietal,
and Temporal
Cortices

Semantic   Syntactic

Wernicke's
Area

Broca's Area

Primary and Secondary
Auditory Cortices

Phonological

Motor and
Premotor
Cortices

Speech Perception

Speech Production

Figure 9.22 Edelman's diagram of the connectivities that subserve the highest linguistic functions. (From Edelman, 1989, with permission.)

external position to ascertain exactly where the internal cycle has been interrupted. Only indirectly and without certainty can this be done.

When the interruption is in the prefrontal links of the cycle because of lesion in prefrontal cortex, then the apparent trouble is characterized by a disorder in the syntagmatic properties of language (see chapter 7). If the lesion is in Broca's area, those properties are disturbed at a relatively low level. The patient's syntax is faulty and sparse because sensorimotor integration fails at a very elementary level. The syntax of linguistical action is disrupted much as that of skeletal action would be by a lesion of the premotor cortex nearby.

If the lesion is in the much larger polar region of dorsolateral prefrontal cortex—that is, within frontal granular cortex proper—then, as noted in chapter 7, the language deficit is much more subtle. Speech has lost spontaneity, richness, and fluidity. On closer analysis, the deficit can easily be ascribed to the failure of active memory and short-term set, the temporal integrative functions of the prefrontal cortex that provide continuity at the top of the cycle.

The spoken language, especially when it is new, complex, and extended in time, makes constant use of those functions of memory and set. As I speak, I need to keep track of what I just said a few moments ago and, at the same time, prepare for saying what is in accord with that. The predicate is dependent on the subject, the verb on the subject and the predicate, the dependent clause on the larger sentence, and so on. All these are, in essence, cross-temporal contingencies, and in speech there is a running reconciliation of these contingencies that constantly change, interleaved and embedded within one another. It is the dorsolateral prefrontal cortex that normally effects that reconciling, with its grasp of the short-term past and the short-term future. The active perceptual and motor memory of prefrontal networks ensures the logical continuity of propositional speech which, when it is original and elaborate, taxes those functions to the maximum as it critically relies on the higher reaches of the perception-action cycle.

10 Phenomenology of Memory

In the human, conscious experience is the essence of remembering, attention, and active memory, the three main aspects of memory dynamics (see chapters 8 and 9). Yet consciousness, per se, is a subject the neuroscientist would rather avoid because it poses insurmountable problems. It can be neither objectified nor measured for it is not directly accessible to the independent observer. (To Carver Mead, the word *consciousness* is, as he says in jest, "reserved"; by definition, the entire subject might rightfully be described that way.) Thus far in this book, I have treated consciousness somewhat obliquely, leaning, for the most part, on the tenuous although widely held assumption that the neural substrate of memory can be explored without dealing at all with mental phenomena. Indeed, a case can be made—and has been made, initially by Ribot (1906)—that conscious awareness is merely an *epiphenomenon*, unnecessary for memory to be formed or retrieved. This certainly is true for much of motor memory. Presumably, therefore, we should be able to learn everything about neural memory by neurobiological methods and with a behaviorist approach that has been sanitized of any trace of mentalism.

Obviously, I have not followed that strategy with rigor. I believe, as does John Searle (1990), that it is an error to dismiss, in principle, conscious phenomena as a source of understanding of cognitive processes. Cognitive science without consciousness is bound to be, if not sterile, of little relevance to human memory. Both the reader and I are interested in the neural basis of human memory and, as we have seen, some of the best evidence for it comes from human neuropsychology and rests on reports of conscious retrieval, or lack thereof. In any event, it is practically impossible to discuss the dynamics of primate memory without reference to conscious experience, whether or not nonhuman primates share it with us. Happily, these animals are beginning to reveal the neural foundation of active memory, a cognitive function with an essential conscious aspect that can be distinctly identified and tested in the human as well as the animal (see chapter 9).

Nevertheless, because phenomenology has not been the essence of my argument, I have relegated it to this last chapter. Here I go back to phenomenal facts mentioned previously only in passing, not to argue for any particular view of neural memory but to highlight those facts and to speculate on the physiology underlying them. My purpose here is not to model mental operations or even to conduct gedankenexperiments on them, as cognitive psychologists ordinarily do. Rather, the purpose is to envision a cortical physiology that not only would be compatible with these operations but that possibly could explain them. With regard to active memory in particular, my reasoning here again may sound tautological, as in the previous chapter I proposed that conscious awareness is an essential attribute of that state of memory. However, the notion that active memory is conscious was treated then, and is treated now, merely as a plausible hypothesis that is consistent with what we know about active or working memory in the human.

In attempting to further examine the phenomenology of memory and its neural implications, I follow the same general order that I have followed in previous chapters and that reflects the natural order, from perception to action. As a whole and in its parts, this chapter is organized to make the discussion flow from the least to the most conscious aspects of memory, from sleep to volition.

SLEEP AND DREAMS

In the course of a night's sleep, the general level of activity of the cerebral cortex, to judge by the electroencephalogram (EEG), is far from steady and uniform. Four different stages or depths of sleep can be distinguished, each characterized by a different pattern of EEG. The organism spends the longest time in slow-wave sleep, with the EEG typically dominated by waves in the alpha and delta frequency ranges. Arousal is accompanied by transition to the low-voltage, high-frequency EEG of the awake state.

Peculiar things happen to our memories during both transitional states, from wakefulness to sleep (hypnagogic state) and vice versa. For one, we may not remember afterward some of the events we have witnessed or the actions we have performed in those states. The amnesia and the less-than-perfect judgment of professionals awakened for telephone consultations has been the cause of embarrassment for more than one of them—and of peril for their clients.

The amnesia for events in the state of transition between sleep and wakefulness may be attributed to absent or incomplete formation of cortical associations. That, in turn, may be due to insufficient tonic activation from the reticular activating system or from the hippocampus, or both. Those hypothetical but plausible conditions may also prevail, to an extreme, after concussion. A severe blow to the head commonly will cause a temporary loss of consciousness with amnesia for the events immediately preceding and succeeding the injury. The precise mechanisms by which the violent shaking of the enclosed brain causes unconsciousness and amnesia are not yet well understood. It is unlikely, however, that the amnesia is solely due to temporary inactivation of memory-making and memory-storing processes, cortical or subcortical. The deficit probably involves also the transient posttraumatic impairment of memory retrieval mechanisms. A clear indication of this is the gradual recovery of memory for events around the time of the trauma, which ordinarily takes place in ensuing days or weeks.

That recovery follows a systematic order: The periods of both retrograde and anterograde amnesia shrink progressively around the time of the trauma. The forgotten events that are temporally most remote from the incident, before and after it, are the first to be recalled. Thereafter, events progressively closer to the incident come back to memory from both temporal directions. Similar amnesia and subsequent order of recovery, though on a lesser scale, may be observed after an electric shock to the head, as for electroconvulsive therapy (ECT). The recovery of memory after concussion or ECT rarely is complete, however, which argues for a memory consolidation deficit in addition to that of retrieval. The consolidation deficit might be the result of a transient obliteration of limbic processes just before and after the causal agent. Memory that was never established cannot be recovered.

On four or five occasions during the night, for a total of 80 to 100 minutes, we lapse into the peculiar stage of so-called REM sleep, a phenomenon first discovered by Aserinsky and Kleitman (1953). That stage is characterized by high-frequency, low-voltage EEG, much as the EEG of the awake state, and for this reason it was called "paradoxical sleep" by Jouvet (1962), the investigator who first explored it in the animal. REM sleep is accompanied by generalized flaccidity of skeletal musculature and rapid eye movements (hence its name).

There is now a large body of literature, from research on animals as well as humans, indicating that REM sleep is important for memory consolidation (Fishbein, 1981; Smith, 1985). Both animals and humans deprived of REM sleep have been reported to have difficulties in acquiring and retaining new information. On the other hand, learning new tasks seems to promote REM sleep (for review, see McGrath and Cohen, 1978, and Smith, 1985). For example, subjects learning the Morse code were noted, after learning sessions, to exhibit increases in the number and duration of REM episodes in their sleep (Mandai et al., 1989). Furthermore, by an obscure mechanism, the learning of the code was facilitated by auditory stimulation (bursts of white noise) during postlearning REM sleep (Guerrien et al., 1989). In the rat, stimulation of the midbrain reticular formation during postlearning REM sleep was noted to improve learning (Hennevin et al., 1989). These observations suggest that the acquisition of new learning depends on some kind of tonic input to the cortex from subcortical nuclei that are active and can be further activated during REM sleep. Neurochemical studies indicate that at least one such subcortical input may be cholinergic and originate in the pontine reticular formation (McCarley and Hobson, 1975).

Somehow related to the phenomena of cortical REM activation may be the finding of oscillatory 40-Hz bioelectrical activity on the scalp of humans in dream state (Llinás and Ribary, 1993). As noted in chapter 5, that kind of activity, in the awake organism, has been ascribed to attention and sensory processing. In more general terms, oscillatory activity of various frequencies may be the expression of the recurrent activity between cortex and thalamus that has been postulated to be essential for the regulation of all sleep stages (Steriade et al., 1993).

In any event, the role of REM sleep in learning needs further study. Thus far, the research that supports it is open to many questions. Good controls are difficult to obtain, and the reported learning-related REM-sleep enhancements seem generally weak, inconsistent and, to a large extent, dependent on the task being learned.

If a human subject is awakened during or immediately after a REM episode, he or she is likely to report a dream. It is now well established that, whereas they can occur in practically any phase of sleep, dreams are most frequent in REM sleep (Hobson 1988). Because REM sleep is accompanied by fast-frequency, low-voltage EEG activity, which is in every respect similar to that of the waking state, it is reasonable to conclude that dreams result from cortical activation or are an epiphen-omenon of it. Without the controls of reality testing and self-awareness that prevail in the waking state, presumably that activation leads to the haphazard and fragmentary mobilization of cortical networks: hence the irrational, fragmented, and chaotic contents of dreams. The concomi-tant, perhaps consequent, activation of limbic structures would provide the conscious experience of the dream with its affective coloring.

After much debate, however, the origin of dreams remains uncertain. Of course, the position just suggested, that dreams are an erratic by-product of neurochemical changes and transactions, is orthogonal to psychoanalytic theory. Freud (1901/1958) never denied neurochemical factors in them, but his belief was that dreams are basically the expres-sion of unconscious wishes and fears and that behind their seemingly arbitrary structure, contorted by substitution, symbolism, and conden-sation, there is the lawful logic of the *id*.

Whatever the physiology and psychology of dreams, there is the incontrovertible fact that they are fundamentally anchored in personal experience, and this is evident even in their superficial structure. For one thing, the protagonist of the dream is almost invariably the dreamer, at least as the emotionally vested observer. For another, practically all the elements of a dream can be traced to the dreamer's personal experience, some of it recent, from the day before. Even the most bizarre, fantastic, and creative dreams are made of elementary sensations with which the subject is familiar. The cast and the scene may be utterly unrecognizable, but many elements of the play can be recognized in both their cognitive and affective aspects, for they are part of the repertoire of personal memories. Thus, it is not far-fetched to construe dreams as the expression of personal memory, of associative memory at that, but in which the associations are new, perhaps formed ad hoc as a result of the simultaneous activation, by subcortical inputs, of two or more cortical networks previously unrelated. Hence, dreams are filled with surprising and grotesque associations.

Only in a speculative vein, for I am unwilling and unable to defend it, shall I mention here the intriguing idea that the archetypal images (e.g., "mandalas," often in color) that recur in the dreams of some people and that C.G. Jung (1968) considered the expression of the collective unconscious, result from nonsensory activation of human phyletic memory. Perhaps in this case, as in LSD-induced dreams and hallucinations, the activated networks are in or near primary visual cortex.

In summary, dreaming is consistent with the activation of cortical memory networks, however refashioned in the absence of guiding reality or critical judgment, under the influence of inputs from subcortical centers and internal receptors. The memory activated in dreams, however, not only is distorted and elaborated, often beyond the recognition of the awakened dreamer, but it lacks a critical attribute of memory in conscious awareness: temporality. The dream, though replete with past experience, is experienced in the present and lacks the phenomenal attributes of past and future. It would appear that without external or internal sensory references, the subject cannot project the events in the dream to any time but the present. Out of sensory inputs and context, the fragmented networks activated in the dream seem to lack the associative links to a time frame, anchored as they are in the present, without time tags and references.

We do not know what kinds of associations provide cortical networks with the time tags that are missing in the dream, but we do know that temporal associations are not the only ones usually missing in it (Hobson, 1988). Ordinarily, associations of smell and taste, for example, are also missing. Most dreams have two major characteristics: They are visual and they contain movement. In addition to moving visual images, somesthetic—especially kinesthetic—sensations are common in dreams, but auditory ones are rare. Olfactory and gustatory sensations are practically unheard of in dreams. Does this order of probability of oneiric experiences reflect the size of cortical territories devoted to the various sensory modalities? It may. In primates, the human included, vision by far takes the largest territory—that is, the conglomerate of striate and extrastriate areas. The cortex of the frontal lobe—motor, premotor, and prefrontal areas included—is, of course, another large territory (more than 30 percent of neocortex in the human). It is, as we now know, mostly devoted to movement and motor memory.

Thus, just on the basis of the magnitude of cortical territory dedicated to visual and motor representations, it is understandable that most dreams are visual and have motion in them. It is as if, in REM sleep, visual and frontal regions of the cortex, because of their large size, attracted the lion's share of brain-stem inputs. The activation of those cortical regions would thus seem to take precedence over that of all other regions and their networks: hence the overpowering access of visual and kinetic representations to a dream.

A final issue is: Why are dreams so difficult to remember? The answer, in all likelihood, lies in their detachment from direct sensory experience. Although made of fragments of prior perceptual and motor memory, they are formed anew and away from the immediate domain of that experience. Their cortical representations, made of old experience and out of conscious awareness, remain isolated from the senses and from awareness even after these have been awakened. Nevertheless, once a dream fragment has been tapped by recall in the awake state, the others usually follow by association, as in the retrieval of any memory, however obscure or remote. The process of dream recall is more laborious, however, because of the frailty and logical inconsistencies of oneiric associations. Crick and Mitchison (1983) offer an additional explanation. According to them, dreams may be subject to a reverse learning mechanism in REM sleep, by which they are actively suppressed and thus consciousness is relieved of unneeded or irrelevant material.

CONSCIOUSNESS AND MEMORY DYNAMICS

Every day of our lives, our brains process a staggering amount of information in unconscious obscurity. Myriad events affect our senses, our thoughts, and our actions without ever reaching awareness. This is both fortunate and necessary, because otherwise our conscious mind would be cluttered with trivia and severely disabled for doing what it does best: attending to critical information, analyzing it, retaining it for subsequent use, and guiding skilled behavior to its goal. In fact, the access of trivia to consciousness can be highly incapacitating—to wit, the patient with obsessive-compulsive disorder.

In the waking state, what has been called the *cognitive unconscious* (Kihlstrom, 1987)—namely, the ensemble of nonconscious cognitive structures and processes—is constantly at work; it never ceases sensing the environment, matching its contents to memory, and constructing appropriate actions in response, all or most all of it outside of consciousness. Whereas we are still far from understanding the neural mechanisms by which all this is accomplished, it is patently obvious that the brain must have at its disposal the means for fast, efficient, and parallel processing that does not rely on conscious awareness. Much of that processing is largely automatized and may occur subcortically, but some undoubtedly involves the cerebral cortex. One of the tenets of this book is that the cerebral cortex is critical for the serial, analytical, and categorical processing that is the basis of selective attention and active memory and that takes place under the limelight of consciousness. One of the book's purposes is to accommodate those two kinds of processing, as postulated by modern information theory, in the framework of cortical neurophysiology. The theoretical approach to cortical memory presented in chapter 5 is consistent with the basic principles of connectionism and parallel distributed processing, while at the same time advocating serial processing for some aspects of memory dynamics, such as conscious retrieval and attention.

Nonetheless, both retrieval and attention also rely substantially on fast parallel processing that occurs at an unconscious level. Again, the apparent objective is efficiency and the conservation of serial, conscious, processing for novel and taxing tasks, for problem-solving tasks that deal with uncertainty and the unexpected and that require decisions. By some curious contrast, it is the conscious awareness of small details of daily experience that reveals to us how very much memory our brain retrieves and processes automatically and out of consciousness. For example, enter a furnished room in your home with which, of course, you are thoroughly familiar and in which someone has displaced an object. The flower vase, say, has been placed on the bookstand instead of on the table. In all probability, you will notice the change. At first, you will be struck by the compelling sensation that something has changed, that something is different in the room, though you cannot tell exactly what. Only after careful scanning of the environment will you find out what it is. Think of how much processing must have taken place in your brain, quickly and unwittingly, from the time you entered the room until the time you spot the flower vase in its new location. Countless memories of your room's objects have been retrieved and matched to reality, or the other way around. It is inconceivable that all that retrieving and processing could have taken place other than through parallel channels, extremely fast, and in the associative areas of your cerebral cortex where perceptual memory resides. Grossberg (1980) has remarked that none of this can be accomplished by conventional linear models of neural encoding and recognition.

The telling detail may be more subtle. For example, I do not ordinarily look at the odometer as I drive my car (I am much less likely to ignore the speedometer). However, almost invariably I notice every change to the next 1000 miles. Now if those three zeroes attract my attention every time they come up, it means that practically every other combination of the last three digits in the mileage counter must be unconsciously registered in peripheral vision while I attend to my driving. But do I really always attend to my driving? I will extend the example to illustrate another point (automobile driving is a curiously fertile source of casual examples for the student of cognition): Automatic and unconscious retrieval and processing apply not only to perceptual memory but to motor memory as well (see later). Indeed, while I am steering my car, changing gears, and obeying traffic lights, my mind may be way off the road, on today's schedule, on last night's concert, or on the amusing antics of one of my monkeys.

Also unconsciously and on a fast track, we are capable of sophisticated retrieval and processing of semantic material—for example, the speed with which we can spot our name on the written page without reading it. Even more amazing is our ability to scan a journal index, without perusal, for articles that interest us.

Subjective observations such as these have been formalized and substantiated by experiment, and the result is a sizeable body of cognitive scientific literature, which will not be reviewed here. The phenomenon of *priming*, formerly discussed in chapters 2 and 8, clearly demonstrates unconscious processing. A prime stimulus (e.g., a word), by virtue of its meaning, can facilitate or bias in some way the cognitive, or even emotional, reaction to a subsequent stimulus (the target) without the subject being aware of the relationships between the two. *Subliminal perception* is another phenomenon of unconscious processing. A tachistoscopic presentation of a message, not consciously perceived by the subject, can appear in his or her dreams or somehow influence his or her subsequent behavior. However, some of the evidence adduced for subliminal perception is of dubious value, and the issue remains controversial and heavily debated, not the least because of its commercial implications.

All these phenomena, subjective or objectifiable, show that mnemonic traces out of consciousness can influence memory retrieval, attention, and consequent behavioral decisions. Thus far here we have dealt primarily with the retrieval and utilization of perceptual memory, including its so-called episodic or declarative contents. The retrieval and enactment of motor memory, however, are also subject to influences from a considerable fund of unconscious knowledge, which has been termed *implicit memory* (Schacter and Graf, 1986). Implicit memory, it will be recalled from chapter 2, is meant to include procedural knowledge as well as the memory of established routines and abstract concepts.

Because implicit memory and its apparent subcomponents, as well as priming, have been found to be unaffected in patients with amnesia from temporal-lobe injury, it has been inferred that this kind of memory, unlike episodic or declarative memory, does not depend on the hippocampus or the cortex of the temporal lobe (Squire, 1986). Even if this inference is correct, however, it does not necessarily follow that implicit memory has a neural topography much different from that of explicit (i.e., episodic, declarative) memory. My position, as explained in previous chapters, is that, with regard to cortical topography, the critical distinction is between perceptual memory and motor memory, respectively represented in postrolandic and prerolandic (frontal) cortex. However, much of motor memory, including habits and conditioned reflexes, is represented in basal ganglia, cerebellum, and other subcortical structures (see chapter 7). Thus, lesions of posterior cortex are more likely to result in perceptual amnesias than frontal lesions are likely to result in motor amnesias. In any event, it is the size and location of a lesion that determines the depth and quality of the amnesia. Semantic memory is anchored in larger networks, with more associations (see chapters 5 and 6), than declarative memory; hence, the latter is more vulnerable to cortical injury than the first. Thus, small posterior lesions may affect only the episodic or declarative aspects of perceptual memory, whereas larger posterior lesions may, in addition, affect the semantic and more abstract memories and knowledge.

By the same reasoning, it is understandable that, under normal circumstances, it is easier to retrieve memories based on many associations (i.e., large cortical networks with many connections) than memories based on only a few (see chapter 6). The reactivation of the large network is facilitated by presence of its numerous access lines. A well-known and often effective maneuver to reach a recondite memory is successively to test in our mind several associative links to it. To retrieve the elusive names of places or persons, it usually helps to recall prior events or contexts of personal contact with them.

As mentioned, in our ordinary contact with the world around us, much memory is retrieved automatically and out of attention or consciousness. However, when our sensory apparatus detects something out of the ordinary, something that does not quite match memory or meet expectations, then attention is mobilized and focused on that something. Otherwise, our attention may be predirected to a given sector of the environment by will, command, or association. In any case, as attention (and consciousness) comes into play, the mode of processing shifts from the parallel and automatic to the serial and methodical mode (see chapter 8). From preconscious preattention, our mind shifts to conscious attention. Within the focus of selective attention, the processing is deployed for the analysis, discrimination, and categorization of the world under the guide of the just-activated memory. While this goes on, however, a substantial amount of other processing continues at a preconscious or unconscious level, quickly and presumably in parallel.

Thus, in the retrieval and activation of memory that go on in ordinary behavior, cortical processing can be conceived to take place along many channels of an extensive network (figure 10.1), with excitation spreading from node to node and elevating neuronal activity above a certain threshold, which we can designate *P-threshold* (*P* for processing). Within that extensive memory network, which is now operational and not just representational, we can conceive a more limited sector of spreading excitation at a higher level yet, above a *C-threshold* (*C* for consciousness). That subsector of cortical network would be the focus of attention, shifting from area to area, within or between hemispheres, and supported, for the most part, by serial processing. Around it there would be a halo of cortex engaged in preconscious parallel processing and, beyond it, an inhibitory halo for filtering and contrast, as hypothesized in chapter 8. Whether, as mentioned there, the thalamus plays a role in the cortical transactions of selective attention is entirely possible but is beyond our present speculation.

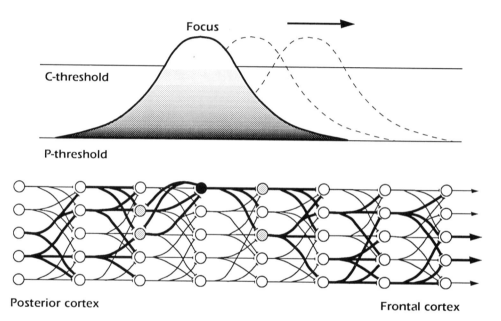

Figure 10.1 Highly schematic and speculative view of the propagation of neural activity through a network linking perceptual cortex to motor cortex. Incoming sensory inputs (entering at left) excite the preconstituted network of interconnected units or cell assemblies (circles), the nodes of the network. As excitation reaches the P-threshold, information is processed within the network, partly in series and partly through interactive parallel channels. The focus of attention, or representation, travels with the processing from one cortical sector to another. As the activation of certain areas surpasses the C-threshold, the focus becomes conscious. If the processing for adaptive behavioral action requires that the focus remain in a given area or group of areas for any length of time, as in active short-term memory, reentry—here symbolized by recurrent connections—temporarily takes precedence and holds the focus in place. Only the part of the network that is in focus at a given time (black unit) would be conscious. Surrounding sectors (gray units) would be preconscious; others (white units) would be unconscious and possibly inhibited.

Very much within current speculation, however, is the idea that consciousness is commonly manifested by high-frequency (approximately 40 Hz oscillatory activity in certain brain structures (Crick and Koch, 1990, 1992). As noted in chapter 5, that kind of activity has been supposed to reflect a correlative neural function important for perceptual binding and attention (Damasio, 1989; Engel et al., 1992; Tiitinen et al., 1993), two psychological functions inextricable from phenomenal experience.

In the transition from perception to action (see the section, Perception-Action Cycle in chapter 9), the spread of excitation takes place, presumably and chiefly, from posterior to frontal cortex, as in the scheme of figure 10.1. The focus of attention is displaced with it when that transition is nonroutine and requires selection and categorization of stimuli and responses. Attention, however, as we have repeatedly noted (see chapters 5, 8) probably is accompanied by a degree of feedback excitation on sensory stages (the network turning on itself). That feedback from frontal to posterior cortex probably is essential when the percept is temporally separate from the action and the intervening time must be bridged with active memory (see chapter 9).

In active memory, the focus of attention has been internalized, no longer directed to external objects but to internal representations; it has become the focus of representation. It is memory in focus, which we experience consciously, though not necessarily continuously; it may be conscious intermittently and rekindled by rehearsal. Nevertheless, despite interruptions and shifts of content, active memory is experienced as a continuous stream of inner awareness and despite the fact that most active memory consists of reactivated long-term memory, it is experienced as an expansion of the present, the "remembered present" of Edelman (1989). As such, it has time tags, but they are recent, in the immediate past. However, I can think of one phenomenon—*déjà vu*—in which these recent tags appear to be lost. Déjà vu is the experience of the present as reenactment of the distant past. It is the compelling sensation that what we are now experiencing we experienced in every detail at another time, although we know with certainty that it cannot have been the case. Some persons experience the phenomenon more than others, at some times in their lives more frequently than at other times, and usually under stress or fatigue.

Déjà vu is difficult to explain neurobiologically. It may be caused by the temporary loss or weakening of the associations that the activated network has with present time references. In the absence of these references, the time references of some old fragments of the network appear to take over and provide the entire network, including its most recent components, with a false (i.e., remote) set of references.

Nonetheless, déja vu is the exception to the rule. To repeat, active memory is experienced as a continuous and coherent flow of representation with recent time references. For this reason, active short-term memory can be considered the quintessential conscious phenomenon. In fact, many writers (e.g., Anderson, 1988; Edelman, 1989; Crick and Koch, 1990, 1992) identify consciousness with this kind of memory. I share their position but differ with those who view active short-term memory as a special and separate structure, cognitive or neural. This is a concept deriving from computer science with dubious neural relevance, for neither consciousness nor active memory has a definite locus in the brain. Consciousness and active memory are where the focus of representation is—where, at a given time, the normal neocortex is most active and above the hypothetical C-threshold. (We are not talking, of course, of the paroxysmal activation of the epileptic seizure.) That cortical field, area, or region varies from moment to moment depending on the needs of the organism, the encounters with the world, and the strivings of creativity.

VOLITION

By its most accepted definition, the act of will is conscious. Nonetheless, just like the act of perception, willful motor action is preceded and accompanied by unconscious processing. There is, in this respect, a remarkable similarity between perception and volition, and this similarity extends to the attentive processes that guide them and, most probably, to their cortical underpinnings. Following the line of reasoning I have tried to develop in previous chapters, it is attractive to explore phenomenologically the parallelism of perceptual and motor attention, although the two affect vastly different spheres of processing. Perceptual attention leads to discrimination and analysis of the sensory world. Motor attention (set) leads to intention and to the willful motor act.

If perceptual attention is the selective categorization of sensory information, motor attention or set is the selective categorization of motor action (see chapter 8). Both are, to a large degree, determined by prior experience (i.e., by perceptual and motor memory, respectively). This implies that in motor attention, in the preparation for the motor act and concomitant with it, much parallel, fast, and unconscious processing takes place, just as in perceptual attention and in retrieval of perceptual memory. Indeed, much of our motility, even in the midst of the most conscious and deliberate behavior, takes place automatically and unconsciously. It is based thoroughly on experience (i.e., on long-term motor memory). Unconscious as it is, it usually serves us well. In fact, as any pianist, typist, or skilled worker will testify to, consciousness can be an impediment to performance. Thus, much motor performance is preorganized and occurs at a preattentive and preconscious level. At the same time, as in the case of perceptual attention, selective motor attention takes place consciously and at least partly in series, setting the motor apparatus for deliberate, usually novel or complex action.

As proposed in chapter 7, the bulk of automatic motility likely is represented, organized, and executed in subcortical structures, including parts of the diencephalon, basal ganglia, and cerebellum. This would be where most of the fast and unconscious processing of motor set takes place. There is, however, neurophysiological evidence to indicate that before a willful act, some of that kind of processing takes place in the cortex. Libet and colleagues (1983a) provided such evidence in a series of ingenious experiments with human subjects carrying scalp electrodes for the recording of slow electrocortical potentials. In one of the experiments, the subject was instructed to self-initiate certain movements while watching the rotating luminous hand of a clocklike display on an oscilloscope screen (a full turn, from 12 to 12 o'clock, in 2.56 seconds). The subject was supposed to report the time at which, before every movement, he or she first felt the awareness of intending to move. The researchers noted that invariably the start of the negative readiness potential, at the vertex, preceded by several hundred milliseconds the reported time of decision. This observation indicates that the voluntary act is preceded by some unconscious processing somewhere in frontal lobe cortex. Thus, frontal activation, of which the subject is unaware, seems to play a role in preattentive motor set. Some investigators (e.g., Deecke and Kornhuber, 1978) have estimated that the readiness potential originates in the supplementary motor area (SMA). I have proposed in chapter 9 that it is part of a larger frontal wave of surface negativity that originates in prefrontal cortex before willful action. In part because of the presumed origin of the readiness potential in the SMA, Eccles (1982) has postulated that this area is the source of voluntary movement.

It seems risky to designate any neural structure, in frontal cortex or elsewhere, as the site of origin of voluntary movement—something akin to a center of will. This kind of reasoning inevitably leads to an infinite regress. Indeed, anyone arguing for the supremacy of prefrontal or premotor cortex in the initiation or execution of action should consider that the frontal, especially prefrontal, cortex is one of the most richly connected regions of the cerebrum (see chapter 4). In addition to receiving afferents from subcortical structures involved in motor control, the prefrontal and premotor cortices receive abundant afferents from limbic and brainstem regions that are clearly implicated in drive and motivation. They also receive profuse connections from a large array of areas of posterior neocortex that we have seen implicated in perception and perceptual memory. It will be remembered that in chapter 5 and subsequent chapters, we reasoned that through those connections the perceptual cortical networks of posterior cortex expand into the frontal lobe and blend there with motor networks. It is through those connections that frontal neuron assemblies are recruited for active memory and for the organization of motor action.

Thus, to assign will to any frontal region obviously begs the question of prior command on that region from another structure; the same question can be asked about that other structure, whatever it may be, and then about its precursor, and so on. Our theoretical construct of the perception-action cycle (see chapter 9) obviates the problem, because it places frontal cortices under the influence of posterior cortices and subcortical structures, within a circular array in which there is no true origin. In that light, the philosophical question of free will versus determinism becomes meaningless. A reasonable neurobiological compromise between the two sides of that much-debated question is the notion that voluntary action is probabilistically determined by resolution of conflict, in frontal cortex, between competing neural influences of diverse origin. Some of them, of course, are at any given time more powerful and peremptory than others. Will is as free as these influences are unconscious and as other seemingly plausible options are available. It should be noted, in closing, that some of those unconscious influences may come from yet unidentified cortical areas that represent our higher values—indeed, from a fund of abstract perceptual and motor memory built by education and the good example of fellow humans.

References

Abeles, M. *Local Cortical Circuits: An Electrophysiological Study.* New York: Springer, 1982.

Abeles, M., Bergman, H., Margalit, E., and Vaadia, E. Spatiotemporal firing patterns in the frontal cortex of behaving monkeys. *J. Neurophysiol.* 70:1629–1638, 1993.

Ackerly, S. S., and Benton, A. L. Report of case of bilateral frontal lobe defect. *Res. Publ. Assoc. Res. Nerv. Ment. Dis.* 27:479–504, 1947.

Adams, J. A. Learning of movement sequences. *Psychol. Bull.* 96:3–28, 1984.

Aertsen, A. M. H. J., Gerstein, G. L., Habib, M. K., and Palm, G. Dynamics of neuronal firing correlation: Modulation of "effective connectivity." *J. Neurophysiol.* 61:900–917, 1989.

Ageranioti-Bélanger, S. A., and Chapman, C. E. Discharge properties of neurones in the hand area of primary somatosensory cortex in monkeys in relation to the performance of an active tactile discrimination task: II. Area 2 as compared to areas 3b and 1. *Exp. Brain Res.* 91:207–228, 1992.

Ahissar, E., and Vaadia, E. Oscillatory activity of single units in a somatosensory cortex of an awake monkey and their possible role in texture analysis. *Proc. Natl. Acad. Sci. U.S.A* 87:8935–8939, 1990.

Aizawa, H., Inase, M., Mushiake, H., Shima, K., and Tanji, J. Reorganization of activity in the supplementary motor area associated with motor learning and functional recovery. *Exp. Brain Res.* 84:668–671, 1991.

Albert, M. L., Goodglass, H., Helm, N. A., Rubens, A. B., and Alexander, M. P. *Clinical Aspects of Dysphasia.* New York: Springer, 1981.

Alexander, G. E. Selective neuronal discharge in monkey putamen reflects intended direction of planned limb movements. *Exp. Brain Res.* 67:623–634, 1987.

Alexander, G. E., and Crutcher, M. D. Preparation for movement: Neural representations of intended direction in three motor areas of the monkey. *J. Neurophysiol.* 64:133–150, 1990a.

Alexander, G. E., and Crutcher, M. D. Neural representations of the target (goal) of visually guided arm movements in three motor areas of the monkey. *J. Neurophysiol.* 64:164–178, 1990b.

Alexander, G. E., and Crutcher, M. D. Functional architecture of basal ganglia circuits: Neural substrates of parallel processing. *Trends Neurosci.* 13:266–271, 1990c.

Alexander, G. E., and Delong, M. R. Microstimulation of the primate neostriatum: II. Somatotopic organization of striatal microexcitable zones and their relation to neuronal response properties. *J. Neurophysiol.* 53:1417–1430, 1985.

Alexander, G. E., Delong, M. R., and Crutcher, M. D. Do cortical and basal ganglia motor areas use "motor programs" to control movement? *Behav. Brain Sci.* 15:656–665, 1992.

Alexander, G. E., and Fuster, J. M. Effects of cooling prefrontal cortex on cell firing in the nucleus medialis dorsalis. *Brain Res.* 61:93–105, 1973.

Alivisatos, B. The role of the frontal cortex in the use of advance information in a mental rotation paradigm. *Neuropsychologia* 30:145–159, 1992.

Alkon, D. L. Calcium-mediated reduction of ionic currents: A biophysical memory trace. *Science* 226:1037–1045, 1984.

Allen, G. I., and Tsukahara, N. Cerebrocerebellar communication system. *Physiol. Rev.* 54:957–997, 1974.

Alvarez-Buylla, A., Kirn, J. R., and Nottebohm, F. Birth of projection neurons in adult avian brain may be related to perceptual or motor learning. *Science* 249:1444–1446, 1990.

Amaral, D. G. Memory: Anatomical organization of candidate brain regions. In *Handbook of Physiology: Nervous System*, vol. 5: *Higher Functions of the Brain* (part 1), edited by F. Plum. Bethesda, MD: American Physiological Society, 1987, pp. 211–294.

Amaral, D. G., and Witter, M. P. The three-dimensional organization of the hippocampal formation: A review of anatomical data. *Neuroscience* 31:571–591, 1989.

Ambros-Ingerson, J., Granger, R., and Lynch, G. Simulation of paleocortex performs hierarchical clustering. *Science* 247:1344–1348, 1990.

Amit, D. J. Attractor neural networks and biological reality: Associative memory and learning. *Future Generat. Comput. Sys.* 6:111–119, 1990.

Andersen, R. A., Asanuma, C., and Cowan, W. M. Callosal and prefrontal associational projecting cell populations in area 7A of the macaque monkey: A study using retrogradely transported fluorescent dyes. *J. Comp. Neurol.* 232:443–455, 1985.

Andersen, R. A., Bracewell, R. M., Barash, S., Gnadt, J. W., and Fogassi, L. Eye position effects on visual, memory, and saccade-related activity in areas LIP and 7a of macaque. *J. Neurosci.* 10:1176–1196, 1990.

Anderson, J. A. *Neural Models with Cognitive Implications*. Hillsdale, NJ: Erlbaum, 1977.

Anderson, J. A., and Hinton, G. E. Models of information processing in the brain. In *Parallel Models of Associative Memory*, edited by G. E. Hinton, and J. A. Anderson. Hillsdale, NJ. Erlbaum, 1981, pp. 9–44.

Anderson, J. A. and Rosenfeld, E., *Neurocomputing*. Cambridge, MA: MIT Press, 1988.

Anderson, J. R. *Cognitive Psychology and Its Implications*. New York: Freeman, 1988.

Aou, S., Woody, C. D., and Dorwin, B. Changes in the activity of units of the cat motor cortex with rapid conditioning and extinction of a compound eye blink movement. *J. Neurosci.* 12:549–559, 1992.

Arbib, M. A. Perceptual structures and distributed motor control. In *Handbook of Physiology: Nervous System*, vol. 2, edited by V. B. Brooks, Bethesda, MD: American Physiological Society, 1981, pp. 1448–1480.

Arikuni, T., Watanabe, K., and Kubota, K. The organization of the connection of the prefrontal cortex with the premotor area in macaque monkeys. *Soc. Neurosci. Abstr.* 12 1440, 1986.

Arnsten, A. F. T., and Goldman-Rakic, P. S. 2-Adrenergic mechanisms in prefrontal cortex associated with cognitive decline in aged nonhuman primates. *Science* 230:1273–1276, 1985.

Asanuma, H. Recent developments in the study of the columnar arrangement of neurons within the motor cortex. *Physiol. Rev.* 55:143–156, 1975.

Asanuma, H. Functional role of sensory inputs to the motor cortex. *Prog. Neurobiol.* 16:241–262, 1981.

Aserinsky, E., and Kleitman, N. Regularly occurring periods of eye motility and concurrent phenomena during sleep. *Science* 118:273–274, 1953.

Ashford, J. W., and Fuster, J. M. Occipital and inferotemporal responses to visual signals in the monkey. *Exp. Neurol.* 90:444–466, 1985.

Atkinson, R. C., and Shiffrin, R. M. Human memory: A proposed system and its control processes. In *The Psychology of Learning and Motivation: Advances in Research and Theory,* vol. 2, edited by Spence, K. W. and Spence, J. T. New York: Academic, 1968, pp. 89–195.

Bachevalier, J., Landis, L. S., Walker, L. C., Brickson, M., Mishkin, M., Price, D. L., and Cork, L. C. Aged monkeys exhibit behavioral deficits indicative of widespread cerebral dysfunction. *Neurobiol. Aging* 12:99–111, 1991.

Bach-y-Rita, P. Neurotransmission in the brain by diffusion through the extracellular fluid: A review. *NeuroReport* 4:343–350, 1993.

Baddeley, A. Working memory. *Philos. Trans. R. Soc. Lond.* [Biol.] 302:311–324, 1983.

Baddeley, A. Cognitive psychology and human memory. *Trends Neurosci.* 4:176–181, 1988.

Bagshaw, M. H., and Pribram, K. H. Cortical organization in gustation. *J. Neurophysiol.* 16:499–508, 1953.

Ballard, D. H. Cortical connections and parallel processing: Structure and function. *Behav. Brain Sci.* 9:67–120, 1986.

Baranyi, A., Szente, M. B., and Woody, C. D. Properties of associative long-lasting potentiation induced by cellular conditioning in the motor cortex of conscious cats. *Neuroscience* 42:321–334, 1991.

Barbas, H. Architecture and cortical connections of the prefrontal cortex in the rhesus monkey. In *Advances in Neurology,* Vol. 57, edited by P. Chauvel, A. V. Delgado-Escueta, E. Halgren, and J. Bancaud. New York: Raven Press, 1992, pp. 91–115.

Barbas, H., and De Olmos, J. Projections from the amygdala to basoventral and mediodorsal prefrontal regions in the rhesus monkey. *J. Comp. Neurol.* 300:549–571, 1990.

Barbizet, J. *Human Memory and Its Pathology.* San Francisco: Freeman, 1970.

Barbizet, J., Duizabo, P., and Flavigny, R. Rôle des lobes frontaux dans le langage. *Rev. Neurol.* (Paris) 131:525–544, 1975.

Barnes, C. A. Memory deficits associated with senescence: A neurophysiological and behavioral study in the rat. *J. Comp. Physiol. Psychol.* 93:74–104, 1979.

Barnes, C. A., and McNaughton, B. L. Physiological compensation for loss of afferent synapses in rat hippocampal granule cells during senescence. *J. Physiol.* 309:473–485, 1980.

Barnes, C. A., and McNaughton, B. L. An age comparison of the rates of acquisition and forgetting of spatial information in relation to long-term enhancement of hippocampal synapses. *Behav. Neurosci.* 99:1040–1048, 1985.

Barnes, C. A., Rao, G., and McNaughton, B. L. Increased electrotonic coupling in aged rat hippocampus: A possible mechanism for cellular excitability changes. *J. Comp. Neurol.* 259:549–558, 1987.

Barrionuevo, G., and Brown, T. H. Associative long-term potentiation in hippocampal slices. *Proc. Natl. Acad. Sci. U.S.A* 80:7347–7351, 1983.

Bartus, R. T. Drugs to treat age-related neurodegenerative problems. *J. Am. Geriatr. Soc.* 38:680–695, 1990.

Basso, A., Capitani, E., and Laiacona, M. Progressive language impairment without dementia: A case with isolated category specific semantic defect. *J. Neurol. Neurosurg. Psychiatry* 51:1201–1207, 1988.

Bates, J. F., and Goldman-Rakic, P. S. Prefrontal connections of medial motor areas in the rhesus monkey. *J. Comp. Neurol.* 336:211–228, 1993.

Bauer, P. J., and Hertsgaard, L. A. Increasing steps in recall of events: Factors facilitating immediate and long-term memory in 13.5- and 16.5-month-old children. *Child Dev.* 64:1204–1223, 1993.

Bauer, P. J., and Mandler, J. M. One thing follows another: Effects of temporal structure on 1- to 2-year-olds' recall of events. *Develop. Psychol.* 25:197–206, 1989.

Bauer, R. H., and Fuster, J. M. Delayed-matching and delayed-response deficit from cooling dorsolateral prefrontal cortex in monkeys. *J. Comp. Physiol. Psychol.* 90:293–302, 1976.

Baylis, G. C., Rolls, E. T., and Leonard, C. M. Functional subdivisions of the temporal lobe neocortex. *J. Neurosci.* 7:330–342, 1987.

Benevento, L. A., Fallon, J., Davis, B. J., and Rezak, M. Auditory-visual interaction in single cells in the cortex of the superior temporal sulcus and the orbital frontal cortex of the macaque monkey. *Exp. Neurol.* 57:849–872, 1977.

Bernstein, N. *The Co-Ordination and Regulation of Movements.* Oxford: Pergamon, 1967.

Betz, W. Anatomischer Nachweis zweier Gehirncentra. *Centralb. Med. Wissensch.* 12:578–580, 1874.

Birbaumer, N., Elbert, T., Canavan, A. G. M., and Rockstroh, B. Slow potentials of the cerebral cortex and behavior. *Physiol. Rev.* 70:1–41, 1990.

Blakemore, C., Garey, L. J., and Vital-Durand, F. The physiological effects of monocular deprivation and their reversal in the monkey's visual cortex. *J. Physiol.* 283:223–262, 1978.

Blakemore, C., and Van Sluyters, C. Reversal of the physiological effects of monocular deprivation in kittens: Further evidence for a sensitive period. *J. Physiol.* 237:195–216, 1974.

Bliss, T. V. P., and Lomo, T. Long-lasting potentiation of synaptic transmission in the dentate area of the anaesthetized rabbit following stimulation of the perforant path. *J. Physiol.* 232:331–356, 1973.

Blum, J. S. Cortical organization in somesthesis: Effects of lesions in posterior associative cortex on somatosensory function in *Macaca mulatta. Comp. Psychol. Monogr.* 20:219–249, 1951.

Bodamer, J. Die Prosop-Agnosie. *Arch. Psychiatr. Nervenkrankheiten* 17:6–53, 1948.

Böhme, G. A., Bon, C., Lemaire, M., Reibaud, M., Piot, O., Stutzmann, J.-M., Doble, A., and Blanchard, J.-C. Altered synaptic plasticity and memory formation in nitric oxide synthase inhibitor-treated rats. *Proc. Natl. Acad. Sci. U.S.A.* 90:9191–9194, 1993.

Bonin, G. von. *Essay on the Cerebral Cortex.* Springfield, IL: Thomas, 1950.

Bonin, G. von, and Bailey, P. *The Neocortex of Macaca Mulatta*, Urbana, IL: University of Illinois Press, 1947.

Bornstein, W. S. Cortical representation of taste in man and monkey. *Yale J. Biol. Med.* 13:133–156, 1940.

Bourgeois, J.-P., Goldman-Rakic, P. S., and Rakic, P. Synaptogenesis in the prefrontal cortex of rhesus monkeys. *Cerebral Cortex* (in press).

Braitenberg, V. Cell assemblies in the cerebral cortex. In *Theoretical Approaches to Complex Systems,* edited by R. Heim, and G. Palm. Berlin: Springer-Verlag, 1978, pp. 171–188.

Braitenberg, V., and Schüz, A. Basic features of cortical connectivity and some consideration on language. In *Language Origin: A Multidisciplinary Approach,* edited by J. Wind, B. Chiarelli, B. Bichakjian, and A. Nocentini, Netherlands: Kluwer Academic, 1992, pp. 89–102.

Breen, R. A., and McGaugh, J. L. Facilitation of maze learning with posttrial injections of picrotoxin. *J. Comp. Physiol. Psychol.* 54:498–501, 1961.

Bressler, S. L., Coppola, R., and Nakamura, R. Episodic multiregional cortical coherence at multiple frequencies during visual task performance. *Nature* 366:153–156, 1993.

Brizzee, K. R., Ordy, J. M., and Bartus, R. T. Localization of cellular changes within multimodal sensory regions in aged monkey brain: Possible implications for age-related cognitive loss. *Neurobiol. Aging* 1:45–52, 1980.

Broadbent, D. E. *Perception and Communication.* New York: Pergamon, 1958.

Broadbent, D. E. The functional approach to memory. *Philos. Trans. R. Soc. Lond. [Biol.]* 302:239–249, 1983.

Broca, P. Remarques sur la siège de la faculté du langage articulé, suivi d'une observation d'aphémie. *Bull. Anat. Soc.* (Paris) 2:330–357, 1861.

Brodmann, K. *Vergleichende Lokalisationslehre der Grosshirnrinde in ihren Prinzipien dargestellt auf Grund des Zellenbaues.* Leipzig: Barth, 1909.

Brody, B. A., Kinney, H. C., Kloman, A. S., and Gilles, F. H. Sequence of central nervous system myelination in human infancy: I. An autopsy study of myelination. *J. Neuropathol. Exp. Neurol.* 46:283–301, 1987.

Brody, H. Organization of the cerebral cortex: III. A study of aging in the human cerebral cortex. *J. Comp. Neurol.* 102:511–556, 1955.

Brooks, D. N., and Baddeley, A. What can amnesic patients learn? *Neuropsychologia* 14:111–122, 1976.

Brooks, V. B. *The Neural Basis of Motor Control.* New York: Oxford University Press, 1986.

Brothers, L., and Ring, B. Mesial temporal neurons in the macaque monkey with responses selective for aspects of social stimuli. *Behav. Brain Res.* 57:53–61, 1993.

Brown, J. W. The microstructure of action. In *The Frontal Lobes Revisited,* edited by E. Perecman. New York: IRBN Press, 1987, pp. 250–272.

Brown, T. H., Kairiss, E. W., and Keenan, C. L. Hebbian synapses: Biophysical mechanisms and algorithms. *Annu. Rev. Neurosci.* 13:475–511, 1990.

Bruce, C., Desimone, R., and Gross, C. G. Visual properties of neurons in a polysensory area in superior temporal sulcus of the macaque. *J. Neurophysiol.* 46:369–384, 1981.

Bruce, C. J., and Goldberg, M. E. Primate frontal eye fields: I. Single neurons discharging before saccades. *J. Neurophysiol.* 53:603–634, 1985.

Bruce, C. J., Goldberg, M. E., Bushnell, M. C., and Stanton, G. B. Primate frontal eye fields: II. Physiological and anatomical correlates of electrically evoked eye movements. *J. Neurophysiol.* 54:714–734, 1985.

Bruner, J. S. Organization of early skilled action. *Child Dev.* 44:1–11, 1973.

Brunia, C. H. M., Haagh, S. A. V. M., and Scheirs, J. G. M. Waiting to respond: Electrophysiological measurements in man during preparation for a voluntary movement. In *Motor Behavior,* edited by H. Heuer, U. Kleinbeck, and K.-H. Schmidt. New York: Springer, 1985.

Bundesen, C. A theory of visual attention. *Psychol. Rev.* 97:523–547, 1990.

Buonomano, D. V., and Byrne, J. H. Long-term synaptic changes produced by a cellular analog of classical conditioning in *Aplysia. Science* 249:420–423, 1990.

Burton, M. J., Rolls, E. T., and Mora, F. Effects of hunger on the responses of neurons in the lateral hypothalamus to the sight and taste of food. *Exp. Neurol.* 51:668–677, 1976.

Buschke, H. Short-term retention, learning, and retrieval from long-term memory. In *Short-Term Memory,* edited by D. Deutsch and J. A. Deutsch. New York: Academic, 1975, pp. 73–106.

Bushnell, M. C., Goldberg, M. E., and Robinson, D. L. Behavioral enhancement of visual responses in monkey cerebral cortex: I. Modulation in posterior parietal cortex related to selective visual attention. *J. Neurophysiol.* 46:755–772, 1981.

Butters, N., and Barton, M. Effect of parietal lobe damage on the performance of reversible operations in space. *Neuropsychologia* 8:205–214, 1970.

Buys, E. J., Lemon, R. N., Mantel, G. W. H., and Muir, R. B. Selective facilitation of different hand muscles by single corticospinal neurones in the conscious monkey. *J. Physiol.* 381:529–549, 1986.

Campbell, A. W. *Histological Studies on the Localization of Cerebral Function.* Cambridge, Engl.: Cambridge University Press, 1905.

Caramazza, A., and Hillis, A. E. Spatial representation of words in the brain implied by studies of a unilateral neglect patient. *Nature* 346:267–269, 1990.

Carew, T. J., Hawkins, R. D., Abrams, T. W., and Kandel, E. A test of Hebb's postulate at identified synapses which mediate classical conditioning in *Aplysia. J. Neurosci.* 4:1217–1224, 1984.

Carlsson, A. Aging and brain neurotransmitters. In *Strategies for the Development of an Effective Treatment for Senile Dementia,* edited by T. Crook and S. Gershon. New Canaan, CT: Mark Powley Associates, 1981, pp. 93–104.

Carpenter, G. A., and Grossberg, S. Normal and amnesic learning, recognition and memory by a neural model of cortico-hippocampal interactions. *Trends Neurosci.* 16:131–137, 1993.

Cavada, C., and Goldman-Rakic, P. S. Posterior parietal cortex in rhesus monkey: I. Parcellation of areas based on distinctive limbic and sensory corticocortical connections. *J. Comp. Neurol.* 287:393–421, 1989a.

Cavada, C., and Goldman-Rakic, P. S. Posterior parietal cortex in rhesus monkey: II. Evidence for segregated corticocortical networks linking sensory and limbic areas with the frontal lobe. *J. Comp. Neurol.* 287:422–445, 1989b.

Cermak, L. S., Lewis, R., Butters, N., and Goodglass, H. Role of verbal mediation in performance of motor tasks by Korsakoff patients. *Percept. Mot. Skills* 37:259–262, 1973.

Cermak, L. S., and O'Connor, M. The anterograde and retrograde retrieval ability of a patient with amnesia due to encephalitis. *Neuropsychologia* 21:213–234, 1983.

Changeux, J. P., and Danchin, A. Selective stabilisation of developing synapses as a mechanism for the specification of neuronal networks. *Nature* 264:705–712, 1976.

Chapman, C. E., and Ageranioti-Bélanger, S. A. Discharge properties of neurones in the hand area of primary somatosensory cortex in monkeys in relation to the performance of an active tactile discrimination task: I. Areas 3b and 1. *Exp. Brain Res.* 87:319–339, 1991.

Chapman, C. E., Spidalieri, G., and Lamarre, Y. Discharge properties of area 5 neurones during arm movements triggered by sensory stimuli in the monkey. *Brain Res.* 309:63–77, 1984.

Chelazzi, L., Miller, E. K., Duncan, J., and Desimone, R. A neural basis for visual search in inferior temporal cortex. *Nature* 363:345–347, 1993.

Cheney, P. D., and Fetz, E. E. Comparable patterns of muscle facilitation evoked by individual corticomotoneuronal (CM) cells and by single intracortical microstimuli in primates: Evidence for functional groups of CM cells. *J. Neurophysiol.* 53:786–804, 1985.

Cherry, E. C. Some experiments on the recognition of speech, with one and with two ears. *J. Acoust. Soc. Am.* 25:975–979, 1953.

Chomsky, N. *Aspects of the Theory of Syntax.* Cambridge, MA: MIT Press, 1965.

Chomsky, N. *Reflections on Language.* New York: Pantheon Books, 1975.

Chomsky, N. *Rules and Representations.* New York: Columbia University Press, 1980.

Chow, K. L. Effects of partial extirpations of the posterior association cortex on visually mediated behavior. *Comp. Psychol. Monogr.* 20:187–217, 1951.

Churchland, P. S. *Neurophilosophy.* Cambridge, MA: MIT Press, 1986.

Churchland, P. S., and Sejnowski, T. J. *The Computational Brain.* Cambridge, MA: MIT Press, 1992.

Coburn, K. L., Ashford, J. W., and Fuster, J. M. Visual response latencies in temporal lobe structures as a function of stimulus information load. *Behav. Neurosci.* 104:62–73, 1990.

Cohen, N. J. Preserved learning capacity in amnesia: Evidence for multiple memory systems. In *Neuropsychology of Memory,* edited by L. R. Squire and N. Butters. New York: Guilford Press, 1984, pp. 83–103.

Cohen, N. J. and Eichenbaum, H. *Memory, Amnesia, and the Hippocampal System.* Cambridge, MA: MIT Press, 1993.

Cohen, N. J., and Squire, L. R. Preserved learning and retention of pattern-analyzing skill in amnesia: Dissociation of knowing how and knowing that. *Science* 210:207–210, 1980.

Colebatch, J. G., Deiber, M.-P., Passingham, R. E., Friston, K. J., and Frackowiak, S. J. Regional cerebral blood flow during voluntary arm and hand movements in human subjects. *J. Neurophysiol.* 65:1392–1401, 1991.

Collingridge, G. L., and Bliss, T. V. P. NMDA receptors—their role in long-term potentiation. *Trends Neurosci.* 10:288–293, 1987.

Collingridge, G. L., Kehl, S. J., and McLennan, H. Excitatory amino acids in synaptic transmission in the Schaffer collateral-commissural pathway of the rat hippocampus. *J. Physiol.* 334:33–46, 1983.

Colombo, M., D'Amato, M. R., Rodman, H. R., and Gross, C. G. Auditory association cortex lesions impair auditory short-term memory in monkeys. *Science* 247:336–338, 1990.

Coltheart, M. Iconic memory. *Philos. Trans. R. Soc. Lond.* [*Biol.*] 302:283–294, 1983.

Conel, J. L. *The Postnatal Development of the Human Cerebral Cortex*, vols. 1–6. Cambridge: Harvard University Press, 1939.

Corbetta, M., Miezin, F. M., Dobmeyer, S., Shulman, G. L., and Petersen, S. E. Attentional modulation of neural processing of shape, color, and velocity in humans. *Science* 248:1556–1559, 1990.

Corbetta, M., Miezin, F. M., Shulman, G. L., and Petersen, S. E. A PET study of visuospatial attention. *J. Neurosci.* 13:1202–1226, 1993.

Corkin, S. Lasting consequences of bilateral medial temporal lobectomy: Clinical course and experimental findings in H. M. *Semin. Neurol.* 4:249–259, 1984.

Corkin, S., Milner, B., and Rasmussen, T. Somatosensory thresholds. *Arch. Neurol.* 23:41–58, 1970.

Cotman, C. W., and Iversen, L. L. Excitatory amino acids in the brain—focus on NMDA receptors. *Trends Neurosci.* 10:263–265, 1987.

Cotman, C. W., Monaghan, D. T., and Ganong, A. H. Excitatory amino acid neurotransmission: NMDA receptors and Hebb-type synaptic plasticity. *Annu. Rev. Neurosci.* 11:61–80, 1988.

Cotman, C. W., Monaghan, D. T., Ottersen, O. P., and Storm-Mathisen, J. Anatomical organization of excitatory amino acid receptors and their pathways. *Trends Neurosci.* 10:273–280, 1987.

Cowan, N. Evolving conceptions of memory storage, selective attention, and their mutual constraints within the human information-processing system. *Psychol. Bull.* 104:163–191, 1988.

Cowey, A. Grasping the essentials. *Nature* 349:102–103, 1991.

Cowey, A., and Gross, C. G. Effects of foveal prestriate and inferotemporal lesions on visual discriminations by rhesus monkeys. *Exp. Brain Res.* 11:128–144, 1970.

Coyle, J. T., Price, D. L., and Delong, M. R. Alzheimer's disease: A disorder of cortical cholinergic innervation. *Science* 219:1184–1190, 1983.

Cragg, B. G. Changes in visual cortex on first exposure of rats to light. *Nature* 215:251–253, 1967.

Cragg, B. G. The density of synapses and neurons in normal, mentally defective and ageing human brains. *Brain* 98:81–90, 1975.

Craik, F. I. M. On the transfer of information from temporary to permanent memory. *Philos. Trans. R. Soc. Lond.* [*Biol.*] 302:341–359, 1983.

Creutzfeldt, O. D. Generality of the functional structure of the neocortex. *Naturwissenschaften* 64:507–517, 1977.

Crick, F. The function of the thalamic reticular complex: The searchlight hypothesis. *Proc. Natl. Acad. Sci.* 81:4586–4590, 1984.

Crick, F., and Koch, C. Towards a neurobiological theory of consciousness. *Seminars in the Neurosciences* 2:263–275, 1990.

Crick, F., and Koch, C. The problem of consciousness. *Sci. Am.* 267:153–159, 1992.

Crick, F., and Mitchison, G. The function of dream sleep. *Nature* 304:111–114, 1983.

Critchley, M. *The Parietal Lobes.* London: Arnold, 1953.

Crutcher, M. D., and Alexander, G. E. Movement-related neuronal activity selectively coding either direction or muscle pattern in three motor areas of the monkey. *J. Neurophysiol.* 64:151–163, 1990.

Crutcher, M. D., and Delong, M. R. Single cell studies of the primate putamen: II. Relations to direction of movement and pattern of muscular activity. *Exp. Brain Res.* 53:244–258, 1984.

Cumin, R., Bandle, E. F., Gamzu, E., and Haefely, W. E. Effects of the novel compound Aniracetam (Ro 13–5057) upon impaired learning and memory in rodents. *Psychopharmacology* 78:104–111, 1982.

Cupp, C. J., and Uemura, E. Age-related changes in prefrontal cortex of *Macaca mulatta*: Quantitative analysis of dendritic branching patterns. *Exp. Neurol.* 69:143–163, 1980.

Damasio, A. R. The brain binds entities and events by multiregional activation from convergence zones. *Neural Comput.* 1:123–132, 1989.

Damasio, A. R. Category-related recognition defects as a clue to the neural substrates of knowledge. *Trends Neurosci.* 13:95–98, 1990a.

Damasio, A. R. Synchronous activation in multiple cortical regions: A mechanism for recall. *Seminars in the Neurosciences* 2:287–296, 1990b.

Damasio, A. R., Eslinger, P. J., Damasio, H., Van Hoesen, G. W., and Cornell, S. Multimodal amnesic syndrome following bilateral temporal and basal forebrain damage. *Arch. Neurol.* 42:252–259, 1985.

Damasio, A. R., Tranel, D., and Damasio, H. Face agnosia and the neural substrates of memory. *Annu. Rev. Neurosci.* 13:89–109, 1990.

Damasio, A. R., and Van Hoesen, G. W. Emotional disturbances associated with focal lesions of the limbic frontal lobe. In *Neuropsychology of Human Emotion,* edited by K. M. Heilman and P. Satz. New York: Guilford Press, 1983, pp. 85–110.

Davidoff, J. B., and Ostergaard, A. L. Colour anomia resulting from weakened short-term colour memory. *Brain* 107:415–431, 1984.

De Renzi, E. *Disorders of Space Exploration and Cognition.* New York: Wiley, 1982.

De Renzi, E., and Scotti, G. Autotopagnosia: Fiction or reality? *Arch. Neurol.* 23:221–227, 1970.

Decker, M. W., and McGaugh, J. L. The role of interactions between the cholinergic system and other neuromodulatory systems in learning and memory. *Synapse* 7:151–168, 1991.

Deecke, L., and Kornhuber, H. H. An electrical sign of participation of the mesial "supplementary" motor cortex in human voluntary finger movement. *Brain Res.* 159:473–476, 1978.

Deiber, M.-P., Passingham, R. E., Colebatch, J. G., Friston, K. J., Nixon, P. D., and Frackowiak, R. S. J. Cortical areas and the selection of movement: A study with positron emission tomography. *Exp. Brain Res.* 84:393–402, 1991.

Delong, M. R., and Georgopoulos, A. P. Motor Functions of the Basal Ganglia. In *Handbook of Physiology,* vol. 2, edited by V. B. Brooks. Bethesda, MD: American Physiological Society, 1981, pp. 1017–1061.

Desimone, R., Albright, T. D., Gross, C. G., and Bruce, C. Stimulus-selective properties of inferior temporal neurons in the macaque. *J. Neurosci.* 4:2051–2062, 1984.

Desimone, R., and Gross, C. G. Visual areas in the temporal cortex of the macaque. *Brain Res.* 178:363–380, 1979.

Deutsch, J. A., and Deutsch, D. Attention: Some theoretical considerations. *Psychol. Rev.* 70:80–90, 1963.

Dewson, J. H. Preliminary evidence of hemispheric asymmetry of auditory function in monkeys. In *Lateralization in the Nervous System,* edited by S. Harnard, R. W. Doty, L. Goldstein, J. Jaynes, and G. Krauthamer. New York: Academic, 1977, pp. 63–71.

Dewson, J. H., Cowey, A., and Weiskrantz, L. Disruptions of auditory sequence discrimination by unilateral and bilateral cortical ablations of superior temporal gyrus in the monkey. *Exp. Neurol.* 28:529–548, 1970.

Diamond, M. C., Law, F., Rhodes, H., Lindner, B., Rosenzweig, M. R., Krech, D., and Bennett, E. L. Increases in cortical depth and glia numbers in rats subjected to enriched environment. *J. Comp. Neurol.* 128:117–126, 1966.

Di Mattia, B. V., Posley, K. A., and Fuster, J. M. Crossmodal short-term memory of haptic and visual information. *Neuropsychologia* 28:17–33, 1990.

Di Pellegrino, G., Fadiga, L., Fogassi, L., Gallese, V., and Rizzolatti, G. Understanding motor events: A neurophysiological study. *Exp. Brain Res.* 91:176–180, 1992.

Di Pellegrino, G., and Wise, S. P. A neurophysiological comparison of three distinct regions of the primate frontal lobe. *Brain* 114:951–978, 1991.

Di Pellegrino, G., and Wise, S. P. Visuospatial versus visuomotor activity in the premotor and prefrontal cortex of a primate. *J. Neurosci.* 3:1227–1243, 1993.

Dingledine, R. N-Methyl aspartate activates voltage-dependent calcium conductance in rat hippocampal pyramidal cells. *J. Physiol.* 343:385–405, 1983.

Donchin, E., and Cohen, L. Averaged evoked potentials and intramodality selective attention. *Electroencephalogr. Clin. Neurophysiol.* 22:537–546, 1967.

Donoghue, J. P., and Sanes, J. N. Peripheral nerve injury in developing rats reorganizes representation pattern in motor cortex. *Proc. Natl. Acad. Sci. U.S.A.* 84:1123–1126, 1987.

Donoghue, J. P., and Sanes, J. N. Organization of adult motor cortex representation patterns following neonatal forelimb nerve injury in rats. *J. Neurosci.* 8:3221–3232, 1988.

Donoghue, J. P., Suner, S., and Sanes, J. N. Dynamic organization of primary motor cortex output to target muscles in adult rats: II. Rapid reorganization following motor nerve lesions. *Exp. Brain Res.* 79:492–503, 1990.

Doty, R. W. Conditioned reflexes elicited by electrical stimulation of the brain in macaques. *J. Neurophysiol.* 28:623–640, 1965.

Drewe, E. A. An experimental investigation of Luria's theory on the effects of frontal lobe lesions in man. *Neuropsychologia* 13:421–429, 1975.

Duara, R., Grady, C., Haxby, J., Ingvar, D., Sokoloff, L., Margolin, R. A., Manning, R. G., Cutler, N. R., and Rapoport, S. I. Human brain glucose utilization and cognitive function in relation to age. *Ann. Neurol.* 16:702–713, 1984.

Duffy, F. H., and Burchfiel, J. L. Somatosensory system: Organizational hierarchy from single units in monkey area 5. *Science* 172:273–275, 1971.

Eason, R. G., Harter, R. M., and White, C. T. Effects of attention and arousal on visually evoked cortical potentials and reaction time in man. *Physiol. Behav.* 4:283–289, 1969.

Eccles, J. C. Circuits in the cerebellar control of movement. *Proc. Natl. Acad. Sci.* 58:336–343, 1967.

Eccles, J. C. The initiation of voluntary movements by the supplementary motor area. *Archiv. Psychiatr. Nervenkrankh.* 231:423–441, 1982.

Eccles, J. C. *Evolution of the Brain: Creation of the Self.* London: Routledge, 1989.

Eckhorn, R., Bauer, R., Jordan, W., Brosch, M., Kruse, W., Munk, M., and Reitboeck, H. J. Coherent oscillations: A mechanism of feature linking in the visual cortex? *Biol. Cyber.* 60:121–130, 1988.

Economo, C. V. *The Cytoarchitectonics of the Human Cerebral Cortex.* London: Oxford University Press, 1929.

Edelman, G. M. *Neural Darwinism.* New York: Basic Books, 1987.

Edelman, G. M. *The Remembered Present.* New York: Basic Books, 1989.

Eichenbaum, H., Fagan, A., Mathews, P., and Cohen, N. J. Hippocampal system dysfunction and odor discrimination learning in rats: Impairment or facilitation depending on representational demands. *Behav. Neurosci.* 102:331–339, 1988.

Engel, A. K., König, P., Kreiter, A. K., and Singer, W. Interhemispheric synchronization of oscillatory neuronal responses in cat visual cortex. *Science* 252:1177–1179, 1991.

Engel, A. K., König, P., Kreiter, A. K., Schillen, T. B., and Singer, W. Temporal coding in the visual cortex: New vistas on integration in the nervous system. *Trends Neurosci.* 15:218–226, 1992.

Errington, M. L., Lynch, M. A., and Bliss, T. V. P. Long-term potentiation in the dentate gyrus: Induction and increased glutamate release are blocked by d(-)aminophosphonovalerate. *Neuroscience* 20:279–284, 1987.

Eskandar, E. N., Richmond, B. J., and Optican, L. M. Role of inferior temporal neurons in visual memory: I. Temporal encoding of information about visual images, recalled images, and behavioral context. *J. Neurophysiol.* 68:1277–1295, 1992.

Ettlinger, G. "Object vision" and "spatial vision": The neuropsychological evidence for the distinction. *Cortex* 26:319–341, 1990.

Ettlinger, G., and Kalsbeck, J. E. Changes in tactile discrimination and in visual reaching after successive and simultaneous bilateral posterior parietal ablations in the monkey. *J. Neurol. Neurosurg. Psychiatry* 25:256–268, 1962.

Evarts, E. V., and Tanji, J. Reflex and intended responses in motor cortex pyramidal tract neurons of monkey. *J. Neurophysiol.* 39:1069–1080, 1976.

Evarts, E. V., and Wise, S. P. Basal ganglia outputs and motor control. In *Functions of the Basal Ganglia (Ciba Foundation Symposium 107)*, edited by D. Evered and M. O'Connor. London: Pitman, 1984, pp. 83–102.

Faglioni, P., Scotti, G., and Spinnler, H. The performance of brain-damaged patients in spatial localization of visual and tactile stimuli. *Brain* 94:443–454, 1971.

Fahy, F. L. Riches, I, P., and Brown, M. W. Neuronal activity related to visual recognition memory: Long-term memory and the encoding of recency and familiarity information in the primate anterior and medial inferior temporal and rhinal cortex, *Exp. Brain Res.* 96:457–472, 1993.

Fair, C.M. *Cortical Memory Functions.* Boston: Birkhäuser, 1992.

Feldman, J. A. A connectionist model of visual memory. In *Parallel Models of Associative Memory,* edited by G. E. Hinton and J. A. Anderson. Hillsdale, NJ: Erlbaum, 1981, pp. 49–81.

Felten, D. L., and Sladek, J. R. Monoamine distribution in primate brain: V. Monoaminergic nuclei: Anatomy, pathways and local organization. *Brain Res. Bull.* 10:171–284, 1983.

Fetz, E. E., and Baker, M. A. Operantly conditioned patterns of precentral unit activity and correlated responses in adjacent cells and contralateral muscles. *J. Neurophysiol.* 36:179–204, 1973.

Fetz, E. E., and Shupe, L. E. Neural network models of the primate motor system. In *Advanced Neural Computers,* edited by R. Eckmiller. North Holland: Elsevier, 1990, pp. 43–50.

Finch, C. E. Age-related changes in brain catecholamines: A synopsis of findings in C57BL/6J mice and other rodent models. *Adv. Exp. Med. Biol.* 113:15–39, 1978.

Fischer, W., Gage, F. H., and Björklund, A. Degenerative changes in forebrain cholinergic nuclei correlate with cognitive impairments in aged rats. *Eur. J. Neurosci.* 1:34–45, 1989.

Fischer, W., Nilsson, O. G., and Björklund, A. In vivo acetylcholine release as measured by microdialysis is unaltered in the hippocampus of cognitively impaired aged rats with degenerative changes in the basal forebrain. *Brain Res.* 556:44–52, 1991.

Fishbein, W., ed. *Sleep, Dreams and Memory.* New York: Spectrum, 1981.

Flechsig, P. Developmental (myelogenetic) localisation of the cerebral cortex in the human subject. *Lancet* 2:1027–1029, 1901.

Flechsig, P. *Anatomie des Menschlichen Gehirns und Rückenmarks auf Myelogenetischer Grundlage.* Leipzig: Thieme, 1920.

Fleischauer, K. Cortical architectonics: The last 50 years and some problems of today. In *Architectonics of the Cerebral Cortex,* edited by M. A. B. Brazier and H. Petsche. New York: Raven Press, 1978, pp.99–117.

Floeter, M. K., and Greenough, W. T. Cerebellar plasticity: Modification of Purkinje cell structure by differential rearing in monkeys. *Science* 206:227–229, 1979.

Fodor, J. A. *The Modularity of Mind.* Cambridge, MA: MIT Press, 1983.

Freeman, W. J. *Mass Action in the Nervous System.* New York: Academic, 1975.

Freeman, W. J. On the fallacy of assigning an origin to consciousness. In *Machinery of the Mind,* edited by E. Roy John. Boston: Birkhäuser, 1990, pp. 14–26.

Freeman, W. J. and Skarda, C. A. Spatial EEG patterns, non-linear dynamics and perception: The neo-Sherringtonian view. *Brain Res. Rev.* 10:147–175, 1985.

French, J. D., Von Amerongen, F. K., and Magoun, H. W. An activating system in brain stem of monkey. *Arch. Neurol. Psychiatry* 68:577–590, 1952.

Freud, S. *A General Introduction to Psychoanalysis.* Garden City, NY: Garden City Publishing Co., 1943.

Freud, S. *On Aphasia* (English translation from the German, *Zur Auffassung der Aphasien,* 1891). London: Imago, 1953.

Freud, S. *On Dreams* (1901), standard edition, vol. 5, London: Hogarth Press, 1958.

Freud, S. *Civilization and Its Discontents (1930)*, standard edition, vol. 21. London: Hogarth Press, 1961.

Fried, I., Katz, A., McCarthy, G., Sass, K. J., Williamson, P., Spencer, S. S., and Spencer, D. D. Functional organization of human supplementary motor cortex studied by electrical stimulation. *J. Neurosci.* 11:3656–3666, 1991.

Friedman, H. R., and Goldman-Rakic, P. S. Activation of the hippocampus and dentate gyrus by working-memory: A 2-deoxyglucose study of behaving rhesus monkeys. *J. Neurosci.* 8:4693–4706, 1988.

Friedman, H. R., Janas, J. D., and Goldman-Rakic, P. S. Enhancement of metabolic activity in the diencephalon of monkeys performing working memory tasks: A 2-deoxyglucose study in behaving rhesus monkeys. *J. Cogn. Neurosci.* 2:18–31, 1990.

Frith, C. D., Friston, K. J., Liddle, P. F., and Frackowiak, R. S. J. A PET study of word finding. *Neuropsychologia* 29:1137–1148, 1991.

Frizzi, T. J. Midbrain reticular stimulation and brightness detection. *Vision Res.* 19:123–130, 1979.

Funahashi, S., Bruce, C. J., and Goldman-Rakic, P. S. Mnemonic coding of visual space in the monkey's dorsolateral prefrontal cortex. *J. Neurophysiol.* 61:331–349, 1989.

Funahashi, S., Bruce, C. J., and Goldman-Rakic, P. S. Visuospatial coding in primate prefrontal neurons revealed by oculomotor paradigms. *J. Neurophysiol.* 63:814–831, 1990.

Funahashi, S., Chafee, M. V., and Goldman-Rakic, P. S. Prefrontal neuronal activity in rhesus monkeys performing a delayed anti-saccade task. *Nature* 365:753–756, 1993.

Fuster, J. M. Effects of stimulation of brain stem on tachistoscopic perception. *Science* 127:150, 1958.

Fuster, J. M. Unit activity in prefrontal cortex during delayed-response performance: Neuronal correlates of transient memory. *J. Neurophysiol.* 36:61–78, 1973.

Fuster, J. M. Behavioral electrophysiology of the prefrontal cortex. *Trends Neurosci.* 7:408–414, 1984.

Fuster, J. M. The prefrontal cortex and temporal integration. In *Cerebral Cortex*, vol. 4, edited by A. Peters and E. G. Jones. New York: Plenum, 1985a, pp. 259–329.

Fuster, J. M. The prefrontal cortex, mediator of cross-temporal contingencies. *Hum. Neurobiol.* 4:169–179, 1985b.

Fuster, J. M. *The Prefrontal Cortex: Anatomy, Physiology, and Neuropsychology of the Frontal Lobe*, 2nd ed. New York: Raven Press, 1989.

Fuster, J. M. Inferotemporal units in selective visual attention and short-term memory. *J. Neurophysiol.* 64:681–697, 1990.

Fuster, J. M. Hippocampal neurons in short-term color memory. *Soc. Neurosci. Abstr.* 17:661, 1991a.

Fuster, J. M. Up and down the frontal hierarchies; whither Broca's area? *Behav. Brain Sci.* 14:558, 1991b.

Fuster, J. M. Frontal lobes. *Curr. Op. Neurobiol.* 3:160–165, 1993.

Fuster, J. M., and Alexander, G. E. Delayed response deficit by cryogenic depression of frontal cortex. *Brain Res.* 20:85–90, 1970.

Fuster, J. M., and Alexander, G. E. Neuron activity related to short-term memory. *Science* 173:652–654, 1971.

Fuster, J. M., and Alexander, G. E. Firing changes in cells of the nucleus medialis dorsalis associated with delayed response behavior. *Brain Res.* 61:79–91, 1973.

Fuster, J. M., and Bauer, R. H. Visual short-term memory deficit from hypothermia of frontal cortex. *Brain Res.* 81:393–400, 1974.

Fuster, J. M., Creutzfeldt, O. D., and Straschill, M. Intracellular recording of neuronal activity in the visual system. *Z. Vergleich. Physiol.* 49:605–622, 1965.

Fuster, J. M., Bauer, R. H., and Jervey, J. P. Effects of cooling inferotemporal cortex on performance of visual memory tasks. *Exp. Neurol.* 71:398–409, 1981.

Fuster, J. M., Bauer, R. H., and Jervey, J. P. Cellular discharge in the dorsolateral prefrontal cortex of the monkey in cognitive tasks. *Exp. Neurol.* 77:679–694, 1982.

Fuster, J. M., Bauer, R. H., and Jervey, J. P. Functional interactions between inferotemporal and prefrontal cortex in a cognitive task. *Brain Res.* 330:299–307, 1985.

Fuster, J. M., Di Mattia, B. V., Posley, K. A., and Shindy, W. W. Deficit in unimodal (tactile) and crossmodal delayed matching from cooling prefrontal cortex. *Soc. Neurosci. Abstr.* 16:1222, 1990.

Fuster, J. M., and Docter, R. F. Variations of optic evoked potentials as a function of reticular activity in rabbits with chronically implanted electrodes. *J. Neurophysiol.* 25:324–336, 1962.

Fuster, J. M., and Jervey, J. P. Inferotemporal neurons distinguish and retain behaviorally relevant features of visual stimuli. *Science* 212:952–955, 1981.

Fuster, J. M., and Jervey, J. P. Neuronal firing in the inferotemporal cortex of the monkey in a visual memory task. *J. Neurosci.* 2:361–375, 1982.

Fuster, J. M., and Uyeda, A. A. Facilitation of tachistoscopic performance by stimulation of midbrain tegmental points in the monkey. *Exp. Neurol.* 6:384–406, 1962.

Fuster, J. M., and Uyeda, A. A. Reactivity of limbic neurons of the monkey to appetitive and aversive signals. *Electroencephalogr. Clin. Neurophysiol.* 30:281–293, 1971.

Gabor, D. Improved holographic model of temporal recall. *Nature* 217:1288–1289, 1968.

Gaffan, D., and Heywood, C. A. A spurious category-specific visual agnosia for living things in normal human and nonhuman primates. *J. Cogn. Neurosci.* 5:118–128, 1993.

Galaburda, A. M., and Pandya, D. N. The intrinsic architectonic and connectional organization of the superior temporal region of the rhesus monkey. *J. Comp. Neurol.* 221:169–184, 1983.

Galambos, R., Sheatz, G., and Vernier, V.G. Electrophysiological correlates of a conditioned response in cats. *Science* 123:376–377, 1955.

Gallagher, M., and Pelleymounter, M. A. An age-related spatial learning deficit: Choline uptake distinguishes "impaired" and "unimpaired" rats. *Neurobiol. Aging* 9:363–369, 1988.

Garcha, H. S., Ettlinger, G., and MacCabe, J. J. Unilateral removal of the second somatosensory projection cortex in the monkey: Evidence for cerebral predominance? *Brain* 105:787–810, 1982.

Garcia, J., and Holder, M. D. Time, space and value. *Hum. Neurobiol.* 4:81–89, 1985.

Geinisman, Y., and Bondareff, W. Decrease in the number of synapses in the senescent brain: A quantitative electron microscopic analysis of the dentate gyrus molecular layer in the rat. *Mech. Ageing Dev.* 5:11–23, 1976.

Georgopoulos, A. P., Kalaska, J. F., Caminiti, R., and Massey, J. T. On the relations between the direction of two-dimensional arm movements and cell discharge in primate motor cortex. *J. Neurosci.* 2:1527–1537, 1982.

Georgopoulos, A. P., Schwartz, A. B., and Kettner, R. E. Neuronal population coding of movement direction. *Science* 233:1416–1419, 1986.

Georgopoulos, A. P., Crutcher, M. D., and Schwartz, A. B. Cognitive spatial-motor processes: III. Motor cortical prediction of movement direction during an instructed delay period. *Exp. Brain Res.* 75:183–194, 1989.

Georgopoulos, A. P., Taira, M., and Lukashin, A. Cognitive neurophysiology of the motor cortex. *Science* 260:47–52, 1993.

Gerstein, G. L. Functional associations of neurons: Detection and interpretation. In *The Neurosciences: Second Study Program,* edited by F. O. Schmitt and F. G. Worden. New York: Rockefeller University Press, 1970, pp. 648–661.

Geschwind, N. Alexia and colour-naming disturbance. In *Functions of the Corpus Callosum,* edited by G. Ettlinger. London: Churchill, 1965a, pp. 95–114.

Geschwind, N. Disconnexion syndromes in animals and man. *Brain* 88:237–274, 1965b.

Geschwind, N. The organization of language and the brain. *Science* 170:940–944, 1970.

Gevins, A. Dynamic functional topography of cognitive tasks. *Brain Topogr.* 2:37–56, 1989.

Gevins, A. S., Bressler, S. L., Morgan, N. H., Cutillo, B. A., White, R. M., Greer, D. S., and Illes, J. Event-related covariances during a bimanual visuomotor task: I. Methods and analysis of stimulus- and response-locked data. *Electroencephalogr. Clin. Neurophysiol.* 74:58–75, 1989a.

Gevins, A. S., Cutillo, B. A., Bressler, S. L., Morgan, N. H., White, R. M., Illes, J., and Greer, D. S. Event-related covariances during a bimanual visuomotor task: II. Preparation and feedback. *Electroencephalogr. Clin. Neurophysiol.* 74:147–160, 1989b.

Gevins, A. S., Bressler, S. L., Cutillo, B. A., Illes, J., Miller, J. C., Stern, J., and Jex, H. R. Effects of prolonged mental work on functional brain topography. *Electroencephalogr. Clin. Neurophysiol.* 76:339–350, 1990.

Ghose, G. M., and Freeman, R. D. Oscillatory discharge in the visual system: Does it have a functional role? *J. Neurophysiol.* 68:1558–1574, 1992.

Gibson, J. J. The capabilities of the haptic-somatic system. In *The Senses Considered as Perceptual Systems.* London: Allen & Unwin, 1966, pp.116–135.

Gibson, K. R. Myelination and behavioral development: A comparative perspective on questions of neoteny, altriciality and intelligence. In *Brain Maturation and Cognitive Development,* edited by K. R. Gibson and A. C. Petersen. New York: Aldine de Gruyter, 1991, pp. 29–63.

Glickman, S. E. Perseverative neural processes and consolidation of the memory trace. *Psychol. Bull.* 58:218–233, 1961.

Globus, A., and Scheibel, A. B. Synaptic loci on visual cortical neurons of the rabbit: The specific afferent radiation. *Exp. Neurol.* 18:116–131, 1967.

Gloor, P. Amygdala. In *Handbook of Physiology. Neurophysiology,* edited by J. Field and H. W. Magoun. Washington, D.C.: American Physiological Society, 1960, pp. 1395–1420.

Godschalk, M., Lemon, R. N., Nijs, H. G. T., and Kuypers, H. G. J. M. Behaviour of neurons in monkey peri-arcuate and precentral cortex before and during visually guided arm and hand movements. *Exp. Brain Res.* 44:113–116, 1981.

Goldberg, E., Antin, S. P., Bilder, R. M., Gerstman, L. J., Hughes, J. E. O., and Mattis, S. Retrograde amnesia: Possible role of mesencephalic reticular activation in long-term memory. *Science* 213:1392–1394, 1981a.

Goldberg, G. Supplementary motor area structure and function: Review and hypotheses. *Behav. Brain Sci.* 567:616, 1985.

Goldberg, G., Mayer, N. H., and Toglia, J. U. Medial frontal cortex infarction and the alien hand sign. *Arch. Neurol.* 38:683–686, 1981.

Goldberg, M. E., and Bruce, C. J. Cerebral cortical activity associated with the orientation of visual attention in the rhesus monkey. *Vision Res.* 25:471–481, 1985.

Goldberg, M. E., and Bushnell, M. C. Behavioral enhancement of visual responses in monkey cerebral cortex: II. Modulation in frontal eye fields specifically related to saccades. *J. Neurophysiol.* 46:773–787, 1981.

Goldman-Rakic, P. S. Circuitry of primate prefrontal cortex and regulation of behavior by representational memory. In *Handbook of Physiology; Nervous System*, vol. 5, *Higher Functions of the Brain* (part 1), edited by F. Plum. Bethesda, MD: American Physiological Society, 1987, pp. 373–417.

Goldman-Rakic, P. S. Topography of cognition: Parallel distributed networks in primate association cortex. *Ann. Rev. Neurosci.* 11:137–156, 1988.

Goldman-Rakic, P. S., and Brown, R. M. Regional changes of monoamines in cerebral cortex and subcortical structures of aging rhesus monkeys. *Neuroscience* 6:177–187, 1981.

Goldman, P. S., and Nauta, W. J. H. An intricately patterned prefrontal-caudate projection in the rhesus monkey. *J. Comp. Neurol.* 171:369–385, 1977.

Goldman-Rakic, P. S., and Schwartz, M. L. Interdigitation of contralateral and ipsilateral columnar projections to frontal association cortex in primates. *Science* 216:755–757, 1982.

Goldstein, K. *Language and Language Disturbances*, New York: Grune & Stratton, 1948.

Goldstein, K. Functional disturbances in brain damage. In: *American Handbook of Psychiatry*, vol. 1, edited by S. Arieti, New York: Basic Books, 1959, pp. 770–794.

Goodale, M. A., Milner, A. D., Jakobson, L. S., and Carey, D. P. A neurological dissociation between perceiving objects and grasping them. *Nature* 349:154–156, 1991.

Goodglass, H., Klein, B., Carey, P., and Jones, K. Specific semantic word categories in aphasia. *Cortex* 2:74–89, 1966.

Gould, H. J., III, Cusick, C. G., Pons, T. P., and Kaas, J. H. The relationship of corpus callosum connections to electrical stimulation maps of motor, supplementary motor, and the frontal eye fields in owl monkeys. *J. Comp. Neurol.* 247:297–325, 1986.

Grafton, S. T., Mazziotta, J. C., Presty, S., Friston, K. J., Frackowiak, R. S. J., and Phelps, M. E. Functional anatomy of human procedural learning determined with regional cerebral blood flow and PET. *J. Neurosci.* 12:2542–2548, 1992a.

Grafton, S. T., Mazziotta, J. C., Woods, R. P., and Phelps, M. E. Human functional anatomy of visually guided finger movements. *Brain* 115:565–587, 1992b.

Gray, C. M., and Singer, W. Stimulus-specific neuronal oscillations in orientation columns of cat visual cortex. *Proc. Natl. Acad. Sci. U.S.A.* 86:1698–1702, 1989.

Greenfield, P. M. Language, tools and brain: The ontogeny and phylogeny of hierarchically organized sequential behavior. *Behav. Brain Sci.* 14:531–595, 1991.

Grillner, S., Wallen, P., Dale, N., Brodin, L., Buchanan, J., and Hill, R. Transmitters, membrane properties and network circuitry in the control of locomotion in lamprey. *Trends Neurosci.* 10:34–41, 1987.

Gross, C.G. Inferotemporal cortex and vision. In *Progress in Physiological Psychology*, vol. 5, edited by E. Stellar and J. M. Sprague. New York: Academic, 1973, pp. 77–123.

Gross, C. G., Rocha-Miranda, C. E., and Bender, D. B. Visual properties of neurons in inferotemporal cortex of the macaque. *J. Neurophysiol.* 35:96–111, 1972.

Grossberg, S. Neural expectation: Cerebellar and retinal analogs of cells fired by learnable or unlearned pattern classes. *Kybernetik* 10:49–57, 1972.

Grossberg, S. How does a brain build a cognitive code? *Psychol. Rev.* 87:1–42, 1980.

Guerrien, A., Dujardin, K., Mandai, O., Sockeel, P., and Leconte, P. Enhancement of memory by auditory stimulation during postlearning REM sleep in human. *Physiol. Behav.* 45:947–950, 1989.

Gustafson, L., Hagberg, B., and Ingvar, D. H. Speech disturbances in presenile dementia related to local cerebral blood flow abnormalities in the dominant hemisphere. *Brain Lang.* 5:103–118, 1978.

Gustavson, C. R., Garcia, J., Hankins, W. G., and Rusiniak, K. W. Coyote predation control by aversive conditioning. *Science* 184:581–583, 1974.

Haberly, L. B., and Bower, J. M. Olfactory cortex: model circuit for study of associative memory? *Trends Neurosci.* 12:258–264, 1989.

Haglund, M. M., Ojemann, G. A., Schwartz, T. W., and Lettich, E. Neuronal activity in human lateral temporal cortex during serial retrieval from short-term memory. *J. Neurosci.* 14:1507–1515, 1994.

Haider, M., Spong, P., and Lindsley, D.B. Attention, vigilance, and cortical evoked-potentials in humans. *Science* 145:180–182, 1964.

Halsband, U., and Freund, H.-J. Premotor cortex and conditional motor learning in man. *Brain* 113:207–222, 1990.

Halsband, U., Ito, N., Tanji, J., and Freund, H.-J. The role of premotor cortex and the supplementary motor area in the temporal control of movement in man. *Brain* 116:243–266, 1993.

Halsband, U., and Passingham, R. E. Premotor cortex and the conditions for movement in monkeys (*Macaca fascicularis*). *Behav. Brain Res.* 18:269–277, 1985.

Hamlyn, L. H. An electron microscope study of pyramidal neurons in the Ammon's horn of the rabbit. *J. Anat.* 97:189–201, 1962.

Harnad, S., Doty, R. W., Goldstein, L., Jaynes, J., and Krauthamer, G., eds. *Lateralization in the Nervous System*. New York: Academic, 1977.

Haug, H., Knebel, G., Mecke, E., Orun, C., and Sass, N.-L. *Eleventh International Congress of Anatomy: Advances in the Morphology of Cells and Tissues*. New York: Alan R. Liss, 1981.

Haug, H., Barmwater, U., Eggers, R., Fischer, D., Kühl, S., and Sass, N.-L. Anatomical changes in aging brain: Morphometric analysis of the human prosencephalon. In *Brain Aging: Neuropathology and Neuropharmacology*, edited by J. Cervós-Navarro and H.-I. Sarkander. New York: Raven Press, 1983, pp. 1–12.

Hawkins, R. D., Abrams, T. W., Carew, T. J., and Kandel, E. R. A cellular mechanism of classical conditioning in *Aplysia*: Activity-dependent amplification of presynaptic facilitation. *Science* 219:400–405, 1983.

Haxby, J. V., Grady, C. L., Horwitz, B., Ungerleider, L. G., Mishkin, M., Carson, R. E., Herscovitch, P., Schapiro, M. B., and Rapoport, S.I. Dissociation of object and spatial visual processing pathways in human extrastriate cortex. *Proc. Natl. Acad. Sci. U.S.A.* 88:1621–1625, 1991.

Hayek, F. A. *The Sensory Order.* Chicago: University of Chicago Press, 1952.

Hayek, F. A. *Studies in Philosophy, Politics and Economics.* Chicago: University of Chicago Press, 1967.

Hebb, D. O. *The Organization of Behavior,* New York: Wiley, 1949.

Hécaen, H., and Ajuriaguerra, J. *Méconnaissances et Hallucinations Corporelles.* Paris: Masson, 1952.

Hedreen, J. C., Struble, R. G., Whitehouse, P. J., and Price, D. L. Topography of the magnocellular basal forebrain system in human brain. *J. Neuropathol. Exp. Neurol.* 43:1–21, 1984.

Heffner, H. E., and Heffner, R. S. Temporal lobe lesions and perception of species-specific vocalizations by macaques. *Science* 226:75–76, 1984.

Heilman, K. M., Pandya, D. N., and Geschwind, N. Trimodal inattention following parietal lobe ablations. In *Transactions of the American Neurological Association,* edited by S. A. Trufant. New York: Springer, 1970, pp. 259–261.

Heilman, K. M., Watson, R. T., and Valenstein, E. Neglect and related disorders. In *Clinical Neuropsychology,* 2nd ed., edited by K. M. Heilman and E. Valenstein. New York: Oxford University Press, 1985, pp. 243–293.

Helmholtz, H. von. *Helmholtz's Treatise on Physiological Optics* (translated from the German by J. P. C. Southall). Menasha, WI: The Optical Society of America, G. Banta, 1925.

Hennevin, E., Hars, B., and Bloch, V. Improvement of learning by mesencephalic reticular stimulation during postlearning paradoxical sleep. *Behav. Neural Biol.* 51:291–306, 1989.

Hernández-Peón, R., Scherrer, H., and Jouvet, M. Modification of electric activity in cochlear nucleus during "attention" in unanesthetized cats. *Science* 123:331–332, 1956.

Hess, R., Negishi, K., and Creutzfeldt, O. The horizontal spread of intracortical inhibition in the visual cortex. *Exp. Brain Res.* 22:415–419, 1975.

Hess, W. R. Teleokinetisches und ereismatisches Kraeftesystem in der Biomotorik. *Helv. Physiol. Pharmacol. Acta* 1:c62–c63, 1943.

Hess, W. R. *Das Zwischenhirn,* Basel: Benno Schwabe, 1954.

Hikosaka, K., Iwai, E., Saito, H., and Tanaka, K. Polysensory properties of neurons in the anterior bank of the caudal superior temporal sulcus of the macaque monkey. *J. Neurophysiol.* 60:1615–1637, 1988.

Hillis, A. E., and Caramazza, A. Category-specific naming and comprehension impairment: A double dissociation. *Brain* 114:2081–2094, 1991.

Hillyard, S. A., Hink, R. F., Schwent, V. L., and Picton, T. W. Electrical signs of selective attention in the human brain. *Science* 182:177–180, 1973.

Hinke, R. M., Hu, X., Stillman, A. E., Kim, S.-G., Merkle, H., Salmi, R., and Ugurbil, K. Functional magnetic resonance imaging of Broca's area during internal speech. *NeuroReport* 4:675–678, 1993.

Hinton, G. E., and Anderson, J. A. *Parallel Models of Associative Memory.* Hillsdale, NJ: Erlbaum, 1981.

Hobson, J. A. *The Dreaming Brain.* New York: Basic Books, 1988.

Hocherman, S., and Wise, S. P. Effects of hand movement path on motor cortical activity in awake, behaving rhesus monkeys. *Exp. Brain Res.* 83:285–302, 1991.

Hockett, C. F. The origin of speech. *Sci. Am.* 203:88–96, 1960.

Hoover, J. E., and Strick, P. L. Multiple output channels in the basal ganglia. *Science* 259:819–821, 1993.

Horel, J. A., and Pytko, D. E. Behavioral effect of local cooling in temporal lobe of monkeys. *J. Neurophysiol.* 47:11–22, 1982.

Horel, J. A., Voytko, M. L., and Salsbury, K. G. Visual learning suppressed by cooling the temporal pole. *Behav. Neurosci.* 98:310–324, 1984.

Horn, D., Sagi, D., and Usher, M. Segmentation, binding, and illusory conjunctions. *Neural Comput.* 3:510–525, 1991.

Horn, G. Physiological and psychological aspects of selective perception. In *Advances in the Study of Behavior,* edited by D. S. Lehrman, R. A. Hinde, and E. Shaw. New York: Academic, 1965, pp. 155–215.

Hörster, W., Rivers, A., Schuster, B., Ettlinger, G., Skreczek, W., and Hesse, W. The neural structures involved in cross-modal recognition and tactile discrimination performance: An investigation using 2-DG. *Behav. Brain Res.* 33:209–227, 1989.

Hubel, D. H., and Wiesel, T. N. Receptive fields, binocular interaction and functional architecture in the cat's visual cortex. *J. Physiol.* 160:106–154, 1962.

Hubel, D. H., and Wiesel, T. N. Receptive fields and functional architecture of monkey striate cortex. *J. Physiol.* (Lond.) 195:215–243, 1968.

Hubel, D. H., and Wiesel, T. N. The period of susceptibility to the physiological effects of unilateral eye closure in kittens. *J. Physiol.* 206:419–436, 1970.

Huttenlocher, P. R. Synaptic density in human frontal cortex—developmental changes and effects of aging. *Brain Res.* 163:195–205, 1979.

Huttunen, M. O. General model for the molecular events in synapses during learning. *Perspect. Biol. Med.* 17:103–108, 1973.

Hyman, B. T., Van Hoesen, G. W., Damasio, A. R., and Barnes, C. L. Alzheimer's disease: Cell-specific pathology isolates the hippocampal formation. *Science* 225:1168–1170, 1984.

Hyvärinen, J., and Poranen, A. Function of the parietal associative area 7 as revealed from cellular discharges in alert monkeys. *Brain* 97:673–692, 1974.

Ingvar, D. H. Serial aspects of language and speech related to prefrontal cortical activity. *Hum. Neurobiol.* 2:177–189, 1983.

Ingvar, D. H. "Memory of the future": An essay on the temporal organization of conscious awareness. *Hum. Neurobiol.* 4:127–136, 1985.

Ingvar, D. H., and Philipson, L. Distribution of cerebral blood flow in the dominant hemisphere during motor ideation and motor performance. *Ann. Neurol.* 2:230–237, 1977.

Ingvar, D. H., and Schwartz, M. S. Blood flow patterns induced in the dominant hemisphere by speech and reading. *Brain* 97:273–288, 1974.

Inoue, M., Oomura, Y., Aou, S., Nishino, H., and Sikdar, S. K. Reward related neuronal activity in monkey dorsolateral prefrontal cortex during feeding behavior. *Brain Res.* 326:307–312, 1985.

Iriki, A., Pavlides, C., Keller, A., and Asanuma, H. Long-term potentiation in the motor cortex. *Science* 245:1385–1387, 1989.

Iwai, E., Aihara, T., and Hikosaka, K. Inferotemporal neurons of the monkey responsive to auditory signal. *Brain Res.* 410:121–124, 1987.

Iwai, E., and Mishkin, M. Further evidence on the locus of the visual area in the temporal lobe of the monkey. *Exp. Neurol.* 25:585–594, 1969.

Iwamura, Y., and Tanaka, M. Postcentral neurons in hand region of area 2: Their possible role in the form discrimination of tactile objects. *Brain Res.* 150:662–666, 1978.

Iwamura, Y., Tanaka, M., and Hikosaka, O. Overlapping representation of fingers in the somatosensory cortex (area 2) of the conscious monkey. *Brain Res.* 197:516–520, 1980.

Iwamura, Y., Tanaka, M., Sakamoto, M., and Hikosaka, O. Functional subdivisions representing different finger regions in area 3 of the first somatosensory cortex of the conscious monkey. *Exp. Brain Res.* 51:315–326, 1983.

Iwamura, Y., Tanaka, M., Sakamoto, M., and Hikosaka, O. Diversity in receptive field properties of vertical neuronal arrays in the crown of the postcentral gyrus of the conscious monkey. *Exp. Brain Res.* 58:400–411, 1985.

Iwamura, Y., Tanaka, M., Sakamoto, M., and Hikosaka, O. Rostrocaudal gradients in the neuronal receptive field complexity in the finger region of the alert monkey's postcentral gyrus. *Exp. Brain Res.* 92:360–368, 1993.

Jackson, J. H. On affections of speech from disease of the brain. *Brain* 38:107–174, 1915.

Jackson, J. H. *Selected Writings.* New York: Basic Books, 1958.

Jacobs, B., and Scheibel, A. B. A quantitative dendritic analysis of Wernicke's area in humans: I. Lifespan changes. *J. Comp. Neurol.* 327:83–96, 1993.

Jacobson, S., and Trojanowski, J. Q. Prefrontal granular cortex of the rhesus monkey: I. Intrahemispheric cortical afferents. *Brain Res.* 132:209–233, 1977a.

Jacobson, S., and Trojanowski, J. Q. Prefrontal granular cortex of the rhesus monkey: II. Interhemispheric cortical afferents. *Brain Res.* 132:235–246, 1977b.

Jäervilehto, T., and Fruhstorfer, H. Differentiation between slow cortical potentials associated with motor and mental acts in man. *Exp. Brain Res.* 11:309–317, 1970.

Jagadeesh, B., Gray, C. M., and Ferster, D. Visually evoked oscillations of membrane potential in cells of cat visual cortex. *Science* 257:552–554, 1992.

James, W. *Principles of Psychology.* New York: Holt, 1890.

Jasper, H., Ricci, G. F., and Doane, B. Patterns of cortical neuronal discharge during conditioned responses in monkeys. In *Neurological Basis of Behavior,* edited by G. E. W. Wolstenholme and C. M. O'Connor. London: Churchill, 1958, pp. 277–294.

Jenkins, W. M., Merzenich, M. M., Ochs, M. T., Allard, T., and Guic-Robles, E. Functional reorganization of primary somatosensory cortex in adult owl monkeys after behaviorally controlled tactile stimulation. *J. Neurophysiol.* 63:82–104, 1990.

John, E. R. *Mechanisms of Memory.* New York: Academic, 1967.

Jones, E. G. Anatomy of cerebral cortex: Columnar input-output organization. In *The Organization of the Cerebral Cortex,* edited by F. O. Schmitt, F. G. Worden, G. Adelman and S. G. Dennis. Cambridge, MA: MIT Press, 1981, pp. 199–235.

Jones, E. G., Coulter, J. D., and Hendry, S. H. C. Intracortical connectivity of architectonic fields in the somatic sensory, motor and parietal cortex of monkeys. *J. Comp. Neurol.* 181:291–348, 1978.

Jones, E. G., and Powell, T. P. S. An anatomical study of converging sensory pathways within the cerebral cortex of the monkey. *Brain* 93:793–820, 1970.

Jonides, J., Smith, E. E., Koeppe, R. A., Awh, E., Minoshima, S., and Mintun, M. A. Spatial working memory in humans as revealed by PET. *Nature* 363:623–625, 1993.

Joseph, J. P., and Barone, P. Prefrontal unit activity during a delayed oculomotor task in the monkey. *Exp. Brain Res.* 67:460–468, 1987.

Jouvet, M. Recherches sur les structures nerveuses et les mécanismes responsables des différentes phases du sommeil physiologique. *Arch. Ital. Biol.* 100:125–206, 1962.

Jung, C. G. *The Archetypes and the Collective Unconscious.* Princeton, NJ: Princeton University Press, 1968.

Kaas, J. H. What, if anything, is S1? Organization of first somatosensory area of cortex. *Physiol. Rev.* 63:206–231, 1983.

Kaas, J. H., Merzenich, M. M., and Killackey, H. P. The reorganization of somatosensory cortex following peripheral nerve damage in adult and developing mammals. *Annu. Rev. Neurosci.* 6:325–356, 1983.

Kaczmarek, B. L. J. Neurolinguistic analysis of verbal utterances in patients with focal lesions of frontal lobes. *Brain Lang.* 21:52–58, 1984.

Kaes, T. *Die Grosshirnrinde des Menschen in ihren Massen und in ihrem Fasengehalt.* Jena, Germany: Fischer, 1907.

Kalaska, J., and Pomeranz, B. Chronic paw denervation causes an age-dependent appearance of novel responses from forearm in "paw cortex" of kittens and adult cats. *J. Neurophysiol.* 42:618–633, 1979.

Kalaska, J. F., Caminiti, R., and Georgopoulos, A. P. Cortical mechanisms related to the direction of two-dimensional arm movements: Relations in parietal area 5 and comparison with motor cortex. *Exp. Brain Res.* 51:247–260, 1983.

Kalaska, J. F., and Crammond, D. J. Cerebral cortical mechanisms of reaching movements. *Science* 20:1517–1523, 1992.

Kalaska, J. F., Cohen, D. A. D., Hyde, M. L., and Prud'homme, M. A comparison of movement direction-related versus load direction-related activity in primate motor cortex, using a two-dimensional reaching task. *J. Neurosci.* 9:2080–2102, 1989.

Kandel, E. *Cellular Basis of Behavior.* San Francisco: Freeman, 1976.

Kapur, N., Ellison, D., Smith, M. P., McLellan, D. L., and Burrows, E. H. Focal retrograde amnesia following bilateral temporal lobe pathology. *Brain* 115:73–85, 1992.

Kartje-Tillotson, G., Neafsey, E. J., and Castro, A. J. Electrophysiological analysis of motor cortical plasticity after cortical lesions in newborn rats. *Brain Res.* 332:103–111, 1985.

Kauer, J. S. Contributions of topography and parallel processing to odor coding in the vertebrate olfactory pathway. *Trends Neurosci.* 14:79–85, 1991.

Keller, A., Arissian, K., and Asanuma, H. Formation of new synapses in the cat motor cortex following lesions of the deep cerebellar nuclei. *Exp. Brain Res.* 80:23–33, 1990.

Kemp, J. M., and Powell, T. P. S. The connexions of the striatum and globus pallidus: Synthesis and speculations. *Philos. Trans. R. Soc. Lond. Biol.* 262:441–457, 1971.

Kesner, R. P., Di Mattia, B. V., and Crutcher, K. A. Evidence for neocortical involvement in reference memory. *Behav. Neural Biol.* 47:40–53, 1987.

Kihlstrom, J. F. The cognitive unconscious. *Science* 237:1445–1452, 1987.

Kimura, D. Some effects of temporal-lobe damage on auditory perception. *Can. J. Psychol.* 15:156–165, 1961.

Kimura, D. Right temporal-lobe damage. *Neurology* 8:264–271, 1963.

Kimura, D. Left-right differences in the perception of melodies. *J. Exp. Psychol. [Gen.]* 16:355–358, 1964.

Kimura, D. Neuromotor mechanisms in the evolution of human communication. In *Neurobiology of Social Communication in Primates: An Evolutionary Perspective,* edited by H. D. Steklis and M. J. Raleigh. New York: Academic, 1979, pp.197–219.

Kimura, M. The role of primate putamen neurons in the association of sensory stimuli with movement. *Neurosci. Res.* 3:436–443, 1986.

Klatzky, R. L. *Human Memory.* San Francisco: Freeman, 1975.

Kleist, K. *Gehirnpathologie.* Leipzig: Barth, 1934.

Klüver, H. *Behavior Mechanisms in Monkeys.* Chicago: Chicago University Press, 1933.

Klüver, H., and Bucy, P. C. An analysis of certain effects of bilateral temporal lobectomy in the rhesus monkey, with special reference to "psychic blindness." *J. Psychol.* 5:33–54, 1938.

Knowlton, B. J., and Squire, L. R. The learning of categories: Parallel brain systems for item memory and category knowledge. *Science* 262:1747–1749, 1993.

Knowlton, B. J., and Thompson, R. F. Conditioning using a cerebral cortical conditioned stimulus is dependent on the cerebellum and brain stem circuitry. *Behav. Neurosci.* 106:509–517, 1992.

Koch, C., and Ullman, S. Shifts in selective visual attention: Towards the underlying neural circuitry. *Hum. Neurobiol.* 4:219–227, 1985.

Koch, K. W., and Fuster, J. M. Unit activity in monkey parietal cortex related to haptic perception and temporary memory. *Exp. Brain Res.* 76:292–306, 1989.

Koh, S., Chang, P., Collier, T. J., and Loy, R. Loss of NGF receptor immunoreactivity in basal forebrain neurons of aged rats: Correlation with spatial memory impairment. *Brain Res.* 498:397–404, 1989.

Kohonen, T. *Associative Memory—A System-Theoretical Approach,* Berlin: Springer-Verlag, 1977.

Kohonen, T. *Self-Organization and Associative Memory.* Berlin: Springer, 1984.

Komatsu, H. Prefrontal unit activity during a color discrimination task with go and no-go responses in the monkey. *Brain Res.* 244:269–277, 1982.

Konishi, M. Birdsong: From behavior to neuron. *Annu. Rev. Neurosci.* 8:125–170, 1985.

Kornhuber, H. H., and Deecke, L. Hirnpotentialanderungen bei Willkurbewegungen und passiven Bewegungen des Menschen: Bereitschaftspotential und reafferent Potentiale. *Pflügers Arch. Gesamte Physiol.* 284:1–17, 1965.

Krasne, F. B. Extrinsic control of intrinsic neuronal plasticity: An hypothesis from work on simple systems. *Brain Res.* 140:197–216, 1978.

Kubota, K., and Funahashi, S. Direction-specific activities of dorsolateral prefrontal and motor cortex pyramidal tract neurons during visual tracking. *J. Neurophysiol.* 47:362–376, 1982.

Kubota, K., Iwamoto, T., and Suzuki, H. Visuokinetic activities of primate prefrontal neurons during delayed-response performance. *J. Neurophysiol.* 37:1197–1212, 1974.

Kubota, K., and Komatsu, H. Neuron activities of monkey prefrontal cortex during the learning of visual discrimination tasks with go/no-go performances. *Neurosci. Res.* 3:106–129, 1985.

Kuhl, D. E., Metter, E. J., Riege, W. H., and Phelps, M. E. Effects of human aging on patterns of local cerebral glucose utilization determined by the [18F] fluorodeoxyglucose method. *J. Cereb. Blood Flow Metab.* 2:163–171, 1982.

Künzle, H. An autoradiographic analysis of the efferent connections from premotor and adjacent prefrontal regions (areas 6 and 9) in *Macaca fascicularis*. *Brain Behav. Evol.* 15:185–234, 1978.

Kurata, K. Somatotopy in the human supplementary motor area. *Trends Neurosci.* 15:159–160, 1992.

Kurata, K. Premotor cortex of monkeys: Set- and movement-related activity reflecting amplitude and direction of wrist movement. *J. Neurophysiol.* 69:187–200, 1993.

Kutas, M., and Donchin, E. Preparation to respond as manifested by movement-related brain potentials. *Brain Res.* 202:95–115, 1980.

Lacalle, S., Iraizoz, I., and Gonzalo, L. M. Differential changes in cell size and number in topographic subdivisions of human basal nucleus in normal aging. *Neuroscience* 43:445–456, 1991.

Lamantia, A. S., and Rakic, P. Cytological and quantitative characteristics of four cerebral commissures in the rhesus monkey. *J. Comp. Neurol.* 291:520–537, 1990.

Lamarre, Y., Busby, L., and Spidalieri, G. Fast ballistic arm movements triggered by visual, auditory, and somesthetic stimuli in the monkey: I. Activity of precentral cortical neurons. *J. Neurophysiol.* 50:1343–1358, 1983.

Larsen, B., Skinhoj, E., and Lassen, N.A. Variation in regional cortical blood flow in the right and left hemispheres during automatic speech. *Brain* 101:193–209, 1978.

Larson, J., Wong, D., and Lynch, G. Patterned stimulation at the theta frequency is optimal for the induction of hippocampal long-term potentiation. *Brain Res.* 368:347–350, 1986.

Lashley, K. S. The effects of strychnine and caffeine upon rate of learning. *Psychobiology* 1:141, 1917.

Lashley, K. S. In search of the engram. *Symp. Soc. Exp. Biol.* 4:454–482, 1950.

Lashley, K. S. The problem of serial order in behavior. In *Cerebral Mechanisms in Behavior*, edited by L. A. Jeffress. New York: Wiley, 1951, pp. 112–146.

Lassen, N. A., and Larsen, B. Cortical activity in the left and right hemispheres during language-related brain functions. *Phonetica* 37:27–37, 1980.

Latto, R. The role of inferior parietal cortex and the frontal eye-fields in visuospatial discriminations in the macaque monkey. *Behav. Brain Res.* 22:41–52, 1986.

Lawler, K. A., and Cowey, A. On the role of posterior parietal and prefrontal cortex in visuo-spatial perception and attention. *Exp. Brain Res.* 65:695–698, 1987.

Lawrence, D. G., and Hopkins, D. A. The development of motor control in the rhesus monkey: Evidence concerning the role of corticomotoneuronal connections. *Brain* 99:235–254, 1976.

Le Bihan, D., Turner, R., Zeffiro, T. A., Cuénod, C. A., Jezzard, P., and Bonnerot, V. Activation of human primary visual cortex during visual recall: A magnetic resonance imaging study. *Proc. Natl. Acad. Sci. U.S.A.* 90:11802–11805, 1993.

Lecas, J.-C., Requin, J., Anger, C., and Vitton, N. Changes in neuronal activity of the monkey precentral cortex during preparation for movement. *J. Neurophysiol.* 56:1680–1702, 1986.

LeDoux, J. E. Cognitive-emotional interactions in the brain. *Cogn. Emot.* 3:267–289, 1989.

LeDoux, J. E. Brain mechanisms of emotion and emotional learning. *Curr. Opin. Neurobiol.* 2:191–197, 1992a.

LeDoux, J. E. Emotion and the amygdala. In *The Amygdala: Neurobiological Aspects of Emotion, Memory, and Mental Dysfunction,* edited by J. P. Aggleton. New York: Wiley-Liss, 1992b, pp. 339–351.

LeDoux, J. E. Emotional memory systems in the brain. *Behav. Brain Res.* 58:69–79, 1993.

Leinonen, L., Hyvärinen, J., Nyman, G., and Linnankoski, I. Functional properties of neurons in lateral part of associative area 7 in awake monkeys. *Exp. Brain Res.* 34:299–320, 1979.

Leinonen, L., Hyvärinen, J., and Sovijarvi, A. R. A. Functional properties of neurons in the temporo-parietal association cortex of awake monkey. *Exp. Brain Res.* 39:203–215, 1980.

Leonard, C. M., Rolls, E. T., Wilson, F. A. W., and Baylis, G. C. Neurons in the amygdala of the monkey with responses selective for faces. *Behav. Brain Res.* 15:159–176, 1985.

Leonard, C. M., and Scott, J. W. Origin and distribution of the amygdalofugal pathways in the rat: An experimental neuroanatomical study. *J. Comp. Neurol.* 141:313–330, 1971.

LeVay, S., and Stryker, M. P. The development of ocular dominance columns in the cat. In *Aspects of Developmental Neurobiology,* edited by J. A. Ferrendelli. Bethesda, MD: Society for Neuroscience, 1979, pp. 83–98.

Levine, D. S. *Introduction to Neural and Cognitive Modeling.* London: Erlbaum, 1991.

Levy, W. B., and Steward, O. Synapses as associative memory elements in the hippocampal formation. *Brain Res.* 175:233–245, 1979.

Lhermitte, F., Deroulsne, J., and Signoret, J. L. Analyse neuropsychologique du syndrome frontal. *Rev. Neurol.* 127:415–440, 1972.

Lhermitte, J., and Ajuriaguerra, J. Asymbolie tactile et hallucinations du toucher. Etude anatomoclinique. *Rev. Neurol.* (Paris) 70:492–495, 1938.

Li, L., Miller, E. K., and Desimone, R. The representation of stimulus familiarity in anterior inferior temporal cortex. *J. Neurophysiol.* 69:1918–1929, 1993.

Libet, B. Unconscious cerebral initiative and the role of conscious will in voluntary action. *Behav. Brain Sci.* 8:529–566, 1985.

Libet, B., Wright, E. W., and Gleason, C. A. Readiness-potentials preceding unrestricted 'spontaneous' vs. pre-planned voluntary acts. *Electroencephalogr. Clin. Neurophysiol.* 54:322–335, 1982.

Libet, B., Gleason, C. A., Wright, E. W., and Pearl, D. K. Time of conscious intention to act in relation to onset of cerebral activity (readiness-potential): The unconscious initiation of a freely voluntary act. *Brain* 106:623–642, 1983a.

Libet, B., Wright, E. W., and Gleason, C. A. Preparation- or intention-to-act, in relation to pre-event potentials recorded at the vertex. *Electroencephalogr. Clin. Neurophysiol.* 56:367–372, 1983b.

Lidow, M. S., Goldman-Rakic, P. S., and Rakic, P. Synchronized overproduction of neurotransmitter receptors in diverse regions of the primate cerebral cortex. *Proc. Natl. Acad. Sci. U.S.A.* 88:10218–10221, 1991.

Liles, S. L. Single-unit responses of caudate neurons to stimulation of frontal cortex, substantia nigra and entopeduncular nucleus in cats. *J. Neurophysiol.* 37:254–265, 1974.

Llinás, R., and Ribary, U. Coherent 40-Hz oscillation characterizes dream state in humans. *Proc. Natl. Acad. Sci. U.S.A.* 90:2078–2081, 1993.

Lorente de Nó, R. Cerebral cortex: Architecture, intracortical connections, motor projections. In *Physiology of the Nervous System,* edited by J. F. Fulton. New York: Oxford University Press, 1938, pp. 291–339.

Lorenz, K. *Studies in Animal and Human Behavior,* vol. 1. Cambridge, MA: Harvard University Press, 1970.

Loveless, N. E., and Sanford, A. J. Slow potential correlates of preparatory set. *Biol. Psychol.* 1:303–314, 1974.

Low, M. D., Borda, R. P., and Kellaway, P. "Contingent negative variation" in rhesus monkeys: An EEG sign of a specific mental process. *Percept. Mot. Skills* 22:443–446, 1966.

Löwel, S., and Singer, W. Selection of intrinsic horizontal connections in the visual cortex by correlated neuronal activity. *Science* 255:209–212, 1992.

Lund, R. D., and Bunt, A. H. Prenatal development of central optic pathways in albino rats. *J. Comp. Neurol.* 165:247–264, 1976.

Luria, A. R. *Higher Cortical Functions in Man.* New York: Basic Books, 1966.

Luria, A. R. *Traumatic Aphasia.* The Hague: Mouton, 1970.

Luria, A. R., and Homskaya, E. D. Disturbance in the regulative role of speech with frontal lobe lesions. In *The Frontal Granular Cortex and Behavior,* edited by J. M. Warren and K. Akert. New York: McGraw-Hill, 1964, pp. 353–371.

Lurito, J. T., Georgakopoulos, T., and Georgopoulos, A. P. Cognitive spatial-motor processes—the making of movements at an angle from a stimulus direction: Studies of motor cortical activity at the single cell and population levels. *Exp. Brain Res.* 87:562–580, 1991.

Lynch, G., and Baudry, M. The biochemistry of memory: A new and specific hypothesis. *Science* 224:1057–1063, 1984.

Lynch, J. C., Mountcastle, V. B., Talbot, W. H., and Yin, T. C. T. Parietal lobe mechanisms for directed visual attention. *J. Neurophysiol.* 40:362–389, 1977.

Mach, E. *Die Analyse der Empfindungen.* Jena: G. Fischer, 1885.

Machado, A. *Campos de Castilla, 1912* (in *Complete Works*). Madrid: Plenitud, 1962.

MacKay, R. P. Toward a neurology of behavior. *Neurology* 4:894–901, 1954.

Mackworth, J. A. *Vigilance and Habituation.* London: Penguin Press, 1970.

Magoun, H. W. *The Waking Brain.* Springfield, IL: Thomas, 1958.

Mahut, H. Effects of subcortical electrical stimulation on discrimination learning in cats. *J. Comp. Physiol. Psychol.* 58:390–395, 1964.

Mamo, H., Meric, P., Luft, A., and Seylaz, J. Hyperfrontal pattern of human cerebral circulation. *Arch. Neurol.* 40:626–632, 1983.

Mandai, O., Guerrien, A., Sockeel, P., Dujardin, K., and Leconte, P. REM sleep modifications following a morse code learning session in humans. *Physiol. Behav.* 46:639–642, 1989.

Mandler, J. M. Recall of events by preverbal children. In *The Development and Neural Bases of Higher Cognitive Functions,* edited by A. Diamond. New York: New York Academy of Sciences, 1990, pp. 485–516.

Mane, A., Sirevaag, E., Coles, M. G. H., and Donchin, E. ERPs and performance under stress conditions. *Proc. Soc. Psychophysiol. Res.* 20:458, 1983.

Mann, S. E., Thau, R., and Schiller, P. H. Conditional task-related responses in monkey dorsomedial frontal cortex. *Exp. Brain Res.* 69:460–468, 1988.

Maren, S., Tocco, G., Standley, S., Baudry, M., and Thompson, R. F. Postsynaptic factors in the expression of long-term potentiation (LTP): Increased glutamate receptor binding following LTP induction in vivo. *Proc. Natl. Acad. Sci. U.S.A.* 90:9654–9658, 1993.

Marler, P. Birdsong: The acquisition of a learned motor skill. *Trends Neurosci.* 4:88–94, 1981.

Marr, D. A theory of cerebellar cortex. *J. Physiol.* 202:437–470, 1969.

Marr, D. A theory for cerebral neocortex. *Proc. R. Soc. Lond. [Biol.]* 176:161–234, 1970.

Marsden, C. D. The mysterious motor function of the basal ganglia: The Robert Wartenberg lecture. *Neurology* 32:514–539, 1982.

Marsh, J. T., Worden, F. G., and Hicks, L. Some effects of room acoustics on evoked auditory potentials. *Science* 137:280–282, 1962.

Masdeu, J. Aphasia after infarction of the left supplementary motor area. *Neurology* 30:359, 1980.

Mayes, A. R. *Human Organic Memory Disorders.* Cambridge, England: Cambridge University Press, 1988.

Mazzoni, P., Andersen, R. A., and Jordan, M. I. A more biologically plausible learning rule for neural networks. *Proc. Natl. Acad. Sci. U.S.A.* 88:4433–4437, 1991.

McAndrews, M. P., and Milner, B. The frontal cortex and memory for temporal order. *Neuropsychologia* 29:849–859, 1991.

McCarley, R. W., and Hobson, J. A. Neuronal excitability modulation over the sleep cycle: A structural and mathematical model. *Science* 189:58–60, 1975.

McCarthy, R. A., and Warrington, E. K. Visual associative agnosia: A clinico-anatomical study of a single case. *J. Neurol. Neurosurg. Psychiatry* 49:1233–1240, 1986.

McClelland, J. L., and Rumelhart, D. E. Distributed memory and the representation of general and specific information. *J. Exp. Psychol. [Gen.]* 114:159–188, 1985.

McCloskey, D. I. Corollary discharges: Motor commands and perception. In *Handbook of Physiology: Nervous System,* edited by V. B. Brooks. Bethesda, MD: American Physiological Society, 1981, pp. 1415–1447.

McGaugh, J. L. Involvement of hormonal and neuromodulatory systems in the regulation of memory storage. *Ann. Rev. Neurosci.* 12:255–287, 1989.

McGaugh, J. L. Neuromodulatory systems and the regulation of memory storage. In *Neuropsychology of Memory*, edited by L. R. Squire and N. Butters. New York: Guilford Press, 1992, pp. 386–401.

McGaugh, J. L., and Herz, M. J. *Memory Consolidation*. San Francisco: Albion, 1972.

McGaugh, J. L., and Petrinovich, L. The effect of strychnine sulphate on maze-learning. *Am. J. Psychol.* 72:99–102, 1959.

McGrath, M. J., and Cohen, D. B. REM sleep facilitation of adaptive waking behavior: A review of the literature. *Psychol. Bull.* 85:24–57, 1978.

McGuire, P. K., Bates, J. F., and Goldman-Rakic, P. S. Interhemispheric integration: I. Symmetry and convergence of the corticocortical connections of the left and the right principal sulcus (PS) and the left and the right supplementary motor area (SMA) in the rhesus monkey. *Cerebral Cortex* 1:390–407, 1991.

McIntosh, A. R., Grady, C. L., Ungerleider, L. G., Haxby, J. V., Rapoport, S. I., and Horwitz, B. Network analysis of cortical visual pathways mapped with PET. *J. Neurosci.* 14:655–666, 1994.

McNaughton, B. L., Douglas, R. M., and Goddard, G. V. Synaptic enhancement in fascia dentata: Cooperativity among coactive afferents. *Brain Res.* 157:277–293, 1978.

Mellah, S., Rispal-Padel, L., and Riviere, G. Changes in excitability of motor units during preparation for movement. *Exp. Brain Res.* 82:178–186, 1990.

Merzenich, M. M., and Kaas, J. H. Principles of organization of sensory-perceptual systems in mammals. *Prog. in Psychobiol. Physiol. Psychol.* 9:1–42, 1980.

Merzenich, M. M., and Kaas, J. H. Reorganization of mammalian somatosensory cortex following peripheral nerve injury. *Trends Neurosci.* 5:434–436, 1982.

Mesulam, M.-M. A cortical network for directed attention and unilateral neglect. *Ann. Neurol.* 10:309–325, 1981.

Mesulam, M.-M., Van Hoesen, G. W., Pandya, D. N., and Geschwind, N. Limbic and sensory connections of the inferior parietal lobule (area PG) in the rhesus monkey: A study with a new method for HRP histochemistry. *Brain Res.* 136:393–414, 1977.

Miceli, G., Silveri, M. C., Villa, G., and Caramazza, A. On the basis for the agrammatic's difficulty in producing main verbs. *Cortex* 20:207–220, 1984.

Mill, J. *Analysis of the Phenomena of the Human Mind*, vol. 1. London: Baldwin and Cradock, 1829.

Miller, E. Verbal fluency as a function of a measure of verbal intelligence and in relation to different types of cerebral pathology. *Br. J. Clin. Psychol.* 23:53–57, 1984.

Miller, E. K., Li, L., and Desimone, R. Activity of neurons in anterior inferior temporal cortex during a short-term memory task. *J. Neurosci.* 13:1460–1478, 1993.

Miller, G. A., and Chomsky, N. Finitary models of language users. In *Handbook of Mathematical Psychology*, edited by R. D. Luce, R. R. Bush and E. Galanter. New York: Wiley, 1963, pp. 419–491.

Miller, R. Designs for a prototype cerebral cortex. In *Cortico-Hippocampal Interplay and the Representation of Contexts in the Brain (Vol. 17: Studies of Brain Function)*, edited by V. Braitenberg, H. B. Barlow, T. H. Bullock, E. Florey, O.-J. Grüsser and A. Peters. New York: Springer-Verlag, 1991, pp. 11–32.

Milner, B. Psychological defects produced by temporal lobe excision. *Res. Publ. Assoc. Nerv. Ment. Dis.* 36:244–257, 1958.

Milner, B. Visual recognition and recall after right temporal-lobe excision in man. *Neuropsychologia* 6:191–209, 1968.

Milner, B. Some cognitive effects of frontal-lobe lesions in man. *Philos. Trans. R. Soc. Lond. [Biol.]* 298:211–226, 1982.

Mishkin, M. Cortical visual areas and their interactions. In *Brain and Human Behavior,* edited by A. G. Karczmar and J. C. Eccles. New York: Springer, 1972, pp. 187–208.

Mishkin, M. Memory in monkeys severely impaired by combined but not by separate removal of amygdala and hippocampus. *Nature* 273:297–298, 1978.

Mishkin, M. Analogous neural models for tactual and visual learning. *Neuropsychologia* 17:139–151, 1979.

Mishkin, M. A memory system in the monkey. *Philos. Trans. R. Soc. Lond. [Biol.]* 298:85–95, 1982.

Mishkin, M., and Petri, H. L. Memories and habits: Some implications for the analysis of learning and retention. In *Neuropsychology of Memory,* edited by L. R. Squire and N. Butters. New York: Guilford Press, 1984, pp. 287–296.

Mistlin, A. J., and Perrett, D. I. Visual and somatosensory processing in the macaque temporal cortex: The role of "expectation." *Exp. Brain Res.* 82:437–450, 1990.

Mitchell, S. J., Richardson, R. T., Baker, F. H., and Delong, M. R. The primate globus pallidus: Neuronal activity related to direction of movements. *Exp. Brain Res.* 68:491–505, 1987.

Miyashita, Y. Neuronal correlate of visual associative long-term memory in the primate temporal cortex. *Nature* 335:817–820, 1988.

Miyashita, Y., and Chang, H. S. Neuronal correlate of pictorial short-term memory in the primate temporal cortex. *Nature* 331:68–70, 1988.

Mogilner, A., Grossman, J. A. I., Ribary, U., Joliot, M., Volkmann, J., Rapaport, D., Beasley, R. W., and Llinás, R. R. Somatosensory cortical plasticity in adult humans revealed by magnetoencephalography. *Proc. Natl. Acad. Sci. U.S.A.* 90:3593–3597, 1993.

Mondadori, C., Ducret, T., and Borkowski, J. How long does "memory consolidation" take? New compounds can improve retention performance, even if administered up to 24 hours after the learning experience. *Brain Res.* 555:107–111, 1991.

Mondadori, C., and Petschke, F. Do piracetam-like compounds act centrally via peripheral mechanisms? *Brain Res.* 435:310–314, 1987.

Moran, J., and Desimone, R. Selective attention gates visual processing in the extrastriate cortex. *Science* 229:782–784, 1985.

Moray, N. Attention in dichotic listening: Affective cues and the influence of instructions. *Q. J. Exp. Psychol.* 11:56–60, 1959.

Morris, R. G. M., Halliwell, R. F., and Bowery, N. Synaptic plasticity and learning: II. Do different kinds of plasticity underlie different kinds of learning? *Neuropsychologia* 27:41–59, 1989.

Moruzzi, G., and Magoun, H. W. Brain stem reticular formation and activation of the EEG. *Electroencephalogr. Clin. Neurophysiol.* 1:455–473, 1949.

Moss, M. B., Rosene, D. L., and Peters, A. Effects of aging on visual recognition memory in the rhesus monkey. *Neurobiol. Aging* 9:495–502, 1988.

Motter, B. C., and Mountcastle, V. B. The functional properties of the light-sensitive neurons of the posterior parietal cortex studied in waking monkeys: Foveal sparing and opponent vector organization. *J. Neurosci.* 1:3–26, 1981.

Mountcastle, V. B. Modality and topographic properties of single neurons of cat's somatic sensory cortex. *J. Neurophysiol.* 20:408–434, 1957.

Mountcastle, V. B. An organizing principle for cerebral function. The unit module and the distributed system. In *The Mindful Brain,* edited by G. M. Edelman and V. B. Mountcastle. New York: Plenum, 1978, pp.7–50.

Mountcastle, V. B., Lynch, J. C., Georgopoulos, A., Sakata, H., and Acuna, C. Posterior parietal association cortex of the monkey: Command functions for operations within extrapersonal space. *J. Neurophysiol.* 38:871–908, 1975.

Mountcastle, V. B., and Powell, T. P. S. Central nervous mechanisms subserving position sense and kinesthesis. *Bull. Johns Hopkins Hosp.* 105:173–200, 1959.

Mountcastle, V. B., Andersen, R. A., and Motter, B. C. The influence of attentive fixation upon the excitability of the light-sensitive neurons of the posterior parietal cortex. *J. Neurosci.* 1:1218–1235, 1981.

Mowbray, G. H. Simultaneous vision and audition: The comprehension of prose passages with varying levels of difficulty. *J. Exp. Psychol.* 46:365–372, 1953.

Muakkasa, K. F., and Strick, P. L. Frontal lobe inputs to primate motor cortex: Evidence for four somatotopically organized "premotor" areas. *Brain Res.* 177:176–182, 1979.

Murdock, B. B. A theory for the storage and retrieval of item and associative information. *Psychol. Rev.* 89:609–626, 1982.

Murray, E. A., and Mishkin, M. Relative contributions of SII and Area 5 to tactile discrimination in monkeys. *Behav. Brain Res.* 11:67–83, 1984.

Murthy, V. N., and Fetz, E. E. Synchronized 25–35 Hz oscillations in sensorimotor cortex of awake monkeys. *Soc. Neurosci. Abstr.* 17:310, 1991.

Mushiake, H., Inase, M., and Tanji, J. Neuronal activity in the primate premotor, supplementary, and precentral motor cortex during visually guided and internally determined sequential movements. *J. Neurophysiol.* 66:705–718, 1991.

Mushiake, H., Inase, M., and Tanji, J. Selective coding of motor sequence in the supplementary motor area of the monkey cerebral cortex. *Exp. Brain Res.* 82:208–210, 1990.

Näätänen, R. Selective attention and evoked potentials in humans—a critical review. *Biol. Psychol.* 2:237–307, 1975.

Naitoh, P., Johnson, L. C., and Lubin, A. Modification of surface negative slow potential (CNV) in the human brain after total sleep loss. *Electroencephalogr. Clin. Neurophysiol.* 30:17–22, 1971.

Nakamura, K., Mikami, A., and Kubota, K. Activity of single neurons in the monkey amygdala during performance of a visual discrimination task. *J. Neurophysiol.* 67:1447–1463, 1992a.

Nakamura, K., Mikami, A., and Kubota, K. Oscillatory neuronal activity related to visual short-term memory in monkey temporal pole. *NeuroReport* 3:117–120, 1992b.

Neisser, U. *Cognitive Psychology.* New York: Appleton-Century-Crofts, 1967.

Neisser, U. *Cognition and Reality: Principles and Implications of Cognitive Psychology.* San Francisco: Freeman, 1976.

Nicoll, R. A., Kauer, J. A., and Malenka, R. C. The current excitement in long-term potentiation. *Neuron* 1:97–103, 1988.

Niki, H. Prefrontal unit activity during delayed alternation in the monkey: I. Relation to direction of response. *Brain Res.* 68:185–196, 1974a.

Niki, H. Prefrontal unit activity during delayed alternation in the monkey. II. Relation to absolute versus relative direction of response. *Brain Res.* 68:197–204, 1974b.

Niki, H. Differential activity of prefrontal units during right and left delayed response trials. *Brain Res.* 70:346–349, 1974c.

Niki, H., Sakai, M., and Kubota, K. Delayed alternation performance and unit activity of the caudate head and medial orbitofrontal gyrus in the monkey. *Brain Res.* 38:343–353, 1972.

Niki, H., and Watanabe, M. Prefrontal unit activity and delayed response: Relation to cue location versus direction of response. *Brain Res.* 105:79–88, 1976.

Nishizawa, Y., Olsen, T. S., Larsen, B., and Lassen, N. A. Left-right cortical asymmetries of regional cerebral blood flow during listening to words. *J. Neurophysiol.* 48:458–466, 1982.

Norman, D. A. Toward a theory of memory and attention. *Psychol. Rev.* 75:522–536, 1968.

Nottebohm, F. Reassessing the mechanisms and origins of vocal learning in birds. *Trends Neurosci.* 14:206–211, 1991.

Nudo, R. J., Jenkins, W. M., and Merzenich, M. M. Repetitive microstimulation alters the cortical representation of movements in adult rats. *Somatosens. Mot. Res.* 7:463–483, 1990.

Ogden, J. A. Autotopagnosia. *Brain* 108:1009–1022, 1985.

Ojemann, G. A. Brain organization for language from the perspective of electrical stimulation mapping. *Behav. Brain Sci.* 6:189–230, 1983.

Ojemann, G. A. Cortical organization of language. *J. Neurosci.* 11:2281–2287, 1991.

Ojemann, G. A., Cawthon, D. F., and Lettich, E. Localization and physiological correlates of language and verbal memory in human lateral temporoparietal cortex. In *Neurobiology of Higher Cognitive Function,* edited by A. B. Scheibel and A. F. Wechsler. New York: Guilford Press, 1990, pp. 185–202.

Ojemann, G. A., and Whitaker, H. A. The bilingual brain. *Arch. Neurol.* 35:409–412, 1978.

Ojemann, J. G., Ojemann, G. A., and Lettich, E. Neuronal activity related to faces and matching in human right nondominant temporal cortex. *Brain* 115:1–13, 1992.

Okano, K. Temporal priority of premotor cortex over nearby areas in receiving visual cues in primates. *NeuroReport* 3:389–392, 1992.

Okano, K., and Tanji, J. Neuronal activities in the primate motor fields of the agranular frontal cortex preceding visually triggered and self-paced movement. *Exp. Brain Res.* 66:155–166, 1987.

O'Leary, D. D. M. Do cortical areas emerge from a protocortex? *Trends Neurosci.* 12:400–406, 1989.

Olton, D. S., Becker, J. T., and Handelmann, G. E. Hippocampus, space, and memory. *Behav. Brain Sci.* 2:313–365, 1979.

Otto, T., Schottler, F., Staubli, U., Eichenbaum, H., and Lynch, G. Hippocampus and olfactory discrimination learning: Effects of entorhinal cortex lesions on olfactory learning and memory in a successive-cue, go-no-go task. *Behav. Neurosci.* 105:111–119, 1991.

Owen, A. M., Downes, J. J., Sahakian, B. J., Polkey, C. E., and Robbins, T. W. Planning and spatial working memory following frontal lobe lesions in man. *Neuropsychologia* 28:1021–1034, 1990.

Paillard, J. Apraxia and the neurophysiology of motor control. *Philos. Trans. R. Soc. Lond. [Biol.]* 298:111–134, 1982.

Palm, G. *Neural Assemblies.* Berlin: Springer-Verlag, 1982.

Pandya, D. N., Hallett, M., and Mukherjee, S. K. Intra- and interhemispheric connections of the neocortical auditory system in the rhesus monkey. *Brain Res.* 14:49–65, 1969.

Pandya, D. N., Dye, P., and Butters, N. Efferent cortico-cortical projections of the prefrontal cortex in the rhesus monkey. *Brain Res.* 31:35–46, 1971.

Pandya, D. N., and Seltzer, B. Intrinsic connections and architectonics of posterior parietal cortex in the rhesus monkey. *J. Comp. Neurol.* 204:196–210, 1982.

Pandya, D. N., and Vignolo, L. A. Intra- and interhemispheric projections of the precentral, premotor and arcuate areas in the rhesus monkey. *Brain Res.* 26:217–233, 1971.

Pandya, D. N., and Yeterian, E. H. Architecture and connections of cortical association areas. In *Cerebral Cortex,* vol. 4, edited by A. Peters and E. G. Jones. New York: Plenum, 1985, pp. 3–61.

Pandya, D. N., and Yeterian, E. H. Architecture and connections of cerebral cortex: Implications for brain evolution and function. In *Neurobiology of Higher Cognitive Function,* edited by A. B. Scheibel and A. F. Wechsler. New York: Guilford Press, 1990, pp. 53–84.

Passingham, R. E. Broca's area and the origins of human vocal skill. *Philos. Trans. R. Soc. Lond. [Biol.]* 292:167–175, 1981.

Passingham, R. E. Premotor cortex: Sensory cues and movement. *Behav. Brain Res.* 18:175–185, 1985.

Passingham, R. E. *The Frontal Lobes and Voluntary Action.* Oxford, UK: Oxford University Press, 1993.

Passingham, R. E., Chen, Y. C., and Thaler, D. Supplementary motor cortex and self-initiated movement. In *Neural Programming,* edited by M. Ito. Tokyo: Japan Scientific Societies, 1989, pp. 13–24.

Patton, H. D. Taste, olfaction and visceral sensation. In *Medical Physiology and Biophysics,* edited by T. C. Ruch and J. F. Fulton. Philadelphia: Saunders, 1960, pp. 369–385.

Paulesu, E., Frith, C. D., and Frackowiak, R. S. J. The neural correlates of the verbal component of working memory. *Nature* 362:342–344, 1993.

Pavlides, C., Miyashita, E., and Asanuma, H. Projection from the sensory to the motor cortex is important in learning motor skills in the monkey. *J. Neurophysiol.* 70:733–741, 1993.

Pei, M. A., and Gaynor, F. *A Dictionary of Linguistics.* New York: Philosophical Library, 1954.

Penfield, W., and Perot, P. The brain's record of auditory and visual experience. *Brain* 86:595–696, 1963.

Penfield, W., and Roberts, L. *Speech and Brain-Mechanisms.* New York: Atheneum, 1966.

Perani, D., Bressi, S., Cappa, S. F., Vallar, G., Alberoni, M., Grassi, F., Caltagirone, C., Cipolotti, L., Franceschi, M., Lenzi, G. L., and Fazio, F. Evidence of multiple memory systems in the human brain. *Brain* 116:903–919, 1993.

Perrett, D. I., Rolls, E. T., and Caan, W. Visual neurones responsive to faces in the monkey temporal cortex. *Exp. Brain Res.* 47:329–342, 1982.

Perrett, D. I., Smith, P. A. J., Mistlin, A. J., Chitty, A. J., Head, A. S., Potter, D. D., Broennimann, R., Milner, A. D., and Jeeves, M. A. Visual analysis of body movements by neurones in the temporal cortex of the macaque monkey: A preliminary report. *Behav. Brain Res.* 16:153–170, 1985.

Petersen, M. R., Beecher, M. D., Zoloth, S. R., Moody, D. B., and Stebbins, W. C. Neural lateralization of species-specific vocalizations by Japanese macaques (*Macaca fuscata*). *Science* 202:324–327, 1978.

Petersen, S. E., Fox, P. T., Snyder, A. Z., and Raichle, M. E. Activation of extrastriate and frontal cortical areas by visual words and word-like stimuli. *Science* 249:1041–1044, 1990.

Peterson, L. R., and Peterson, M. J. Short-term retention of individual verbal items. *J. Exp. Psychol.* 58:193–198, 1959.

Petrides, M. Deficits on conditional associative-learning tasks after frontal- and temporal-lobe lesions in man. *Neuropsychologia* 23:601–614, 1985.

Petrides, M. The effect of periarcuate lesions in the monkey on the performance of symmetrically and asymmetrically reinforced visual and auditory go, no-go tasks. *J. Neurosci.* 6:2054–2063, 1986.

Petrides, M. Functional specialization within the primate dorsolateral frontal cortex. *Adv. Neurol.* 57:379–388, 1992.

Petrides, M., Alivisatos, B., Evans, A. C., and Meyer, E. Dissociation of human mid-dorsolateral from posterior dorsolateral frontal cortex in memory processing. *Proc. Natl. Acad. Sci. U.S.A.* 90:873–877, 1993a.

Petrides, M., Alivisatos, B., Meyer, E., and Evans, A. C. Functional activation of the human frontal cortex during the performance of verbal working memory tasks. *Proc. Natl. Acad. Sci. U.S.A.* 90:878–882, 1993b.

Piaget, J. *The Origins of Intelligence in the Child.* London: Routledge & Kegan Paul, 1952.

Pitts, W., and McCulloch, W. S. How we know universals: The perception of auditory and visual forms. *Bull. Math. Biophys.* 9:127–147, 1947.

Pohl, W. Dissociation of spatial discrimination deficits following frontal and parietal lesions in monkeys. *J. Comp. Physiol. Psychol.* 82:227–239, 1973.

Pons, T. P., Garraghty, P. E., Cusick, C. G., and Kaas, J. H. A sequential representation of the occiput, arm, forearm and hand across the rostrocaudal dimension of areas 1, 2 and 5 in macaque monkeys. *Brain Res.* 335:350–353, 1985.

Pons, T. P., Garraghty, P. E., Friedman, D. P., and Mishkin, M. Physiological evidence for serial processing in somatosensory cortex. *Science* 237:417–420, 1987.

Pons, T. P., Garraghty, P. E., Ommaya, A. K., Kaas, J. H., Taub, E., and Mishkin, M. Massive cortical reorganization after sensory deafferentation in adult macaques. *Science* 252:1857–1860, 1991.

Pons, T. P., Garraghty, P. E., and Mishkin, M. Serial and parallel processing of tactual information in somatosensory cortex of rhesus monkeys. *J. Neurophysiol.* 68:518–527, 1992.

Posner, M. I. Structures and functions of selective attention. In *Clinical Neuropsychology and Brain Function*, edited by T. Boll and B. K. Bryant. Washington, DC: American Psychological Association, 1988, pp. 173–202.

Posner, M. I., and Boies, S. J. Components of attention. *Psychol. Rev.* 78:391–408, 1971.

Posner, M. I., Petersen, S. E., Fox, P. T., and Raichle, M. E. Localization of cognitive operations in the human brain. *Science* 24:1627–1631, 1988.

Powell, T. P. S., and Mountcastle, V. B. Some aspects of the functional organization of the cortex of the postcentral gyrus of the monkey: A correlation of findings obtained in a single unit analysis with cytoarchitecture. *Bull. Johns Hopkins Hosp.* 105:133–162, 1959.

Pribram, K. H. The neurophysiology of remembering. *Sci. Am.* 220:73–86, 1969.

Pulvermüller, F., and Preissl, H. A cell assembly model of language. *Network* 2:455–468, 1991.

Pumain, R., and Heinemann, U. Stimulus- and amino acid-induced calcium and potassium changes in rat neocortex. *J. Neurophysiol.* 53:1–16, 1985.

Pysh, J. J., and Weiss, G. M. Exercise during development induces an increase in Purkinje cell dendritic tree size. *Science* 206:230–232, 1979.

Quintana, J., and Fuster, J. M. Mnemonic and predictive functions of cortical neurons in a memory task. *NeuroReport* 3:721–724, 1992.

Quintana, J., and Fuster, J. M. Spatial and temporal factors in the role of prefrontal and parietal cortex in visuomotor integration. *Cerebral Cortex* 3:122–132, 1993.

Quintana, J., Yajeya, J., and Fuster, J. M. Prefrontal representation of stimulus attributes during delay tasks: I. Unit activity in cross-temporal integration of sensory and sensory-motor information. *Brain Res.* 474:211–221, 1988.

Quintana, J., Fuster, J. M., and Yajeya, J. Effects of cooling parietal cortex on prefrontal units in delay tasks. *Brain Res.* 503:100–110, 1989.

Rakic, P. Prenatal development of the visual system in rhesus monkey. *Philos. Trans. R. Soc. Lond.* 278:245–260, 1977.

Rakic, P., Bourgeois, J. P., Eckenhoff, M. F., Zecevic, N., and Goldman-Rakic, P. S. Concurrent overproduction of synapses in diverse regions of the primate cerebral cortex. *Science* 232:232–235, 1986.

Ramier, A. M., and Hécaen, H. Les déficits au test de "fluence verbale" chez les sujets gauchers avec lésions hémisphériques unilatérales. *Rev. Neurol.* 133:571–574, 1977.

Ramón y Cajal, S. *Textura del Sistema Nervioso del Hombre y de los Vertebrados*, vol. 2. Madrid: Moya, 1904.

Ramón y Cajal, S. *Recuerdos de mi Vida*. Madrid: Pueyo, 1923.

Rapp, P. R. Visual discrimination and reversal learning in the aged monkey (*Macaca mulatta*). *Behav. Neurosci.* 104:876–884, 1990.

Recanzone, G. H., Jenkins, W. M., Hradek, G. T., and Merzenich, M. M. Progressive improvement in discriminative abilities in adult owl monkeys performing a tactile frequency discrimination task. *J. Neurophysiol.* 67:1015–1030, 1992a.

Recanzone, G. H., Merzenich, M. M., and Jenkins, W. M. Frequency discrimination training engaging a restricted skin surface results in an emergence of a cutaneous response zone in cortical area 3a. *J. Neurophysiol.* 67:1057–1070, 1992b.

Recanzone, G. H., Schreiner, C. E., and Merzenich, M. M. Plasticity in the frequency representation of primary auditory cortex following discrimination training in adult owl monkeys. *J. Neurosci.* 13:87–103, 1993.

Reinoso-Suárez, F. Connectional patterns in parietotemporooccipital association cortex of the feline cerebral cortex. In *Cortical Integration*, edited by F. Reinoso-Suárez and C. Ajmone-Marsan. New York: Raven Press, 1984, pp. 255–273.

Reinoso-Suárez, F., and Fuster, J. M. Effects of subcortical lesions on the potentials evoked in the visual pathway by light stimuli and geniculate shock. *Excerpta Medica, International Congress Series* 37:215–216, 1961.

Renaud, L. P., and Kelly, J. S. Identification of possible inhibitory neurons in the pericruciate cortex of the cat. *Brain Res.* 79:9–28, 1974.

Ribot, T. *Les Maladies de le Mémoire.* Paris: F. Alcan, 1906.

Richmond, B. J., and Optican, L. M. Temporal encoding of two-dimensional patterns by single units in primate inferior temporal cortex: II. Quantification of response waveform. *J. Neurophysiol.* 57:147–161, 1987.

Richmond, B. J., and Sato, T. Enhancement of inferior temporal neurons during visual discrimination. *J. Neurophysiol.* 58:1292–1306, 1987.

Ridley, R. M., and Ettlinger, G. Further evidence of impaired tactile learning after removals of the second somatic sensory projection cortex (SII) in the monkey. *Exp. Brain Res.* 31:475–488, 1978.

Riehle, A. Visually induced signal-locked neuronal activity changes in precentral motor areas of the monkey: Hierarchical progression of signal processing. *Brain Res.* 540:131–137, 1991.

Riehle, A., and Requin, J. Monkey primary motor and premotor cortex: Single-cell activity related to prior information about direction and extent of an intended movement. *J. Neurophysiol.* 61:534–549, 1989.

Riehle, A., and Requin, J. The predictive value for performance speed of preparatory changes in neuronal activity of the monkey motor and premotor cortex. *Behav. Brain Res.* 53:35–49, 1993.

Rizzolatti, G., Matelli, M., and Pavesi, G. Deficits in attention and movement following the removal of postarcuate (area 6) and prearcuate (area 8) cortex in macaque monkeys. *Brain* 106:655–673, 1983.

Rizzolatti, G., Camarda, R., Fogassi, M., Gentilucci, M., Luppino, G., and Matelli, M. Functional organization of inferior area 6 in the macaque monkey. *Exp. Brain Res.* 71:491–507, 1988.

Robinson, C. J., and Burton, H. Somatic submodality distribution within the second somatosensory (SII), 7b, retroinsular, postauditory, and granular insular cortical areas. *J. Comp. Neurol.* 192:93–108, 1980.

Robinson, D. L., Goldberg, M. E., and Stanton, G. B. Parietal association cortex in the primate: Sensory mechanisms and behavioral modulations. *J. Neurophysiol.* 41:910–932, 1978.

Rockland, K. S., and Pandya, D. N. Laminar origins and terminations of cortical connections of the occipital lobe in the rhesus monkey. *Brain Res.* 179:3–20, 1979.

Roe, A. W., Pallas, S. L., Hahm, J., and Sur, M. A map of visual space induced in primary auditory cortex. *Science* 250:818–820, 1990.

Roland, P. E. Astereognosis: Tactile discrimination after localized hemispheric lesions in man. *Arch. Neurol.* 33:543–550, 1976.

Roland, P. E. Somatotopical tuning of postcentral gyrus during focal attention in man. A regional cerebral blood flow study. *J. Neurophysiol.* 46:744–754, 1981.

Roland, P. E. Cortical organization of voluntary behavior in man. *Hum. Neurobiol.* 4:155–167, 1985.

Roland, P. E., and Friberg, L. Localization of cortical areas activated by thinking. *J. Neurophysiol.* 53:1219–1243, 1985.

Roland, P. E., Larsen, B., Lassen, N. A., and Skinhoj, E. Supplementary motor area and other cortical areas in organization of voluntary movements in man. *J. Neurophysiol.* 43:118–136, 1980a.

Roland, P. E., Skinhoj, E., Lassen, N. A., and Larsen, B. Different cortical areas in man in organization of voluntary movements in extrapersonal space. *J. Neurophysiol.* 43:137–150, 1980b.

Roland, P. E., Gulyás, B., Seitz, R. J., Bohm, C., and Stone-Elander, S. Functional anatomy of storage, recall, and recognition of a visual pattern in man. *NeuroReport* 1:53–56, 1990.

Roland, P. E., and Larsen, B. Focal increase of cerebral blood flow during stereognostic testing in man. *Arch. Neurol.* 33:551–558, 1976.

Rolls, E. T. Information processing in the taste system of primates. *J. Exp. Biol.* 146:141–164, 1989.

Rolls, E. T., Baylis, G. C., Hasselmo, M. E., and Nalwa, V. The effect of learning on the face selective responses of neurons in the cortex in the superior temporal sulcus of the monkey. *Exp. Brain Res.* 76:153–164, 1989a.

Rolls, E. T., Sienkiewicz, Z. J., and Yaxley, S. Hunger modulates the responses to gustatory stimuli of single neurons in the caudolateral orbitofrontal cortex of the macaque monkey. *Eur. J. Neurosci.* 1:53–60, 1989b.

Romo, R., and Schultz, W. Neuronal activity preceding self-initiated or externally timed arm movement in area 6 of monkey cortex. *Exp. Brain Res.* 67:656–662, 1987.

Romo, R., and Schultz, W. Role of primate basal ganglia and frontal cortex in the internal generation of movements. *Exp. Brain Res.* 91:396–407, 1992.

Roney, K. J., Scheibel, A. B., and Shaw, G. L. Dendritic bundles: Survey of anatomical experiments and physiological theories. *Brain Res. Rev.* 1:225–271, 1979.

Rosenkilde, C. E., Bauer, R. H., and Fuster, J. M. Single cell activity in ventral prefrontal cortex of behaving monkeys. *Brain Res.* 209:375–394, 1981.

Rosenzweig, M. R. Experience, memory, and the brain. *Am. Psychol.* 39:365–376, 1984.

Routtenberg, A. Protein kinase C activation leading to protein F1 phosphorylation may regulate synaptic plasticity by presynaptic terminal growth. *Behav. Neural Biol.* 44:186–200, 1985.

Rovee-Collier, C. The "memory system" of prelinguistic infants. In *The Development and Neural Bases of Higher Cognitive Functions*, edited by A. Diamond. New York: New York Academy of Sciences, 1990, pp. 517–542.

Rubens, A. B. Anatomical asymmetries of human cerebral cortex. In *Lateralization in the Nervous System*, edited by S. Harnad, R. W. Doty, L. Goldstein, J. Jaynes and G. Krauthamer. New York: Academic, 1977, pp. 503–516.

Rumelhart, D. E., Hinton, G. E., and Williams, R.J. Learning representations by back-propagating errors. *Nature* 323:533–536, 1986.

Sakai, K., and Miyashita, Y. Neural organization for the long-term memory of paired associates. *Nature* 354:152–155, 1991.

Sakai, M. Prefrontal unit activity during visually guided lever pressing reaction in the monkey. *Brain Res.* 81:297–309, 1974.

Sakamoto, T., Porter, L. L., and Asanuma, H. Long-lasting potentiation of synaptic potentials in the motor cortex produced by stimulation of the sensory cortex in the cat: A basis of motor learning. *Brain Res.* 413:360–364, 1987.

Sakata, H., Takaoka, Y., Kawarasaki, A., and Shibutani, H. Somatosensory properties of neurons in the superior parietal cortex (area 5) of the rhesus monkey. *Brain Res.* 64:85–102, 1973.

Sakata, H., Shibutani, H., and Kawano, K. Spatial properties of visual fixation neurons in posterior parietal association cortex of the monkey. *J. Neurophysiol.* 43:1654–1672, 1980.

Sanes, J. N., Suner, S., and Donoghue, J. P. Dynamic organization of primary motor cortex output to target muscles in adult rats: I. Long-term patterns of reorganization following motor or mixed peripheral nerve lesions. *Exp. Brain Res.* 79:479–491, 1990.

Sanes, J. N., Wang, J., and Donoghue, J. P. Immediate and delayed changes of rat motor cortical output representations with new forelimb configurations. *Cerebral Cortex* 2:141–152, 1992.

Sanghera, M. K., Rolls, E. T., and Roper-Hall, A. Visual responses of neurons in the dorsolateral amygdala of the alert monkey. *Exp. Neurol.* 63:610–626, 1979.

Sanides, F. The cyto-myeloarchitecture of the human frontal lobe and its relation to phylogenetic differentiation of the cerebral cortex. *J. Hirnforsch.* 6:269–282, 1964.

Sarter, M., and Markowitsch, H. J. Involvement of the amygdala in learning and memory: A critical review, with emphasis on anatomical relations. *Behav. Neurosci.* 99:342–380, 1985.

Sato, K. C., and Tanji, J. Digit-muscle reponses evoked from multiple intracortical foci in monkey precentral motor cortex. *J. Neurophysiol.* 62:959–969, 1989.

Sato, T. Effects of attention and stimulus interaction on visual responses of inferior temporal neurons in macaque. *J. Neurophysiol.* 60:344–364, 1988.

Sawaguchi, T., and Goldman-Rakic, P. S. D1 dopamine receptors in prefrontal cortex: Involvement in working memory. *Science* 251:947–951, 1991.

Sawaguchi, T., and Goldman-Rakic, P. S. The role of D1-dopamine receptor in working memory: Local injections of dopamine antagonists into the prefrontal cortex of rhesus monkeys performing an oculomotor delayed-response task. *J. Neurophysiol.* 71:515–528, 1994.

Sawaguchi, T., Matsumura, M., and Kubota, K. Effects of dopamine antagonists on neuronal activity related to a delayed response task in monkey prefrontal cortex. *J. Neurophysiol.* 63:1401–1412, 1990.

Schacter, D. L., and Graf, P. Effects of elaborative processing on implicit and explicit memory for new associations. *J. Exp. Psychol.* 12:432–444, 1986.

Scheibel, M. E., Lindsay, R. D., Tomiyasu, U., and Scheibel, A. B. Progressive dendritic changes in aging human cortex. *Exp. Neurol.* 47:392–403, 1975.

Scheibel, M. E., and Scheibel, A. B. Structural substrates for integrative patterns in the brain stem reticular core. In *Reticular Formation of the Brain*, edited by H. H. Jasper, L. D.

Proctor, R. S. Knighton, W. C. Noshay, and R. T. Costello. Boston: Little, Brown, 1958, pp. 31–55.

Scheibel, M. E., and Scheibel, A. B. Elementary processes in selected thalamic and cortical subsystems—the structural substrates. In *The Neurosciences: Second Study Program*, edited by F. O. Schmitt and F. G. Worden. New York: Rockefeller University Press, 1970, pp. 443–457.

Schmidt, E. M., McIntosh, J. S., Durelli, L., and Bak, M. J. Fine control of operantly conditioned firing patterns of cortical neurons. *Exp. Neurol.* 61:349–369, 1978.

Schneider, R. J., Friedman, D. P., and Mishkin, M. A modality-specific somatosensory area within the insula of the rhesus monkey. *Brain Res.* 621:116–120, 1993.

Schnider, A., Landis, T., Regard, M., and Benson, F. Dissociation of color from object in amnesia. *Arch. Neurol.* 49:982–985, 1992.

Schnider, A., Regard, M., and Landis, T. Anterograde and retrograde amnesia following bitemporal infarction. *J. Behav. Neurol.* (in press).

Schulhoff, C., and Goodglass, H. Dichotic listening, side of brain injury and cerebral dominance. *Neuropsychologia* 7:149–160, 1969.

Schultz, W., and Romo, R. Role of primate basal ganglia and frontal cortex in the internal generation of movements: I. Preparatory activity in the anterior striatum. *Exp. Brain Res.* 91:363–384, 1992.

Schuman, E. M., and Madison, D. V. Locally distributed synaptic potentiation in the hippocampus. *Science* 263:532–536, 1994.

Schwartz, A. B., Kettner, R. E., and Georgopoulos, A. P. Primate motor cortex and free arm movements to visual targets in three-dimensional space: I. Relations between single cell discharge and direction of movement. *J. Neurosci.* 8:2913–2927, 1988.

Schwartz, E. L., Desimone, R., Albright, T. D., and Gross, C. G. Shape recognition and inferior temporal neurons. *Proc. Natl. Acad. Sci. U.S.A.* 80:5776–5778, 1983.

Schwartz, M. L., and Goldman-Rakic, P. S. Callosal and intrahemispheric connectivity of the prefrontal association cortex in rhesus monkey: Relation between intraparietal and principal sulcal cortex. *J. Comp. Neurol.* 226:403–420, 1984.

Scott, T. R., Yaxley, S., Sienkiewicz, Z. J., and Rolls, E. T. Gustatory responses in the nucleus tractus solitarius of the alert cynomolgus monkey. *J. Neurophysiol.* 55:182–200, 1986a.

Scott, T. R., Yaxley, S., Sienkiewicz, Z. J., and Rolls, E. T. Gustatory responses in the frontal opercular cortex of the alert cynomolgus monkey. *J. Neurophysiol.* 56:876–890, 1986b.

Scoville, W. B., and Milner, B. Loss of recent memory after bilateral hippocampal lesions. *J. Neurol. Neurosurg. Psychiatry* 20:11–21, 1957.

Seal, J., and Commenges, D. A quantitative analysis of stimulus- and movement-related responses in the posterior parietal cortex of the monkey. *Exp. Brain Res.* 58:144–153, 1985.

Searle, J. R. Consciousness, explanatory inversion, and cognitive science. *Behav. Brain Sci.* 13:585–642, 1990.

Seitz, R. J., Roland, P. E., Bohm, C., Greitz, T., and Stone-Elander, S. Motor learning in man: A positron emission tomographic study. *NeuroReport* 1:57–66, 1990.

Sejnowski, T. J. On the stochastic dynamics of neuronal interaction. *Biol. Cybern.* 22:203–211, 1976.

Sejnowski, T. J. Skeleton filters in the brain. In *Parallel Models of Associative Memory*, edited by G. E. Hinton and J. A. Anderson. Hillsdale, NJ: Erlbaum, 1981, pp. 189–212.

Selemon, L. D., and Goldman-Rakic, P. S. Common cortical and subcortical target areas of the dorsolateral prefrontal and posterior parietal cortices in the rhesus monkey: A double label study of distributed neural networks. *J. Neurosci.* 8:4049–4068, 1988.

Seltzer, B., and Pandya, D. N. Further observations on parieto-temporal connections in the rhesus monkey. *Exp. Brain Res.* 55:301–312, 1984.

Semmes, J. A non-tactual factor in astereognosis. *Neuropsychologia* 3:295–315, 1965.

Senden, M. von. *Space and Sight.* London: Methuen, 1960.

Sergent, J., Zuck, E., Terriah, S., and MacDonald, B. Distributed neural network underlying musical sight-reading and keyboard performance. *Science* 257:106–109, 1992.

Shallice, T. Specific impairments of planning. *Philos. Trans. R. Soc. Lond. [Biol.]* 298:199–209, 1982.

Shallice, T. *From Neuropsychology to Mental Structure.* New York: Cambridge University Press, 1988.

Shallice, T. Précis of "From Neuropsychology to Mental Structure." *Behav. Brain Sci.* 14:429–469, 1991.

Shaw, G. L., and Palm, G., eds. *Brain Theory* (reprint vol.). Singapore: World Scientific Publishing, 1988.

Shaw, G. L., Silverman, D. J., and Pearson, J. C. Model of cortical organization embodying a basis for a theory of information processing and memory recall. *Proc. Natl. Acad. Sci. U.S.A.* 82:2364–2368, 1985.

Shaw, T. G., Mortel, K. F., Meyer, J. S., Rogers, R. L., Hardenberg, J., and Cutaia, M. M. Cerebral blood flow changes in benign aging and cerebrovascular disease. *Neurology* 34:855–862, 1984.

Shenoy, K. V., Kaufman, J., McGrann, J. V., and Shaw, G. L. Learning by selection in the trion model of cortical organization. *Cerebral Cortex* 3:239–248, 1993.

Sherry, D. F., and Schacter, D. L. The evolution of multiple memory systems. *Psychol. Rev.* 94:439–454, 1987.

Shindy, W. W., Posley, K. A., and Fuster, J. M. Reversible deficit in haptic delay tasks from cooling prefrontal cortex. *Cerebral Cortex* (in press).

Sierra-Paredes, G., and Fuster, J. M. Auditory-visual association task impaired by cooling prefrontal cortex. *Soc. Neurosci. Abstr.* 19:801, 1993.

Smith, C. Sleep states and learning: A review of the animal literature. *Neurosci. Behav. Rev.* 9:157–168, 1985.

Smith, C. B. Aging and changes in cerebral energy metabolism. *Trends Neurosci.* 7:203–208, 1984.

Smyrnis, N., Taira, M., Ashe, J., and Georgopoulos, A. P. Motor cortical activity in a memorized delay task. *Exp. Brain Res.* 92:139–151, 1992.

Soechting, J. F., and Flanders, M. Moving in three-dimensional space: Frames of reference, vectors, and coordinate systems. *Annu. Rev. Neurosci.* 15:167–191, 1992.

Sparks, R., Goodglass, H., and Nickel, B. Ipsilateral versus contralateral extinction in dichotic listening resulting from hemisphere lesions. *Cortex* 6:249–260, 1970.

Sperling, G. The information available in brief visual presentations. *Psychol. Monogr.* 74:1–29, 1960.

Sperry, R. Some effects of disconnecting the cerebral hemispheres. *Science* 217:1223–1226, 1982.

Sperry, R. W. Lateral specialization in the surgically separated hemispheres. In *The Neurosciences: Third Study Program,* edited by F. O. Schmitt and F. G. Worden. Cambridge, MA: MIT Press, 1974, pp. 5–19.

Sperry, R. W., Gazzaniga, M. S., and Bogen, J. E. Interhemispheric relationships: The neocortical commissures; syndromes of hemisphere disconnection. In *Handbook of Clinical Neurology,* edited by P. J. Vinken and G. W. Bruyn. Amsterdam: North-Holland, 1969, pp. 273–290.

Spitzer, H., and Richmond, B. J. Task difficulty: Ignoring, attending to, and discriminating a visual stimulus yield progressively more activity in inferior temporal neurons. *Exp. Brain Res.* 83:340–348, 1991.

Spong, P., Haider, M., and Lindsley, D. B. Selective attentiveness and cortical evoked responses to visual and auditory stimuli. *Science* 148:395–397, 1965.

Sporns, O., Gally, J. A., Reeke, G. N., and Edelman, G. M. Reentrant signaling among simulated neuronal groups leads to coherency in their oscillatory activity. *Proc. Natl. Acad. Sci. U.S.A.* 86:7265–7269, 1989.

Squire, L. R. Mechanisms of memory. *Science* 232:1612–1619, 1986.

Squire, L. R. *Memory and Brain.* New York: Oxford University Press, 1987.

Squire, L. R., and Zola-Morgan, S. Memory: Brain systems and behavior. *Trends Neurosci.* 11:170–175, 1988.

Staubli, U., Fraser, D., Kessler, M., and Lynch, G. Studies on retrograde and anterograde amnesia of olfactory memory after denervation of the hippocampus by entorhinal cortex lesions. *Behav. Neural Biol.* 46:432–444, 1986.

Staubli, U., Kessler, M., and Lynch, G. Aniracetam has proportionately smaller effects on synapses expressing long-term potentiation: Evidence that receptor changes subserve LTP. *Psychobiology* 18:377–381, 1990.

Stein, B. E., and Meredith, M.A. *The Merging of the Senses.* Cambridge, MA: MIT Press, 1993.

Steinmetz, J. E., Lavond, D. G., Ivkovich, D., Logan, C. G., and Thompson, R. F. Disruption of classical eyelid conditioning after cerebellar lesions: Damage to a memory trace system or a simple performance deficit? *J. Neurosci.* 12:4403–4426, 1992.

Stent, G. S. A physiological mechanism for Hebb's postulate of learning. *Proc. Natl. Acad. Sci. U.S.A.* 70:997–1001, 1973.

Steriade, M., McCormick, D. A., and Sejnowski, T.J. Thalamocortical oscillations in the sleeping and aroused brain. *Science* 262:679–685, 1993.

Sterman, M. B., and Fairchild, M. D. Modification of locomotor performance by reticular formation and basal forebrain stimulation in the cat: Evidence for reciprocal systems. *Brain Res.* 2:205–217, 1966.

Stroessner-Johnson, H. M., Rapp, P. R., and Amaral, D. G. Cholinergic cell loss and hypertrophy in the medial septal nucleus of the behaviorally characterized aged rhesus monkey. *J. Neurosci.* 12:1936–1944, 1992.

Stryker, M. P. Temporal associations. *Nature* 354:108–109, 1991.

Stuss, D. T., and Benson, D. F. *The Frontal Lobes.* New York: Raven Press, 1986.

Sur, M., Pallas, S. L., and Roe, A. W. Cross-modal plasticity in cortical development: Differentiation and specification of sensory neocortex. *Trends Neurosci.* 13:227–233, 1990.

Suzuki, H., and Azuma, M. Prefrontal neuronal activity during gazing at a light spot in the monkey. *Brain Res.* 126:497–508, 1977.

Swanson, L. W., Teyler, T. J., and Thompson, R. F. Hippocampal long-term potentiation: Mechanisms and implications for memory. *Neurosci. Res. Program Bull.* 20:613–764, 1982.

Swartz, B. E., Halgren, E., Fuster, J. M., Simpkins, F., Gee, M., and Mandelkern, M. Cortical metabolic activation in humans during a visual memory task. *Cerebral Cortex,* 1994 (in press).

Szentágothai, J. The neuron network of the cerebral cortex: A functional interpretation. *Proc. R. Soc. Lond. [Biol.]* 201:219–248, 1978a.

Szentágothai, J. Specificity versus (quasi-)randomness in cortical connectivity. In *Architectonics of the Cerebral Cortex,* edited by M. A. B. Brazier and H. Petsche. New York: Raven Press, 1978b, pp. 77–117.

Szentágothai, J. The modular architectonic principle of neural centers. *Rev. Physiol. Biochem. Pharmacol.* 98:11–61, 1983.

Tanabe, T., Yarita, H., Iino, M., Ooshima, Y., and Takagi, S. F. An olfactory area in the prefrontal lobe. *Brain Res.* 80:127–130, 1974.

Tanabe, T., Iino, M., and Takagi, S. F. Discrimination of odors in olfactory bulb, pyriform-amygdaloid areas, and orbitofrontal cortex of the monkey. *J. Neurophysiol.* 38:1284–1296, 1975a.

Tanabe, T., Yarita, H., Iino, M., Ooshima, Y., and Takagi, S. F. An olfactory projection area in orbitofrontal cortex of the monkey. *J. Neurophysiol.* 38:1269–1283, 1975b.

Tanaka, K. Neuronal mechanisms of object recognition. *Science* 262:685–688, 1993.

Tanila, H., Carlson, S., Linnankoski, I., Lindroos, F., and Kahila, H. Functional properties of dorsolateral prefrontal cortical neurons in awake monkey. *Behav. Brain Res.* 47:169–180, 1992.

Tanji, J., and Kurata, K. Comparison of movement-related activity in two cortical motor areas of primates. *J. Neurophysiol.* 48:633–653, 1982.

Tanji, J., and Kurata, K. Contrasting neuronal activity in supplementary and precentral motor cortex of monkeys: I. Responses to instructions determining motor responses to forthcoming signals of different modalities. *J. Neurophysiol.* 53:129–141, 1985.

Tanji, J., and Kurata, K. Changing concepts of motor areas of the cerebral cortex. *Brain Dev.* 11:374–377, 1989.

Tanji, J., Taniguchi, K., and Saga, T. Supplementary motor area: Neuronal response to motor instructions. *J. Neurophysiol.* 43:60–68, 1980.

Tanzi, E. I fatti e le induzioni nell'odierna istologia del sistema nervoso. *Riv. Sper. Freniatr. Med. Leg. Alienazioni Ment.* 19:419–472, 1893.

Terry, R. D., Deteresa, R., and Hansen, L. A. Neocortical cell counts in normal human adult aging. *Ann. Neurol.* 21:530–539, 1987.

Terzian, H., and Dalle Ore, G. Su di un caso di ablazione bilaterale dei lobi temporali realizzante nell'uomo la sindrome di Klüver e Bucy. *Chirurgia* 9:249–255, 1954.

Teuber, H.-L. Unity and diversity of frontal lobe functions. *Acta Neurobiol. Exp.* (Warsz.) 32:625–656, 1972.

Teyler, T. J., Perkins, A. T., and Harris, K. M. The development of long-term potentiation in hippocampus and neocortex. *Neuropsychologia* 27:31–39, 1989.

Thach, W. T. Correlation of neural discharge with pattern and force of muscular activity, joint position, and direction of intended next movement in motor cortex and cerebellum. *J. Neurophysiol.* 41:654–676, 1978.

Thaler, D. E., Rolls, E. T., and Passingham, R. E. Neuronal activity of the supplementary motor area (SMA) during internally and externally triggered wrist movements. *Neurosci. Lett.* 93:264–269, 1988.

Thompson, R. F. The neurobiology of learning and memory. *Science* 233:941–947, 1986.

Thomson, A. M., West, D. C., and Lodge, D. An N-methylaspartate receptor-mediated synapse in rat cerebral cortex: A site of action of ketamine? *Nature* 313:479–481, 1985.

Thorpe, S. J., Rolls, E. T., and Maddison, S. The orbitofrontal cortex: Neuronal activity in the behaving monkey. *Exp. Brain Res.* 49:93–115, 1983.

Tiitinen, H., Sinkkonen, J., Reinikainen, K., Alho, K., Lavikainen, J., and Näätänen, R. Selective attention enhances the auditory 40-Hz transient response in humans. *Nature* 364:59–60, 1993.

Tinbergen, N. *The Study of Instinct.* Oxford: Oxford University Press, 1951.

Toledo-Morrell, L., Morrell, F., and Fleming, S. Age-dependent deficits in spatial memory are related to impaired hippocampal kindling. *Behav. Neurosci.* 98:902–907, 1984.

Tononi, G., Sporns, O., and Edelman, G.M. Reentry and the problem of integrating multiple cortical areas: Simulation of dynamic integration in the visual system. *Cerebral Cortex* 2:310–335, 1992.

Tranel, D., Damasio, A. R., and Damasio, H. Intact recognition of facial expression, gender, and age in patients with impaired recognition of face identity. *Neurology* 38:690–696, 1988.

Treisman, A., and Geffen, G. Selective attention: Perception or response? *Q. J. Exp. Psychol.* 19:1–17, 1967.

Treisman, A., and Gormican, S. Feature analysis in early vision: Evidence from search asymmetries. *Psychol. Rev.* 95:15–48, 1988.

Treisman, A. M. Contextual cues in selective listening. *Q. J. Exp. Psychol.* 12:242–248, 1960.

Treisman, A. M. Selective attention in man. *Br. Med. Bull.* 20:12–16, 1964.

Tulving, E. *Elements of Episodic Memory.* Oxford: Clarendon Press, 1983.

Tulving, E. Multiple memory systems and consciousness. *Hum. Neurobiol.* 6:67–80, 1987.

Tulving, E., and Schacter, D.L. Priming and human memory systems. *Science* 247:301–306, 1990.

Tulving, E., Schacter, D. L., and Stark, H. A. Priming effects in word-fragment completion are independent of recognition memory. *J. Exp. Psychol. [Learn. Mem. Cogn.]* 8:336–342, 1982.

Turner, B. H., Mishkin, M., and Knapp, M. Organization of the amygdalopetal projections from modality-specific cortical association areas in the monkey. *J. Comp. Neurol.* 191:515–543, 1980.

Uemura, E. Age-related changes in prefrontal cortex of *Macaca mulatta*: Synaptic density. *Exp. Neurol.* 69:164–172, 1980.

Uemura, E., and Hartmann, H. A. RNA content and volume of nerve cell bodies in human brain: I. Prefrontal cortex in aging normal and demented patients. *J. Neuropathol. Exp. Neurol.* 37:487–496, 1978.

Ungerleider, L. G. The corticocortical pathways for object recognition and spatial perception. In *Pattern Recognition Mechanisms,* edited by C. Chagas, R. Gattass and C. G. Gross. Vatican City: Pontifical Academy of Sciences, 1985, pp. 21–37.

Ungerleider, L. G., and Mishkin, M. Two cortical visual systems. In *Analysis of Visual Behavior,* edited by D. J. Ingle, M. A. Goodale and R. J. W. Mansfield. Cambridge, MA: MIT Press, 1982, pp. 549–586.

Valverde, F. Rate and extent of recovery from dark rearing in the visual cortex of the mouse. *Brain Res.* 33:1–11, 1971.

Van der Loos, H., and Woolsey, T. Somatosensory cortex: Structural alterations following early injury to sense organs. *Science* 179:395–398, 1973.

Van Essen, D. C. Functional organization of primate visual cortex. In *Cerebral Cortex,* vol. 3, edited by A. Peters and E. G. Jones. New York, Plenum, 1985, pp. 259–329.

Van Essen, D. C., and Maunsell, J. H. R. Hierarchical organization and functional streams in the visual cortex. *Trends Neurosci.* 6:370–375, 1983.

Van Hoesen, G. W. The differential distribution, diversity and sprouting of cortical projections to the amygdala in the rhesus monkey. In *The Amygdaloid Complex,* edited by Y. Ben-Ari. Amsterdam: Elsevier/North-Holland Biomedical, 1981, pp. 77–90.

Van Hoesen, G. W. The parahippocampal gyrus. *Trends Neurosci.* 5:345–350, 1982.

Villa, A. E. P., and Fuster, J. M. Temporal correlates of information processing during visual short-term memory. *NeuroReport* 3:113–116, 1992.

Villa, G., Gainotti, G., De Bonis, C., and Marra, C. Double dissociation between temporal and spatial pattern processing in patients with frontal and parietal damage. *Cortex* 26:399–407, 1990.

Vogt, C., and Vogt, O. Allgemeine Ergebnisse unserer Hirnforschung. *J. Psychol. Neurol.* 25:279–462, 1919.

Von der Malsburg, C. Nervous structures with dynamical links. *Berl. Bunsenges. Phys. Chem.* 89:703–710, 1985.

Wall, J. T. Variable organization in cortical maps of the skin as an indication of the lifelong adaptive capacities of circuits in the mammalian brain. *Trends Neurosci.* 11:549–557, 1988.

Walsh, K. W. *Neuropsychology.* Edinburgh: Churchill Livingstone, 1978.

Walter, W. G., Cooper, R., Aldrige, V. J., McCallum, W. C., and Winter, A. L. Contingent negative variation: An electric sign of sensori-motor association and expectancy in the human brain. *Nature* 203:380–384, 1964.

Walters, E. T., and Byrne, J. H. Associative conditioning of single sensory neurons suggests a cellular mechanism for learning. *Science* 219:405–408, 1983.

Warrington, E. K., and Duchen, L. W. A re-appraisal of a case of persistent global amnesia following right temporal lobectomy: A clinico-pathological study. *Neuropsychologia* 30:437–450, 1992.

Warrington, E. K., and McCarthy, R. A. Categories of knowledge: Further fractionations and an attempted integration. *Brain* 110:1273–1296, 1987.

Watanabe, M. Prefrontal unit activity during delayed conditional go/no-go discrimination in the monkey: I. Relation to the stimulus. *Brain Res.* 382:1–14, 1986a.

Watanabe, M. Prefrontal unit activity during delayed conditional go/no-go discrimination in the monkey: II. Relation to go and no-go responses. *Brain Res.* 382:15–27, 1986b.

Watanabe, M. Frontal units of the monkey coding the associative significance of visual and auditory stimuli. *Exp. Brain Res.* 89:233–247, 1992.

Webster, J. C., and Thompson, P. O. Responding to both of two overlapping messages. *J. Acoust. Soc. Am.* 26:396–402, 1954.

Weinrich, M., and Wise, S. P. The premotor cortex of the monkey. *J. Neurosci.* 2:1329–1345, 1982.

Weizsäcker, V. von. *Der Gestaltkreis.* Stuttgart: Thieme, 1950.

Werbos, P. J. *Beyond regression: New tools for prediction and analysis in the behavioral sciences.* Unpublished doctoral dissertation, Harvard University, 1974.

Westbrook, G. L., and Jahr, C. E. Glutamate receptors in excitatory neurotransmission. *Semin. Neurosci.* 1:103–114, 1989.

White, G., Levy, W. B., and Steward, O. Spatial overlap between populations of synapses determines the extent of their associative interaction during the induction of long-term potentiation and depression. *J. Neurophysiol.* 64:1186–1198, 1990.

Whitehouse, P. J., Price, D. L., Struble, R. G., Clark, A. W., Coyle, J. T., and Delong, M. R. Alzheimer's disease and senile dementia: Loss of neurons in the basal forebrain. *Science* 215:1237–1239, 1982.

Whiteley, A. M., and Warrington, E. K. Prosopagnosia: A clinical, psychological, and anatomical study of three patients. *J. Neurol. Neurosurg. Psychiatry* 40:394–430, 1977.

Whitsel, B. L., Dreyer, D. A., and Roppolo, J. R. Determinants of body representation in postcentral gyrus of macaques. *J. Neurophysiol.* 34:1018–1034, 1971.

Wickelgren, W. A. The long and the short of memory. In *Short-Term Memory,* edited by D. Deutsch and J. A. Deutsch. New York: Academic, 1975, pp. 41–63.

Wiesel, T. N. Postnatal development of the visual cortex and the influence of environment. *Nature* 299:583–591, 1982.

Wiesel, T. N., and Hubel, D. H. Comparison of the effects of unilateral and bilateral eye closure and cortical unit responses in kittens. *J. Neurophysiol.* 28:1029–1040, 1965.

Wiesendanger, M. Organization of secondary motor areas of cerebral cortex. In *Handbook of Physiology,* edited by S. R. Geiger. Bethesda, MD: American Physiological Society, 1981, pp. 1121–1147.

Wigstrom, H., and Gustafsson, B. Facilitation of hippocampal long-lasting potentiation by GABA antagonists. *Acta Physiol. Scand.* 125:159–172, 1985.

Wilkins, A. J., Shallice, T., and McCarthy, R. Frontal lesions and sustained attention. *Neuropsychologia* 25:359–365, 1987.

Willshaw, D. Holography, associative memory, and inductive generalization. In *Parallel Models of Associative Memory,* edited by G. E. Hinton and J. A. Anderson. Hillsdale, NJ: Erlbaum, 1981, pp. 83–104.

Wilson, D. A., Sullivan, R. M., and Leon, M. Single-unit analysis of postnatal olfactory learning: Modified olfactory bulb output response patterns to learned attractive odors. *J. Neurosci.* 7:3154–3162, 1987.

Wilson, M., Stamm, J. S., and Pribram, K. H. Deficits in roughness discrimination after posterior parietal lesions in monkeys. *J. Comp. Physiol. Psychol.* 53:535–539, 1960.

Wise, S. P., and Jones, E. G. The organization and postnatal development of the commissural projection of the rat somatic sensory cortex. *J. Comp. Neurol.* 168:313–344, 1976.

Wise, S. P., and Mauritz, K.-H. Set-related neuronal activity in the premotor cortex of rhesus monkeys: Effects of changes in motor set. *Proc. R. Soc. Lond. [Biol.]* 223:331–354, 1985.

Withers, G. S., and Greenough, W. T. Reach training selectively alters dendritic branching in subpopulations of layer II–III pyramids in rat motor-somatosensory forelimb cortex. *Neuropsychologia* 27:61–69, 1989.

Woodruff-Pak, D. S., Conway, L. P., and Li, Y.-T. Nefiracetam (DM-9384): An effective cognition-enhancing agent in NM classical conditioning in older rabbits. *Soc. Neurosci. Abstr.* 19:1234, 1993.

Woody, C. D. *Memory, Learning, and Higher Function.* New York: Springer, 1982.

Worden, F. G., and Marsh, J. T. Amplitude changes of auditory potentials evoked at cochlear nucleus during acoustic habituation. *Electroencephalogr. Clin. Neurophysiol.* 15:866–881, 1963.

Yajeya, J., Quintana, J., and Fuster, J. M. Prefrontal representation of stimulus attributes during delay tasks: II. The role of behavioral significance. *Brain Res.* 474:222–230, 1988.

Yakovlev, P. I., and Lecours, A. R. The myelogenetic cycles of regional maturation of the brain. In *Regional Development of the Brain in Early Life,* edited by A. Minkowski. Oxford: Blackwell, 1967, pp. 3–70.

Yamatani, K., Ono, T., Nishijo, H., and Takaku, A. Activity and distribution of learning-related neurons in monkey (*Macaca fuscata*) prefrontal cortex. *Behav. Neurosci.* 104:503–531, 1990.

Yaxley, S., Rolls, E. T., and Sienkiewicz, Z. J. Gustatory responses of single neurons in the insula of the macaque monkey. *J. Neurophysiol.* 63:689–700, 1990.

Young, M. P., and Yamane, S. Sparse population coding of faces in the inferotemporal cortex. *Science* 256:1327–1331, 1992.

Zatorre, R. J., and Jones-Gotman, M. Human olfactory discrimination after unilateral frontal or temporal lobectomy. *Brain* 114:71–84, 1991.

Zatorre, R. J., Jones-Gotman, M., Evans, A. C., and Meyer, E. Functional localization and lateralization of human olfactory cortex. *Nature* 360:339–340, 1992.

Zatorre, R. J., and Samson, S. Role of the right temporal neocortex in retention of pitch in auditory short-term memory. *Brain* 114:2403–2417, 1991.

Zhou, Y., and Fuster, J. M. Unit discharge in monkey's parietal cortex during perception and mnemonic retention of tactile features. *Soc. Neurosci. Abstr.* 18:706, 1992.

Zipser, D. Identification models of the nervous system. *Neuroscience* 47:853–862, 1992.

Zipser, D., Kehoe, B., Littlewort, G., and Fuster, J. A spiking network model of short-term active memory. *J. Neurosci.* 13:3406–3420, 1993.

Zola-Morgan, S., and Squire, L. R. Preserved learning in monkeys with medial temporal lesions: Sparing of motor and cognitive skills. *J. Neurosci.* 4:1072–1085, 1984.

Zola-Morgan, S., and Squire, L. R. Medial temporal lesions in monkeys impair memory on a variety of tasks sensitive to human amnesia. *Behav. Neurosci.* 99:22–34, 1985.

Zola-Morgan, S., and Squire, L. R. The primate hippocampal formation: Evidence for a time-limited role in memory storage. *Science* 250:288–290, 1990.

Zola-Morgan, S., and Squire, L. R. Neuroanatomy of memory. *Annu. Rev. Neurosci.* 16:547–563, 1993.

Zola-Morgan, S., Squire, L. R., Amaral, D. G., and Suzuki, W. A. Lesions of perirhinal and parahippocampal cortex that spare the amygdala and hippocampal formation produce severe memory impairment. *J. Neurosci.* 9:4355–4370, 1989.

Zola-Morgan, S., Squire, L. R., Alvarez-Royo, P., and Clower, R. P. Independence of memory functions and emotional behavior: Separate contributions of the hippocampal formation and the amygdala. *Hippocampus* 1:181–194, 1991.

Index

Aphasia. *See also* Language; Speech
  Broca's, 192
  disconnection, 279
  prefrontal, 193–194, 280–281
  premotor, 193
  semantic, 141–142, 278
Architecture of the cortex, 47–52
  cytoarchitectonic maps, 60, 62
Arousal, 219, 284. *See also* Alertness
  neurotransmitter systems in, 219
  reticular formation in, 219
Artificial intelligence, 86
Association, essence of memory, 2, 4, 10–
  11, 90, 199
Associative memory, 2, 11, 85
Astereognosia, 129. *See also* Stereognosis
Attention, 217–235
  amygdala in, 222
  categorization, 217–218, 224, 227
  definition, 217–218
  evoked potentials in, 219, 221, 226
  filter theory, 225
  focus, 107, 156, 218, 225, 291–293
  frontal cortex in, 233 (*see also* Frontal cor-
    tex, in motor set)
  hippocampus in, 222
  inhibition in, 225–226
  interaction with memory, 198, 217
  IT neurons in, 226–230
  mechanisms, 217–235
  modulation of cortical neurons, 227
  motor, 218, 232–236, 272, 294 (*see also*
    Motor set)
  network activation, 224–225
  neurotransmitters in, 216
  parallel processing, 225, 230, 289–292
  parietal neurons in, 227
  perceptual vs. motor, 232–233
  prefrontal neurons in, 227
  qualitative, 224, 227–232
  reticular activating system in, 219–221
  selective, 14, 217–218, 224–236, 289 (*see
    also* Attention, focus)
  serial processing, 230, 289, 291–292
  shift from parallel to serial processing,
    291
  short-term memory buffer, 225
  spatial, 129–131, 137, 224, 226–227, 230,
    232
  spotlight theory, 226–227
  tactile, 230, 232, 251
  transfer from perceptual to motor, 235,
    271–272

unconscious processing, 225
  visual, 129–131, 226–231
Attractors, fixed point, 257, 259–260
Auditory agnosia, 140–142
Auditory cortex, 140
  reorganization, 57
  stimulation, 145
Auditory discrimination, 57, 147
Auditory memory, 139–149
  deficits from temporal lesions, 142, 147
  prefrontal cooling on, 241
Auditory short-term memory, 142
Autoradiography, 252
Autotopagnosia, 129

Backpropagation, 91–92, 254, 257, 272
Basal ganglia, 3, 166–167. *See also* Striatum
  in automatic acts and habits, 167
Behavior. *See also* Motor behavior; Percep-
  tion-action cycle; Temporal organization
  of behavior
  classifying and selectivity in, 169
  temporal structure, 225, 238
Bereitschaftspotential, 183, 273, 295
Binding, perceptual, 102, 120, 293
Bird song, 55
Blindsight, 113
Braitenberg's model, 104–105
Broca's aphasia 192. *See also* Speech
Broca's area, 145, 192, 280
  imaging, 192

Caffeine, 44
Callosal connections, 64, 80
Categorical memory, 97, 99, 158. *See also*
  Semantic memory
  auditory, 146
  retrieval, 103
  visual, 120
  widespread distribution, 128
Categorization, 90, 95, 97, 99, 127, 155–
  156, 159, 218
  attention, 217–218, 224, 227
  language, 278
  motor, 169, 184, 218, 232–233, 294
  perception, 102–103, 114, 218
  speech, 191
  visual, 117, 127–128, 230
Caudate, 166. *See also* Basal ganglia;
  Striatum
Central motor aphasia, 194
Cerebellum, 3, 106, 163–165
  conditioning of eye-blink reflex, 163

cortex, 63–164
  in motor coordination, 163–164
  in motor memory, 163
  nucleus interpositus, 163
  plasticity, 55
  synaptic facilitation in, 163
Chemical enhancement of memory. *See*
  Enhancement of memory, chemical
Cholinergic system, 40–41, 45, 214–216
  in Alzheimer's disease, 41, 45, 215–216
  in REM sleep, 286
  involution in aging, 214–215
Chomsky's universality of grammar, 192
CNV, 183, 221–222, 273
  fatigue and, 221–222
Coding
  ensemble, 187
  frequency, 101
Cognitive neuroscience, 85
Coincidence detectors, 101
Color anomia, 144
Columns, cortical, 49, 92
  interdigitation, 73
  ocular dominance, 53
Command neurons, 135, 137
Competition of inputs, 53, 57–59
Computational models, 6, 34, 85–86, 90–
  94, 99, 153–156, 247, 254–261, 272
Conceptual memory, 98, 158, 160. *See also*
  Semantic memory
Concussion amnesia, 284
  recovery, 285
Conditional association, 183
Conditioned reflexes, 163
Conditioning. *See also* Learning
  classical, 3, 11, 21, 163
  defensive reflexes, 163
  instrumental, 11
  invertebrate, 25
  motor neurons, 59, 163
  synchronous convergence in, 163
Congenital cataracts, 52
Connectionism, 83, 85, 101
Connections. *See also* Corticocortical
  connections
  afferent to cortex from cortex, 47–51
  afferent to cortex from thalamus, 47–51
  between amygdala and association cor-
    tex, 222
  between hippocampus and midtemporal
    cortex, 38
  between limbic structures and associa-
    tion cortex, 37–38, 222

between posterior parietal and frontal
  cortex, 71, 73–75
between prefrontal and premotor cortex,
  77
between sensory association and frontal
  cortex, 71, 73–75, 263–264, 267
convergent, 33, 63
development, 213 (*see also* Critical developmental periods; Myelination; Ontogenetic gradients)
divergent, 33, 63
individual variability, 81
Consciousness, 13, 283–296
  as active memory, 294
  40-cycle oscillations, 293
  memory dynamics, 288–294
  stream of, 107, 293
Consolidation of memory, 15, 100. *See also*
  Network(s), growth
  hippocampus in, 36–44
  interference with, 36
  limbic system in, 36–40
  neurotransmitters in, 40–44
  REM sleep, 285
Consolidation period, 36
Constancy
  motor, 170
  perceptual, 119, 155
Contingent negative variation. *See* CNV
Co-occurrence. *See* Temporal coincidence
Cooling, 109–110, 239
  IT cortex, 239–240, 267–268
  prefrontal cortex, 241–244, 267–270
Cooperativity principle, 29
Corollary discharge, 149, 276–277, 279
Corpus callosum, 64, 80
Correlation of potentials
  in attention, 293
  in perception, 100–102, 293
  in retrieval, 201–204
Cortex (cerebral)
  architectural uniformity, 5, 47
  architecture, 47–52
  area 4, 59, 97
  area 5, 69, 132–136, 148
  area 6, 78, 182
  area 7, 69, 130, 132–134, 137
  area 8, 181, 277
  area 9, 37, 78, 265
  area 10, 265
  area 19, 37, 57, 69, 132–133
  area 20, 37, 69, 132–133, 148
  area 21, 37, 115

Cortex (cerebral) (cont.)
  area 35, 39, 57, 69, 132–133
  area 36, 39
  area 44, 192
  area 45, 192
  area 46, 37, 59, 78, 265
  area FB, 182
  area FD, 172, 177
  area Ig, 69–70
  area MI, 77, 187–188, 192
  area MII, 182
  area PEm, 136
  area PG, 126, 130, 147
  area SI, 69, 132, 250
  area SII, 69–70, 132
  area STP, 147
  area TE, 67, 115
  area TPO, 120, 147
  area Tpt, 147
  area V1, 67, 249–250
  area V2, 67
  area V3, 67
  area V4, 67, 226
  association, 6, 11, 38, 64, 95
  auditory, 57, 140
  connective heterogeneity, 5, 47, 50
  cytoarchitectonic maps, 60, 62
  entorhinal, 38–39, 71, 153
  evolution, 67, 174
  frontal (*see* Frontal cortex)
  hierarchical organization, 20, 60–80
  horizontal fiber arrays, 48
  inferotemporal (*see* Inferotemporal cortex)
  LTP in, 30, 59
  maturation, 64 (*see also* Development; Myelination; Ontogenetic gradients)
  modular organization, 37, 49, 128
  motor (*see* Motor cortex)
  NMDA, 44
  olfactory, 76, 152
  orbitofrontal, 76, 150–152
  parahippocampal (*see* Parahippocampal cortex)
  paralimbic, 71, 76
  parietal (*see* Parietal cortex)
  perirhinal, 38–39
  piriform, 152
  plasticity (*see* Plasticity)
  polymodal (*see* Polymodal cortex)
  posterior parietal (*see* Posterior parietal cortex)
  prefrontal (*see* Prefrontal cortex)
  prepiriform, 77
  supragranular layers, 48, 64, 268
  temporal (*see* Temporal cortex)
  vertical fiber arrays, 48–49
  visual (*see* Visual cortex)
Cortical ablation, limitations, 109, 192, 239. *See also* Reversible cortical lesion, cooling
Cortical deafness, 140
Cortical maps (cytoarchitectonic), 60, 62
Cortical motor representation, 173–195. *See also* Motor memory
Corticocortical connections, 47–50, 71–73, 263–264
  reciprocity, 62, 68, 77, 79–80, 133, 260, 276
  supragranular origin and termination, 50, 62, 215, 268
  topological order, 71, 77
Corticothalamic circuits in sleep, 286
Creativity, 174–176
Crick's searchlight hypothesis of attention, 226–227
Critical developmental periods, 52–55
Cross-modal interaction, 148–149, 152–153, 205–209, 250
Cross-temporal contingency, 174, 176, 235, 246, 263, 267
  prefrontal cortex in, 79, 174, 176, 263
  in speech, 281
Cross-temporal integration, 14
C-threshold, 292, 294

Damasio's model, 103
Declarative memory, 3, 16–20, 160, 291. *See also* Episodic memory; Explicit memory; Perceptual memory; Nondeclarative memory; Semantic memory
  in neocortex, 19
  and perceptual memory, 20
  vs. nondeclarative memory, 16–20
Decussation (crossover) of fibers, 80
Defensive reflexes, 163
Déjà vu, 293
Delay activation (of discharge), 243, 245–246, 271. *See also* Memory cells
Delay inhibition (of discharge), 245
Delay tasks, 110, 136, 147, 172, 189, 238–251, 264–273. *See also* Delayed matching to sample; Delayed nonmatching to sample; Delayed response; Delayed tone-matching

cross-temporal contingency, 263
deficits from hippocampal lesions, 19,
  38–40
deficits from prefrontal lesions, 176, 189–
  190
memory cells, 177, 243, 244–261
procedural memory in, 172
properties, 189
short-term memory in, 172
temporal structure, 238
working memory tests, 238
Delayed matching to sample, 121, 125,
  201, 239, 241, 247, 265
haptic, 242–243, 250–251
Delayed nonmatching to sample, 19, 39
Delayed response, 239–241, 245
Delayed tone-matching, 147
Dendrites
apical, 48
basal, 48
branching in enriched environment, 56
bundles, 48
involution in aging, 215
Development. *See also* Critical developmental periods; Myelination; Ontogenetic gradients; Synaptogenesis
of cortical connectivity, 213
of memory, 212–213
Dichotic listening, 142
Disconnection aphasia, 279
Disconnection syndromes, 142, 144, 279
Discrimination, 106, 114, 132, 155–156,
  198, 225
auditory, 57, 147
gustatory, 150
olfactory, 152
tactile, 132
visual, 115–116, 240
Dopamine, 41
Dopamine receptors, 181
Dorsolateral prefrontal cortex, 172. *See also*
  Prefrontal cortex; Sulcus principalis
in short-term memory, 174, 263, 280–281
in short-term motor set, 174, 263, 280–281
Dorsolateral prefrontal lesion, recovery
  from, 172
Dreams, 284–288
archetypal, 287
40-cycle oscillations, 286
memory in, 286–288
movement in, 287–288
phyletic memory in, 287
psychoanalytic theory, 286

recall, 288
in REM sleep, 286
smell in, 287
sound in, 287
taste in, 287
timelessness, 287
vision in, 287–288

Edelman's group selection theory and
  model, 56, 90–91
neural darwinism, 33, 91, 93
Efferent copy, 106, 149, 276. *See also*
  Corollary discharge
Electroconvulsive shock, 36
Electroshock amnesia, 285
Emotion and memory, 39–40, 159, 212
Endocranial casts, 67
Engram, 15, 170, 177. *See also* Network(s)
Enhancement of memory, chemical, 44–46
amphetamine, 45
monoaminergic agonists, 45
nootropics, 45–46
physostigmine, 45
picrotoxin, 44
strychnine, 44
Ensemble code, 187
Entorhinal cortex, 38–39, 71, 153
Episodic memory, 17. *See also* Declarative
  memory
Ethology of motor behavior, 54–55
Evoked potentials
in attention, 219, 221, 226
coherence in retrieval, 201–204
in discrimination, 201
fatigue and, 221–223
Evolution. *See also* Phyletic memory
cortex, 67, 174
memory systems, 10, 32, 52
Explicit memory, 17. *See also* Declarative
  memory
Eye-blink reflex, 163

Face cells, 118–120
Fatigue, 221–223
Filter theory of attention, 225. *See also*
  Inhibition
Fixed point attractors, 257, 259–260
Flavor, 153
Focus of attention, 107, 156, 218, 225,
  291–293. *See also* Attention, selective
Focus of representation, 5, 18, 107, 225,
  237, 247, 253, 293–294. *See also* Atten-
  tion, focus

Motor memory (cont.)
unconscious retrieval and processing, 288–290
vs. perceptual memory, 3–4, 20–22
Motor neurons
conditioning, 59, 163
in motor set, 272
in movement execution, 186
Motor programs, 162, 169–173. *See also* Motor schemata; Planning
vs. computer programs, 170
instinctual, 165
novel, in prefrontal cortex, 189
Motor schemata, 106, 165, 168, 263; *See also* Motor programs
Motor set, 204, 218, 232–233, 294–295. *See also* Motor attention
frontal cortex in, 78–79, 177–195, 181, 232–235, 270–274, 277
frontal eye field in, 277
motor cortex in, 272
preattentive, 295
prefrontal cortex in, 174–181, 234–236, 263–266, 270–274
premotor cortex in, 79, 182–183, 265–266, 272
speech, 280
in volition, 294
Motor skills, 21. *See also* Procedural memory
Mountcastle's columnar concepts, 254
Movement. *See also* Motor behavior
automatic, 167, 172, 183, 189, 263, 276
multiple neural representations, 171
templates, 54
unlearned, 54–55
voluntary, 172–173, 189, 274, 294–296
Musical memory, 141–142
Myelination, 64, 66–67. *See also* Ontogenetic gradients

Neglect from parietal lesions, 129
Network(s). *See also* Network activation
conceptual, 98
cooperation, 242, 246, 266–270
dynamics 99–107
growth, 87–96
language, 278–281
local, 254
memory, 2, 11–12, 14–15, 35–38, 83–111, 237
motor, 97, 106–107, 266–274 (*see also* Motor cortical hierarchy)

nodes 97, 101
perceptual, 97, 266–270 (*see also* Sensory cortical hierarchies)
properties, 96–107
shape, 98
size, 98
spontaneous activity, 99
structure, 96–99
turning on itself, 99, 106, 225, 293
Network activation. *See also* Active memory; Attention; Network(s); Retrieval
in active memory, 16, 36–37, 99, 104, 247–270, 293
in attention, 224–225
in behavior, 224–225, 233
C-threshold, 292, 294
LSD, 287
in memory acquisition, 105–106
in perception, 100–105
P-threshold, 292
in retrieval, 204–211, 224–225, 291
in short-term memory, 15–16, 36, 99, 104–105
threshold, 104, 238, 270
in working memory, 104
Neural memory. *See also* Memory
robustness, 86
special aspects of, 9
Neuroscience of networks
aware and behaving animals in, 109
computer modeling in, 111
connectivity studies in, 109
cortical lesions in, 109
delay tasks in, 110
discrimination behavior in, 110
functional brain imaging in, 111
microelectrode methods in, 110
molecular neurobiology in, 108
reversible cortical lesions (e.g., cooling) in, 109
Neurotransmitter receptors. *See also* Dopamine receptors; Glutamate receptors; Neurotransmitters; NMDA receptors
development, 52, 66
involution, 215
Neurotransmitters. *See also* Neurotransmitter receptors
acetylcholine, 41 (*see also* Cholinergic system)
in aging, 215
AMPA, 43
in arousal, 219
dopamine, 41

Perception
  categorization, 87–88, 102–103, 114, 218
  interaction with memory, 89, 113
  network activation, 100–105
Perception-action cycle, 106, 137, 208, 225,
    233, 246–247, 250, 274–281, 296. *See also*
    Temporal organization of behavior; Mo-
    tor behavior
  corollary discharge, 276
  definition, 274
  haptic, 276
  neuroanatomy, 275
  neurobiology of behavior, 276
  prefrontal cortex in, 276–277
  spoken language, 277–281
Perceptual attention, vs. motor, 232–233
Perceptual binding, 102, 120, 293
Perceptual constancy, 119, 155
Perceptual memory, 2–3, 20–23, 88, 113–
    114, 160. *See also* Auditory memory;
    Conceptual memory; Declarative mem-
    ory; Episodic memory; Explicit memory;
    Gustatory memory; Olfactory memory;
    Polymodal memory; Semantic memory;
    Tactile memory; Visual memory
  activation, 247–266, 271
  and declarative memory, 20
  definition, 21
  hierarchical organization, 88, 156–160
  vs. motor memory, 3–4, 20–22
  phyletic, 21
  polymodal, 156–160
  in posterior cortex, 3, 20, 22
Perceptual representational system (PRS),
    21
Perirhinal cortex, 38–39
PET, 152, 173, 209, 230, 264–266. *See also*
    Imaging
Phyletic memory, 2–3, 9–10, 20, 35, 52–56,
    89, 97
  in brain stem and spinal cord, 163
  in dreams, 287
  in hypothalamus, 165
  vs. individual memory, 6, 9–12
  motor, 54–56, 165, 187
  in primary (sensory and motor) cortex,
    9–10
  sensory, 52–54
  synchronous convergence in, 32–33
Physostigmine, 45
Picrotoxin, 44
Piriform cortex, 152
Planning, 174, 176, 233. *See also* Motor set

Plans (strategies, etc.). *See* Behavior, tem-
    poral structure; Motor programs; Motor
    schemata; Planning
Plasticity, 6, 52–59, 82, 94–95
  adult (cortical), 56–59
  in auditory cortex, 57
  in cerebellum, 55
  cross-modal, 56–57
  in motor cortex, 55–59, 188
  in olfactory cortex, 54
  in premotor cortex, 186–187
  in primary (sensory and motor) cortex,
    52–59
  in somatosensory cortex, 54, 57–58
Polymodal cortex, 71, 98, 120, 141, 147–
    148, 191, 246, 264, 278
Polymodal integration, 127
Polymodal memory, 156–160, 208. *See also*
    Categorical memory; Conceptual mem-
    ory; Semantic memory
Positron emission tomography. *See* PET
Posterior parietal cortex, 69, 126–132,
    138
  in stereognostic memory, 139
  in tactile discrimination, 132
Preattentive processing, 225, 230, 291,
    294–295
Prefrontal cooling, 241–244, 267–270. *See
    also* Prefrontal lesions
  on auditory memory, 241
  delay-task deficits from, 177
  and IT neurons, 267–270
  and tactile memory, 241–244
  and visual memory, 241–244, 267–270
Prefrontal cortex, 174–181. *See also* Orbito-
    frontal cortex; Prefrontal cooling; Pre-
    frontal lesions; Prefrontal neurons;
    Sulcus principalis
  in active memory, 79, 172–181, 264 (*see
    also* in short-term memory)
  in creativity, 174–179
  dopamine receptors, 181
  in haptics, 241
  imaging, 181, 194, 264–266
  in mediation of cross-temporal contin-
    gencies, 174, 176, 263–264, 280–281
  in motor memory, 106, 174–181, 263
  in motor processing, 78–79
  in motor set, 174–181, 234–236, 263–266,
    272–274
  in perception-action cycle, 275–276
  in planning, 174–176, 181
  in representation of movement, 181

in short-term memory, 174–179, 181,
189–190, 241–244, 277 (*see also* in active
memory)
in speech, 193–194, 280–281
in temporal integration, 14
in temporal organization of behavior,
127, 174–176, 194, 277
Prefrontal lesions. *See also* Prefrontal
cooling
aphasia from, 193–194, 280–281
delay-task deficits from, 176, 189–190
planning deficit from, 174–176, 194
recovery from, 172
and short-term motor memory, 174–176
Prefrontal neurons
in attention, 227
in cross-temporal contingency, 177
delay activation, 264
in delay tasks, 177–180, 245–246, 264
IT cooling on, 267–268
in learning, 177
motor-coupled, 179, 235, 271
in motor memory, 264
in motor set, 177–181, 234–236, 272–274
polymodal convergence on, 264
sensory-coupled, 179, 234, 271
in short-term memory, 177–179, 264, 270,
277
Prefrontal speech disorders, 193–194, 280
Premotor aphasia, 193
Premotor cortex, 182–187, 190. *See also*
Premotor lesions; Premotor neurons;
SMA
in automatic movement, 183
imaging, 183, 187, 193, 264–266
in motor memory, 106, 182–187
in motor processing, 78
in motor set, 79, 182–183, 265–266, 272
plasticity, 186–187
teleokinetic neurons, 184
Premotor hierarchy, 184–185
Premotor lesions
aphasia from, 193
and conditional association, 183
and execution of motor sequences, 183
and motor rhythm, 184
and self-initiation of movement, 183
Premotor neurons
directional tuning, 184–185
kinematic representation, 184
in motor set, 182, 272
in movement sequences, 184
in visually guided movement, 186

Premotor speech disorders, 193
Prepiriform cortex, 77
Primary memory, 5, 13, 237. *See also*
Active memory
Priming, 18, 199, 211, 290. *See also* Uncon-
scious processing
Probabilism vs. determinism in memory,
6, 86
Procedural memory, 17–20, 161, 189. *See
also* Habit; Motor memory; Motor skills
vs. declarative memory, 3
in delay tasks, 172
and motor memory, 21
Processing and representation
common cortical substrate, 35, 82, 89, 95
intertwined in memory, 21, 35
Prosopagnosia, 120
Protein metabolism
LTP in, 43
NMDA in, 43
Protocortex, 57
Provisional memory. *See* Working memory
Psychoanalysis, 165–166, 211–212, 286
Psychophysics, 84, 113, 155
P-threshold, 292
PTO cortex, 141–142, 191
Putamen, 166. *See also* Basal ganglia;
Striatum
Pyramidal cells, 14, 48–51, 187–188, 243

Qualitative attention, 224, 227–232

Random firing (Poisson-like process), 256
Readiness potential, 183, 273, 295
Recall, 103, 199. *See also* Retrieval
Receptive field reorganization, 57–58
Recognition, 105, 199, 201. *See also*
Retrieval
Recurrent collaterals, 48, 99
Reentry, 99, 102–105, 252–253, 257, 260–
261, 267, 269, 272. *See also* Reverberat-
ing circuits
Reference memory, 19
Reflex arcs, 163
Rehearsal, 13
REM sleep, 285
cholinergic system, 286
consolidation of memory, 285
dreams, 286
40-cycle oscillations, 286
learning, 285–286
unlearning, 288
Remembering, 199. *See also* under Retrieval

DATE DUE